Current Surgical Practice Volume 1

Edited on behalf of the Royal College of Surgeons of England by

John Hadfield, TD, MS, FRCS

Surgeon, Stoke Mandeville Hospital, Aylesbury; Member of the Council and Court of Examiners, Royal College of Surgeons of England

and

Michael Hobsley, TD, PhD, MChir, FRCS

Professor of Surgical Science, The Middlesex Hospital Medical School; Surgeon, The Middlesex Hospital and Acton Hospital, London; Penrose May Tutor, Royal College of Surgeons of England

with a Foreword by
Sir Rodney Smith, KBE, MS, PRCS

Surgeon, St George's Hospital, London; President of the Royal College of Surgeons of England

Edward Arnold

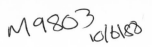

First published 1976 by
Edward Arnold (Publishers) Ltd
41 Bedford Square WC1B 3DQ
Reprinted 1979, 1981

Boards ISBN: 0 7131 4281 2
Paper ISBN: 0 7131 4282 0

Printed in Great Britain by
Butler & Tanner Ltd, Frome and London

Contributors

J. Alexander-Williams, MD, ChM, FRCS
   Surgeon, United Birmingham Hospitals; Member of External Scientific
   Staff, Medical Research Council

P. S. Boulter, FRCS, FRCSEd
   Surgeon, Guildford Hospitals; Hon. Tutor, Department of Surgery, Guy's
   Hospital Medical School, London; Reader in Clinical Subjects, Department
   of Biological Sciences, University of Surrey

M. D. Cameron, FRCS, FRCOG
   Obstetric and Gynaecological Surgeon, St Thomas' Hospital, London

H. P. Cook, FDSRCS
   Dental Surgeon, The Middlesex Hospital, and The Royal Dental Hospital,
   London

H. A. F. Dudley, ChM, FRCSEd, FRCS, FRACS
   Professor of Surgery, St Mary's Hospital Medical School; Director of Surgical Unit, St Mary's Hospital, London

H. H. G. Eastcott, MS, FRCS
   Surgeon, St Mary's Hospital, London; Consultant in Surgery and Vascular
   Surgery to the Royal Navy; Member of the Council and Court of Examiners,
   Royal College of Surgeons of England

A. J. Gunning, MA, FRCS, DLO
   Surgeon, United Oxford Hospitals

G. J. Hadfield, TD, MS, FRCS
   Surgeon, Stoke Mandeville Hospital, Aylesbury; Member of the Council
   and Court of Examiners, Royal College of Surgeons of England

B. H. Hand, MS, FRCS
   Surgeon, Ipswich and East Suffolk Hospitals

M. Hobsley, TD, PhD, MChir, FRCS
  Professor of Surgical Science, The Middlesex Hospital Medical School;
  Hon. Surgeon, The Middlesex Hospital, and Acton Hospital; Penrose May
  Surgical Tutor, Royal College of Surgeons of England

A. G. Horsburgh, FRCS
  Surgeon, Watford General Hospital and Bushey and District Hospital;
  Member of the Court of Examiners, Royal College of Surgeons of England

D. Johnston, MD, ChM, FRCSEd, FRCSGlas
  Professor of Surgery, University of Bristol; Honorary Surgeon, Bristol
  Royal Infirmary

J. E. Lennard-Jones, MD, FRCP
  Gastroenterologist, St Mark's Hospital, London; Reader in Medicine, The
  London Hospital Medical College

L. P. Le Quesne, DM, MCh, FRCS, FRACS (Hon.)
  Professor of Surgery, The Middlesex Hospital Medical School; Surgeon,
  The Middlesex Hospital, London; Member of the Court of Examiners,
  Royal College of Surgeons of England

H. H. Nixon, FRCS, FAAP (Hon.)
  Surgeon, The Hospital for Sick Children, Great Ormond Street, and The
  Children's Hospital, Paddington Green, London

Sir Thomas Holmes Sellors, DM, MCh, FRCP, FRCS
  Emeritus Surgeon, The Middlesex Hospital, London; Consulting Surgeon,
  National Heart Hospital, London, London Chest Hospital, and Harefield
  Hospital, Middlesex; Past President of the Royal College of Surgeons of Eng-
  land

J. E. Trapnell, MD, FRCS
  Surgeon, Royal Victoria Hospital, Bournemouth

D. Innes Williams, MD, MChir, FRCS
  Surgeon, St Peter's Hospital, London; Dean, Institute of Urology, Univer-
  sity of London; Genitourinary Surgeon, The Hospital for Sick Children,
  Great Ormond Street, London; Member of the Council, Royal College of
  Surgeons of England

Foreword

A not unreasonable ambition for a young would-be surgeon is to become a Fellow of the Royal College of Surgeons of England and a not unreasonable ambition for the College is to help him to do it.

Rightly concentrating upon the training rather than the examination, the College appointed, some 15 years ago, a Penrose May Surgical Tutor and, as part of the training programme which evolved, a regular course of lectures became established which made no attempt to cover the whole of surgery but tried instead to highlight those areas in which some important advance or change in philosophy had occurred during the preceding year or two. These lectures rapidly became popular and it soon became obvious that their content contained much that was of value not only to those embarking upon a surgical career but also to any surgeon, whatever his age or seniority, who wished to keep fully in touch with the growing edge of surgery.

So much is easily understood. What is difficult to understand is why the relatively simple step of publishing the lectures together in book form has not, up till now, been taken. The number of those who can personally attend a course at Lincoln's Inn Fields is limited. The number of those who could benefit from the lectures is almost unlimited.

What a waste!

Mr John Hadfield and Professor Michael Hobsley are to be congratulated on their industry in compiling a volume which to surgeons cannot fail to be of an absorbing interest, for the topics which are selected for the lecture courses are always those which particularly attract discussion and argument. The salesman's cliché 'no one can afford to be without this book' is very nearly right! Certainly any surgeon who does not take steps to read it is missing something which is both absorbing and highly instructive.

London   Rodney Smith
1976

Preface

For the last fifteen years, since our Fellowship class was started by the first Penrose May Tutor, Sir Rodney Smith, the evening lectures have been a popular feature. The subjects of these lectures were chosen for their interest and educational value and reflected changing views and accents on the topics of surgical interest and sometimes controversy at that time. Our lectures are picked from a nationwide field of contributors. Many were reviews of knowledge by a surgeon with a special interest in the subject, and for that reason obviously contained his own views as well.

On many occasions in the past, regret was expressed that there was no way of recording a larger number of these lectures than could be accommodated in existing journals. The present book, a selection of lectures given recently at the College, is an attempt to remedy this deficiency. The Council of the College asked us to prepare this as the first volume of a possible series.

In presenting this, the Editors have tried to produce a book which will interest surgeons of all grades and bring this aspect of the work and life of the College nearer to those who are not able to attend the lectures. The emphasis is on current practice: each author describes his own present approach to the practical solution of the particular problem.

As this is a book of lectures on totally different subjects and each one is self-sufficient, editing has been minimal. The author's personal style has therefore been maintained and each chapter becomes an entity within itself.

It is not the purpose of this book to compete with journals. Its role is quite different and complementary rather than competitive. In this context Professor Harding Rains has been generous with his advice and help to the editors. Two of the contributions, those of Hobsley and Cameron, were originally published in the *Annals of the Royal College of Surgeons of England*, but Cameron's is presented here in a modified and expanded form. We are grateful to the Editors of the *Annals* for their use.

Throughout the preparation of the book our publishers have given a combination of hard work, understanding and enthusiasm; for this we are most grateful.

We are grateful to our contributors whose co-operation has made this venture possible. The President, members of Council, the Board of Surgical Training in the College and the Regional Advisers and Tutors have all in various ways contributed to the course and hence to this book. To them all, we offer our thanks.

A great deal of organization is needed to bring any book to presentation. Final and special thanks are due to Mr R. S. Johnson-Gilbert for his invaluable advice on administrative matters and to Miss Diana Readhead at the Royal College of Surgeons who has helped with much of this secretarial work.

London   John Hadfield
1976   Michael Hobsley

Contents

1

The Aims of Postgraduate Surgical Education: a Personal View*

M. Hobsley, TD, PhD, MChir, FRCS

The Penrose May Tutor is responsible for organizing the College course for candidates for the Final Fellowship examination. Since I have assumed this office, the present seems a good moment to define my attitude to the task. I must emphasize that the opinions I shall detail are entirely my own; they are set out here to encourage discussion and argument and as a basis for modification—not as immutable dogma.

The Diploma of Fellowship signifies not that a practitioner is a fully qualified surgeon, but that he is ready to proceed to the final stages of training. The factors that are involved in making this decision obviously include intelligence and a knowledge of the basic sciences and of clinical surgery, but the natural selection of earlier examinations, including the Primary, should have eliminated most candidates who are unsuitable from the first two points of view by the time that the Final examination occurs. In that case, why do some candidates have difficulty in passing the Final examination, often having to make several attempts?

I believe that only rarely is the cause a lack of knowledge. The examination should be seen as a crisis of confidence. The candidate has to impress the examiners that he deserves to be trusted with the immediate responsibility for patients. The phrase 'immediate care' implies not necessarily that he can handle all surgical situations himself, but that he can deal with the commoner emergency and routine problems and can be trusted to summon aid should he find himself out of his depth. The ideal way for the examiners to establish that the candidate merits their confidence would be to assess his work as their registrar for a period of several weeks, but such an arrangement would hardly be practicable. Nevertheless, the essence of the examination is practical; the question the examiners are asking all the time is, Can this candidate be trusted to handle surgical problems *in practice*?

How can an examination consisting of written papers and the artificially contrived situations of clinical and viva voce tests achieve an assessment of the candidate's practical ability? The answer to this question lies in the analysis of how a surgeon (or indeed any doctor) tackles the problems presented by a patient. There are three aspects to be considered, and it is worth emphasizing that all

*Reprinted from *Annals of the Royal College of Surgeons of England*, Vol. 53, pp. 258–263.

three aspects have featured in the undergraduate curriculum but must be further developed at postgraduate level.

Data-collection

First, data must be collected from the patient. The skills of data-collection—history-taking, clinical examination, and special investigations—occupy a large and fundamental part of undergraduate medical education. At a higher level of expertise and accuracy, and with a concentration of experience in those areas of medicine particularly important to the surgeon, data-collection remains the simplest yardstick by which the postgraduate surgical aspirant must be judged. Clearly, this is the aspect of surgical ability mainly tested by the clinical part of the examination. No wealth of experience or mass of reading can possibly compensate for a poor performance in collecting data.

Having collected his information, the surgeon's next concern is to establish a working diagnosis. I suspect that many experienced clinicians, to whom making a diagnosis in most of the situations they meet is simply a matter of attaching a well worn label to a familiar problem, have stopped thinking consciously about the processes involved. The making of a working diagnosis is, however, the crux of the clinician's problem, and perhaps one can best approach the factors involved by considering the part played in the process by knowledge.

Data-storage

The acquisition of knowledge by the student is the second great concern of undergraduate medical education. In the modern jargon, this process might be called data-storage and data-retrieval. Again, in those areas of concern to the surgeon, the Fellowship candidate must build on the foundations he has established in his undergraduate period, so that he acquires a solid body of factual knowledge about disease (and treatment). Clearly, in all parts of the examination the size, accuracy and depth of the knowledge possessed by the candidate are being assessed. However, there are certain features about this 'solid body of factual knowledge' which render it less than perfect as a test of whether a candidate should be permitted to become a surgeon. For example, while most authorities would agree about a few facts that a candidate must know in order to pass the examination, most facts cannot be classified simply as essential or non-essential knowledge. In any case, examiners are well aware that today's 'fact' may turn out to be tomorrow's discarded hypothesis or exploded theory.

Quite apart from these considerations, no surgeon can possibly carry in his head all the knowledge that he might need to deal with problems in his clinical practice. An important part of his postgraduate education, therefore, might well be training in how to look up facts in the medical literature. However, as far as I am aware, no one has as yet been asked in the Final Examination how he would search for articles on a specific subject through the *Index Medicus*!

Problem-solving

Data-collection and data-storage are not in themselves sufficient for making a working diagnosis. In some way the clinician must marry up the picture he has constructed of the patient's situation with the picture in his data-store that corresponds most closely to it. This aspect of clinical science—problem-solving—is the one that the inexperienced doctor finds most difficult. As an undergraduate he gets plenty of teaching on ward rounds and in outpatient clinics designed to strengthen his data-collecting skills, and help from lectures and textbooks in the task of absorbing a systematic knowledge of disease. However, by comparison the emphasis his teachers lay on problem-solving is relatively small. Then he qualifies and is pitchforked into clinical work, where the patient presents as a problem in terms of complaints and physical signs and the disease causing this picture may not be immediately apparent. The young doctor may feel overwhelmed with the difficulties of making a diagnosis. To reduce his problem to absurdity, must he, in order to achieve a diagnosis, thumb through every page of the textbook constituted by his data-store till he finds one that perfectly describes the situation of his patient?

We are all aware that clinical practice is not conducted along these lines; such a procedure would be laughably exhausting and time-consuming. Processes that permit a logical progression towards the diagnosis in a reasonably short time must be developed. To continue the analogy of the textbook, at the very outset one can usually decide that the clinical situation must be due to a disease in one out of relatively few chapters; discriminatory tests are then applied which yield results that lead one towards one or other subgroup of these possible chapters. Further handling of the patient's problem, whether through more tests or actual treatment, will depend on the answers to the first tests, and at each stage the patient's diagnosis has been defined more accurately until a final solution of his problems has been achieved or some or all are found to be insoluble. The working diagnosis has altered at each stage and is indeed often not expressed in pathological terms until a late stage. Perhaps the important point to stress is that one should not think about 'the diagnosis' of a patient's troubles so much as about the 'working diagnosis'—that is, a diagnosis sufficient to determine the clinician's next step in management.

If the argument of the preceding paragraph seems obscure, the following example may help. A woman presents in the outpatient clinic complaining of an otherwise symptomless lump in the breast. The process of data-collection by history-taking and physical examination is undertaken, the presence of the lump is confirmed, and the surgeon then considers the question of diagnosis. The inexperienced student tends to think along the lines—What pathological lesions may produce a lump in the breast? Certainly it is possible to construct a list of differential diagnoses ranging from fat necrosis to Hodgkin's disease that *could* be present. The experienced surgeon, however, does not try to answer the impossibly difficult question, what is the pathology of this lump? He simply asks, into which of the following categories does the patient fall?

1. The lump is clinically benign.
2. The lump is not definitely benign.

Placement in one of these two categories constitutes a working diagnosis because it decides the surgeon's next step. If he is confident that the lump is benign, this is probably because he has diagnosed it as a cyst or a fibroadenoma.

He then recommends the appropriate management—usually needle-aspiration for a cyst and excision-biopsy for a fibroadenoma. If the surgeon cannot be certain that the lump is benign, he assumes that it is malignant and advises (in the first instance) urgent excision-biopsy. This is a slightly over-simplified, but not altogether inaccurate, analysis of the situation.

The Final examination

How is the candidate in Finals to be tested for his ability to analyse a surgical situation in terms like these? Certainly the examiners have a chance to lead him into suitable discussion in the oral part of the examination, but the written papers are the great opportunity, both for the examiners to test the candidate and for the candidate to impress his examiners.

Only rarely are the questions set in the written papers primarily aimed at testing the store of knowledge possessed by the candidate. Not often will there be a question couched in terms such as 'Describe the symptoms, signs, and treatment ...' of a disease; such a question can of course be easily answered by quoting the appropriate pages of any good textbook. Usually the questions will be phrased 'Discuss the management of ...' a certain clinical presentation.

Reverting to our previous example, the question may read 'Discuss the management of a woman presenting with an otherwise symptomless lump in her breast'. The inexperienced candidate describes the clinical features of a carcinoma and outlines his scheme of treatment for carcinoma of the breast. Then he describes the characteristic features of fat necrosis and it may occur to him as an uncomfortable thought that there may be no way of distinguishing the one lump from the other. None the less, his plan for answering the question forces him to continue with the characteristic signs of all the possible breast lumps and the treatment of each. Yet he and his examiners know both that all the signs may be misleading and that the initial treatment for nearly all lumps in the breast is excision-biopsy. This way of describing the management of a patient with a lump in the breast is time-consuming and repetitive; and even if the candiate writes it all down correctly, the examiner may say to himself, 'Yes, he knows all the textbook stuff; but can he really be trusted to handle the clinical problem as it presents in the outpatient clinic?'

The best way to handle questions like these is to forget about the textbook descriptions of individual diseases and to try to think oneself into the situation as one meets it in clinical practice. This is surely the simplest way to persuade the examiners that in practice one could cope with the situation. The method requires a reorientation of thinking about examination questions, and of course practice in the writing of answers along these lines.

Two useful rules can be laid down to help with this approach. The first is analogous to the scheme that many generations have used to aid their memory and ensure that no important pathological cause of a clinical state has been left out. If one thinks in terms of pathology, one goes through the classification of congenital or acquired, traumatic, inflammatory, degenerative, metabolic or neoplastic. In terms of the approach by situation, the analogous aide mémoire is the list of possible geographical sites at which a surgeon may meet a situation—for example, in the field (that is, at the site of an accident), the outpatient clinic, the wards, the operating theatre, etc. It should thus be possible to avoid such embarrassing errors as answering a question about retention of urine without mentioning post-operative retention, or one on the management of blood loss without mentioning bleeding during elective surgical operations!

The second rule that may give useful guidance in planning the answer to a question is this: always deal first with the emergency aspects of any situation. Clearly an ability to deal with the urgent problem, when there is no time to summon aid, is the most important of the surgical skills that the examiner is seeking in the candidate, so the latter should make sure that he gives plenty of time to the emergency aspects rather than sketching them in hastily at the end of a long answer.

The College course

The preceding discussion may be summarized as follows: the Final Fellowship examination aims to test a candidate's practical ability in handling surgical situations. The three components of such ability are data-collection (tested by the clinical part), data-storage (tested by all parts, but particularly the oral interviews in surgery and pathology), and problem-solving (again tested throughout, but particularly in the written papers). The written answers are usually better constructed as analyses of how to deal with a clinical presentation rather than as textbook descriptions of diseases.

The course organized by the College for candidates for the Final Fellowship has always strongly emphasized the importance of data-collection. Participants each visit 16 hospitals, where the instruction is mainly concentrated upon data-collection by history-taking and clinical examination. The candidates' data-store should benefit from the evening lectures on surgical subjects of topical interest, from the Saturday morning tutorials, and from clinical presentations that occupy some of the time at the hospital sessions. Finally, problem-solving, with special reference to writing answers, is the concern of the tutors, who take small groups of students for several hours on the four Wednesdays of the course and correct their written answers to model questions. Problem-solving is an aspect which many young surgeons may feel has not been adequately emphasized in their earlier education, and it is hoped that further aid to thinking in terms of situations rather than in terms of diseases may be afforded by the evening speakers if they cast their lectures in this mould.

Finally, I would greatly value comments on and criticisms of this chapter.

2

A Review of Cardiac Surgery for the General Surgeon

Sir Thomas Holmes Sellors, DM, MCh, FRCP, FRCS

Introduction

The general surgeon who has had limited experience of heart surgery can well be at a loss when faced with a patient who has had a heart operation, and has now to face an operation elsewhere. On many occasions the records and documentation are sufficient for the surgeon and anaesthetist to weigh up the operative and post-operative problems, but in an emergency there may be genuine difficulties.

Patients who have undergone major open-heart operations, such as valve replacement or coronary artery bypass, have a regime which may include anticoagulants, beta-blockers, diuretics, and so on. The effect of these and other agents on the circulation and other body systems may well influence the decision that has to be taken. There are additional hazards and potential complications that arise from the presence, say, of an indwelling pacemaker if there is any question of electrical equipment being used in the operating theatre. On the other hand, there are a number of heart operations which, if successful, involve a minimal risk: atrial and ventricular septal defects, persistent ductus arteriosus and congenital valve stenosis can be instanced in this connection. Obviously, if there has been a prior gross overload of either ventricle the state of the myocardium has to be taken into account, and in such lesions as coarctation a permanently high blood pressure is not unexpected and should be handled accordingly.

Cardiac surgery is one of the newer and dramatic developments in medicine, and whereas many of its procedures have become standardized and are regarded as routine, there is still considerable flexibility and its future is unpredictable. By the circumstances of evolution, heart operations are generally undertaken in units where an expert team of physicians, surgeons and people from other branches can be concentrated to deal with the complex technology required for investigation, the actual operation and its sequel. This inevitably accounts for a certain degree of isolation or separation from the general stream of surgery.

The original cardiovascular procedures were mainly concerned with the great vessels—occluding a persistent ductus or resecting a coarctation. The next phase was 'closed' or 'blind' approaches to stenosed valves and, since open-heart surgery became practical and sufficiently safe, most operations on valves have become replacements with prostheses or grafts. Finally and currently, myocardial ischaemia due to atherosclerosis of the coronary system is being treated by providing a bypass from the aorta or internal mammary arteries into a distal patent coronary vessel.

The complications and difficulties in providing satisfactory apparatus for open-heart surgery have been largely overcome, and comparatively simple heart–lung machines with a low priming volume can maintain an extracorporeal circulation while the heart is 'out of circuit'. Inevitably there are differences in points of technique, but the principle of maintaining adequate perfusion of the vital organs during and after operation is inviolable.

Whereas extracorporeal circulation is by a long way the most favoured method used in open-heart work, the advantages of hypothermia should not be ignored. So-called conventional 30°C hypothermia induced by surface cooling allows the heart to be excluded from the circulation for 10–12 minutes before there is any risk of brain damage. This enables a simple pulmonary valvotomy or closure of a secundum atrial septal defect to be undertaken without the complexities of heparinization and multiple cannulation. For example, the writer closed 300 septal defects with a 4 per cent mortality, and in selected or 'good' cases with a death rate of 0·5 per cent.

Deep hypothermia, introduced by Drew et al. (1959), lowered the temperature with the use of cannulae and heat exchangers to a much lower extent—20°C and even as low as 15°C, producing heart arrest and allowing the surgeon anything from half to 1 hour with an open heart before rewarming was introduced to restart the circulation.

Until or if a reversible agent which can arrest the body's metabolism is discovered, open-heart surgery looks like being dependent on the pump oxygenator in whatever form is found most efficient. The question as to whether cooling should or should not be used as a protective supplement is one for individual choice. Protection of the myocardium during aortic valve surgery can be effected by additional perfusion of the coronary arteries with cooled blood. In open-heart operations on the very young, surface-induced hypothermia plus perfusion is held to produce good results.

Assessment of a patient who may require operation usually involves detailed investigations. Some lesions can be studied by two-plane cardioangiography and/or catheter pressure or gas estimations comparatively simply, but volumetric estimations of regurgitation through valves may require cine-cardioangiography and a number of highly technical investigations such as ballistocardiography. In the study of coronary artery disease, coronary angiography has to be carried out. In all these important advanced investigations there is an element, even though small, of risk. Assessment is, therefore, quite a formidable though necessary undertaking before any decision to operate is made, and in major open-heart procedures the post-operative handling is no less exacting. Carefully monitoring with ECG and estimations of arterial and venous pressures, blood gases and chemistry, and urine output, are added to the more usual observations on respiration, blood and fluid loss, and so on. As a measure of comparison of what it means from the patient's point of view, it can be assumed that a patient 'surfaces' within 24 hours after an abdominal operation, a closed-heart operation takes about twice as long and a valve replacement may take 3 to 4 days before continuous monitoring can be abandoned.

The procedures that are used for different forms of heart disorders vary somewhat according to the views of the individual surgeons, but the variations are largely those of detail and not principle. What is being treated is either an obstruction in the tortuous channels of the cardiac complex or a leak through its valves or between its chambers. An obstruction can be relieved by division or reconstruction; a leak can be closed by suture or patch and, in the case of a valve, the defective unit replaced. In addition, there are possibilities in the way of reconstructing by patch or tube conduit some of the more complicated malformations. One of the major advances and advantages has been the introduction of foreign body prostheses in the form of patches, tubes or non-return valves. Surprisingly, these have been accepted by the tissues far more readily than one would have expected in continually moving surroundings. Artificial valves are a case in point, and, though the caged ball valve is haemodynamically nothing like as efficient as the human cusped valve, it is gratifying to see how frequently it is tolerated.

Though the Starr–Edwards ball valve prosthesis has achieved a high measure of success, artificial valves based on flap and disc are continually being tried out and, to avoid the problem of using foreign body material, homografts, heterografts and valves made from autogenous material (fascia lata) have been successfully used.

Common congenital cardiac conditions requiring operative treatment

Persistent ductus arteriosus

This condition is usually symptomless, uncomplicated and acyanotic until well into adult life. Patients are liable to develop pulmonary hypertension and in neonatal life it can be a cause of severe heart failure. In any event, if recognized before school age, the channel should be obliterated by ligature or division and suture, the former being suitable for young children. The approach is via a standard left thoracotomy and there is little danger apart from inadvertent damage to ductus or pulmonary artery—in which case haemorrhage can be very difficult to control. The results are excellent and no restrictions to a normal existence are required. The patient, as with all congenital conditions, must have antibiotic cover if any infection (dental abscess) develops.

Coarctation of the aorta

This is a common cause of undiagnosed hypertension in young adults who are robust with arm span greater than height and the muscular torso well developed—in other words, the ideal amateur boxer type. The degree of hypertension in the upper extremity may be considerable, and absent or delayed pulse in the lower limbs gives the diagnosis. It should be noted that the mean arterial pressures above and below the coarctation are equal in spite of lack of pulsation. There is a vast collateral network in the intercostal and internal mammary areas distally.

These patients, even though symptomless, should be treated without undue delay as structural ('berry') aneurysms may be present at the point where tortuous and dilated intercostals join the post-stenotic enlarged aorta.

Treatment consists of mobilizing the aorta above and below the coarctation area which is usually just distal to the point of entry of the ligamentum arteriosum. The aorta is clamped above and below the stricture and a narrow segment is resected prior to performing a single-layer end-to-end junction. Alternatively, a wedge can be excised to include two-thirds to three-quarters of the stricture and the gap closed with a small Dacron patch. Where a section more than 2–3 cm has to be removed, it may not be possible to bring the ends together and here a Dacron tube graft can be used to bridge the deficiency.

The results are highly satisfactory and, though the blood pressure may never return to normal limits, it is reduced sufficiently to avoid the worst risks of hypertension (Sellors and Hobsley, 1963).

Pulmonary stenosis

Isolated pulmonary stenosis may be quite symptomless and indeed of no major significance if the right ventricular pressure is not severely raised. Cardiac catheterization is necessary to determine the level of right ventricular strain. Operation consists of dividing the commissures of the pulmonary valve after incising the base of the pulmonary artery.

Pulmonary stenosis is also part of the complex tetralogy of Fallot, but is more usually associated with gross muscle hypertrophy of the right infundibular outflow tract. The handling of this disabling condition has been an important part of the history of cardiac surgery. Prior to safe open-heart surgery, considerable relief was obtained by Blalock's operation in which a shunt from a systemic artery into the pulmonary circuit can give great improvement in oxygenation. Other anastomoses—Potts (Potts et al., 1946) and Waterston (1962)—follow the same principle, but all such operations are only palliative procedures. Pulmonary valvotomy and infundibular resection (Sellors, 1948; Brock 1948) constituted a more direct approach to the problem, but radical cure of this complex deformity had to be postponed until open-heart surgery became practicable. Then at the same operation the ventricular septal defect is closed by a patch and the right outflow tract freely opened by freeing the pulmonary valve stenosis and excising the considerable mass of muscle that occludes the infundibulum. Successful operation gives a dramatic result, but there are still considerable hazards in operating on very young children (Sade et al, 1975). Many units prefer to perform the palliative Blalock (1947) or Waterston (1962) procedure on babies and very young, and defer the total correction till later.

Septal defects

Atrial septal defects (ASD) are of two varieties. The simple secundum type is simply a hole in the septal partition, but the primum defect is complicated by malformation of the septal leaflet of the mitral valve. The secundum ASD can be closed by simple suture after incising the right atrium. Patching is not necessary and, as has been said, the closure can be achieved using conventional 30°C hypothermia, though extracorporeal circulation is now more commonly used. The results are highly satisfactory.

Primum ASD requires full bypass techniques as the mitral valve has to be reconstructed and a patch used to close the extensive defect. The AV node, close to the suture line, is recognized as a potential hazard and, if the conducting system is damaged, heart-block will ensue.

Ventricular septal defects (VSD) are varied and, in addition to congenital forms, may include deficiencies following infarction and perforation of the septum. Again, when closure is being carried out the conducting mechanism of the AV bundle is open to injury. Direct closure by suture for small defects may be possible, but, if it produces any distortion, the seating of the aortic valves may be affected and regurgitation follow.

In some cases of VSD, particularly in the young, the high resistance in the pulmonary vessels puts so much strain on the right ventricle as to make closure of the defect highly dangerous. In such cases 'banding' of the pulmonary artery can be carried out, tightening the obstructing band until the pressures in the ventricles are equalized. If and when the situation is stabilized—a matter of years rather than months—closure of the defect can be considered.

Transposition of the great vessels

Until quite recently, treatment of transposition of the great vessels was impractical, but, with advances in paediatric cardiac surgery, considerable success has been achieved. An initial and relatively simple procedure is to enlarge or produce an atrial defect which allows freer mixing of red and blue blood at that level. A balloon catheter is introduced via the femoral vein into the right atrium and under radiographic vision the catheter is passed through the foramen ovale and the balloon inflated. The catheter is then withdrawn (with some force) so that the balloon bursts through the septum and leaves an appreciable defect.

A more definite procedure which attempts to restore functional if not literal anatomy is to insert a spiral- or cochlear-shaped septum so that the venous blood is deflected into the pulmonary ventricle and the arterial blood into the systemic ventricle (Mustard et al., 1964). Dramatic successes have been achieved, but, as might be anticipated, the operation is not without hazards.

Other complicated congenital conditions—single ventricle, truncus arteriosus, Epstein's deformity, coronary artery fistula—tax the ingenuity of the investigating team to work out the exact type and extent of deformity before coming to a decision whether anything mechanical can be done to improve the position.

Acquired heart disease

Often an end-result of rheumatic infection, this group constitutes the major part of the cardiac surgeon's activities. Mitral stenosis and regurgitation and aortic stenosis and regurgitation alone or in combination have to be carefully analysed before deciding an operation. Occasionally, patients in acute heart failure have an obstructive or regurgitant lesion that cries out for relief, but usually there is a period of preparation and adjustment involving the extensive use of drugs to provide the optimum conditions of circulatory and myocardial efficiency that is possible.

Angiocardiography is particularly valuable in assessing the degree of regurgitation which may well influence the operative decision to perform a local repair or a total valve replacement.

Mitral valve surgery was, in the first instance, carried out as a closed operation splitting the stenosed valve with finger or valvotome. This procedure had a high measure of success in selected cases as long as there was little or no regurgitation. With a heavily calcified and regurgitant valve, open operation gives an opportunity to determine if plastic repair by dividing the commissures, excising calcified plaques, etc., will give a sufficiently competent valve or whether in the long term replacement is preferable. Prostheses of the ball valve or flap type or reversed homograft aortic valves are most commonly used. The homograft or even a heterograft aortic valve supported on a specially designed frame and covered by Teflon fabric is then carefully sutured into the atrioventricular ring. Many modifications have been employed, but if it is possible to repair the existing valve cusps without removing and replacing them a more favourable outlook can be anticipated.

Aortic valve surgery

The valve is approached from above through the ascending aorta and not as originally with a valvotome through the left ventricle. The chief problem in open operations on this valve is the state of the left ventricle, whose muscle is grossly hypertrophied and in the case of stenosis the capacity of the ventricular chamber is grossly reduced. The coronary artery blood flow is invariably poor and the risk of ventricular fibrillation in an advanced case is considerable. In consequence, protection of the myocardium by cooling and/or coronary perfusion during operation is necessary. Normally, as soon as the aorta is incised under bypass coronary artery cannulae are inserted and maintained in position as a preliminary to any manipulation on the valve.

Here again, circumstances dictate the procedure, but most operations on the valve tend to consist of replacement. Division of commissures in cases of stenosis and local patching or suturing of a leaking valve have only a limited place.

The most commonly used prosthesis is the ball valve type whose basal ring covered by cloth is held in place below the coronary orifices by multiple sutures. When this frame is securely anchored and all the sutures firmly tied, a catheter or tube is passed into the ventricle chamber and the ball pressed into the cage. The aortic incision is sutured but not finally closed till all air has been removed from the interior of the heart; again, before the cross-clamp of the aorta distal to the incision is released, a small tube or needle is inserted into the apex of the ventricle to ensure no potential air emboli remain.

As an alternative to prostheses, homograft valves have been and are being used with considerable success. A reconstituted cadaver aortic valve with a rim of aorta carefully shaped for ease of securing is inserted into the position of the excised valve. Valves constructed of autologous fascia lata have also been used (Senning, 1968), but fibrotic contracture and subsequent regurgitation have been noted. In short, there is no standardization in the actual method of replacement, and innovations and modifications to avoid damage to blood cells and prevent thrombosis appear continuously.

In severe cases or when both valves have had to be dealt with, the take-over of the heart from bypass can be slow. Arrhythmias, particularly fibrillation, can occur and may require repeated high voltage shocks to restore normal rhythm and a reasonable cardiac output. Bleeding in this, as in all heparinized patients, can be a problem, not so much on the operating table as in the early post-operative period, and an appreciable number of patients have to be returned to the theatre for haemostasis. With experience, however, this complication becomes less frequent.

Post-operative patients with valve replacements require most careful observation and monitoring. Heart arrest or arrhythmias can occur and the cardiac output and the blood volume may fall to a dangerous extent. Pressor agents and many varieties of drugs may have to be used and massive blood transfusions may be required to replace blood loss at and after operations.

Antibiotic cover is essential in all open-heart operations, particularly with valves, and has to be continued over a prolonged period, but the major point of contention is the role of anticoagulants. A valve replacement, even with a homograft, involves a great deal of foreign body tissue within the heart and aorta and the risk of clotting is always present. No follow-up is lacking in incidence of embolism following clot formation on the prosthesis. One sinister and late complication that has been observed is the development of fungus infections in the valve or holding sutures.

In spite of the technical and biological problems, valve replacement surgery has achieved an important place in medicine, and in the long term the results are proving increasingly gratifying.

Coronary artery disease

Atherosclerosis of the coronary artery system is responsible for ischaemia of the myocardium, and a sudden occlusion of a major artery may precipitate a catastrophe by triggering ventricular fibrillation before the actual heart muscle dies. Early efforts at revascularizing the myocardium through anastomotic channels developing within adhesions produced on the heart surface proved inadequate, as did an arterial shunt directed from the aorta into the coronary venous sinuses (Beck, 1935).

Vineberg (1946) introduced a more direct approach by implanting an artery into the deep layers of the myocardium. The internal mammary artery was mobilized and its divided and open end inserted into the myocardium in the area of ischaemia.

With the wider introduction of selective coronary artery angiography, obstructions due to atheroma or occlusion by thrombosis could be identified. If these were localized, direct operation (endarterectomy) became a possibility. It would also be possible to bypass the obstruction by using a graft between a systemic artery and the coronary artery distal to the obstruction.

The mobilized and divided internal mammary arteries have been used for this purpose, but more commonly the bypass is performed between the ascending aorta and the coronary artery distal to the obstruction, using an isolated segment of the internal saphenous vein. If there is more than one occluded coronary artery a second or even a third bypass can be used.

The technical side of the operation requires considerable technical expertise, particularly in performing the oblique anastomosis between the vein graft and the coronary vessel.

The philosophy behind this approach is simple. If the bypass remains patent, the damaged area supplied by that coronary vessel will receive additional blood supply. This may reduce the threat of the trigger mechanism that might at any time set off ventricular fibrillation.

What is not always fully appreciated is that atherosclerosis of the coronary vessels is not confined to the main trunks or larger branches, but that it is a generalized process involving also finer channels which cannot be demonstrated on angiography.

This form of bypass surgery has achieved a large measure of popularity and success, but several years will have to lapse before a realistic appraisal of its worth can be made.

The selection of patients suitable for operation is variable. At one extreme the incapacitated victim of several coronary artery attacks with a localized and demonstrable occluded vessel and with a poor prognosis may gain considerable relief. At the other end there is a comparatively fit individual who has positive ECG and radiographic evidence of myocardial ischaemia and who is operated on as an insurance policy against a 'heart attack'. In Britain the approach is much more conservative than in some clinics in North America—and time alone will demonstrate the scope of this form of operation (Achuff et al., 1975; Effler, 1975).

The advances in cardiac surgery which have made such an impact in recent years have been parallelled by advances in medicine, radiology and anaesthesia. The study of cardiology is an intricate combined operation involving all branches working together in full understanding of each other's problems—problems that are often complex and not always soluble.

References

ACHUFF S. C., GRIFFITH L. S. C., CONTI C. R., HUMPHRIES J. O'N., BRAWLEY R. K., GOTT V. L. and ROSS R. S. (1975) The angina producing myocardial segment: an approach to the interpretation of results of coronary by-pass surgery. *Am. J. Cardiol.* **36**, 723–733.

BECK C. S. (1935) The development of a new blood supply to the heart by operation. *Ann. Surg.* **102**, 801–813.

BLALOCK A. (1947) The technique of creation of an artificial ductus arteriosus in the treatment of pulmonic stenosis. *J. Thorac. Surg.* **16**, 244–257.

BROCK R. C. (1948) Pulmonary valvulotomy for the relief of congenital pulmonary stenosis. *Br. Med. J.* **1**, 1121–1126.

DREW C. E., KEEN G. and BENAZON D. B. (1959) Profound hypothermia. *Lancet* **1**, 745–747.

EFFLER D. B. (1975) Myocardial revascularisation: current state of the art. *Am. J. Cardiol.* **36**, 849–851.

MUSTARD W. T., KEITH J. D., TRUSLER G. A., FOWLER R. and KIDD L. (1964) The surgical management of transposition of the great vessels. *J. Thorac. Cardiovasc. Surg.* **48**, 953–958.

POTTS W. J., SMITH S. and GIBSON S. (1946) Anastomosis of the aorta to a pulmonary artery. *JAMA* **132**, 627–631.

ROSS D. N. (1967) Homograft replacement of the aortic valve. *Br. J. Surg.* **54**, 165–168.

SADE, R. M., WILLIAMS R. G. and CASTENADA A. R. (1975) Corrective surgery for congenital cardiovascular defects in early infancy. *Am. Heart J.* **90,** 656–663.

SELLORS T. H. (1948) Surgery of pulmonary stenosis. *Lancet* **1,** 988–989.

SELLORS T. H. (1963) Coarctation of the aorta. Effect of operation on blood pressure. *Lancet* **1,** 1387–1391.

SENNING A. (1968) Results of fascia lata reconstruction of the aortic valve. *J. Cardiovasc. Surg.*, Suppl. 28.

VINEBERG A. M. (1946) Development of anastomosis between coronary vessels and transplanted internal mammary artery: a preliminary report. *Can. Med. Assoc. J.* **55,** 117–119.

WATERSTON D. J. (1962) The treatment of Fallot's tetralogy in infants under the age of one year. *Rozhl. Chir.* **41,** 181–183.

3

The Principles Underlying the Management of the Seriously Injured Patient

H. A. F. Dudley, ChM, FRCSEd, FRCS, FRACS

The early management of those who are the victims of trauma has become so efficient that there is not apparently a pressing need to review the subject again. Yet the very increase in skills, the lavish expenditure of medical and other resources and the frequency of trauma in our violent world make it imperative that all concerned have a grasp of the principles. Without such organization, there is always a risk that standards will not be sustained and that opportunities to save lives and reduce morbidity will be lost. This paper deals with *organization*, not in terms of disaster planning, but in relation to how the surgeon should see himself and systematize his thinking about small groups of casualties or individually injured patients with whom he is confronted. Details of surgery for particular areas can be found in a recent excellent review series (Gray and Coppel, 1975).

At the site

Organization of first aid

We may begin by dividing medical activities into those possible and desirable at the scene of an incident and those carried out definitively. Both in war and in peace the utility of highly skilled medical attention at the point of injury, while questionable, is also limited. Those who should dominate the scene are usually the rescue, demolition or defensive experts. Occasionally, and particularly where there is a need to take a decision about the worth of evacuating an injured person or on the allocation of individual resources, a surgeon may have to adjudicate. Occasionally also, as the London tube-train disaster of 1974 has shown, urgent surgery may be required to free a trapped victim, but such occasions are rare. Medical men unconsciously feel they have a monopoly on expertise; they should remember that ambulance crews, police, firemen, soldiers and heavy rescue personnel have, more likely than not, a far greater experience of dealing with the problems set by the release and evacuation of casualties.

This is not to deny that a medical team sent to the site of an accident can make considerable contributions to our understanding of the problems. Snook (1974) has made a special study of this and has shown that, by skilled intervention, he can reduce mortality. Nevertheless, most of the things he recommends can be passed on to other skilled non-medical people.

The compromise that emerges is that there should be a means whereby surgeons can be rapidly summoned to the scene of an accident and arrive there ready for any eventuality that may present. Integrated radio networks, a standard feature of war, are slowly becoming part of the apparatus of peace and, with careful planning of duty rosters and availability of staff, a necessary feature of good hospital practice.

Medical problems

Summoned to the scene of an accident or faced with the task of training others who will be, the medical problems that must be confronted are chiefly those of first aid: the restoration and maintenance of airway, adequate respiratory excursion, the diagnosis of rapidly progressing intracranial compression and the identification and control of external bleeding. All these may have to be played out against a background of local danger, the needs of others not injured and problems such as traffic congestion or the progress of a battle. In addition, the distance to the nearest point for definitive treatment and the type and efficacy of evacuation to it must always be in the back of the mind. For example, there is a great difference in the management of the patient who has been exsanguinated by a massive injury if transfusion facilities and an operating theatre are within a stone's throw, by contrast with the situation where only a long, difficult evacuation route can be followed to some distant point.

Airway

The restoration and maintenance of airway is such a basic principle that we need not dwell upon it at length. Nevertheless, the very complex facial and neck injuries that can result from high-speed deceleration or short-range gunshot wounds may make essential decisive action to insert a wide airway, to detail an individual to support the jaw, to put the patient into the 'tonsillar' semi-prone position and *very occasionally* to perform emergency tracheostomy. The last is best done as a temporary subglottic procedure, in effect a laryngotomy, through the cricopharyngeal membrane; it should certainly be in the repertoire of the surgeon at the scene of an incident but, equally, should rarely be required. The restoration of an airway is no guarantee that the patient will breathe. A rapid review for mechanical impediment such as multiple fractured ribs, pneumothorax, a sucking chest wound or the recognition of a severe brain-stem injury should permit appropriate action. Sucking wounds are covered with a large pad; in the presence of an undoubted pneumothorax a flutter valve should, if possible, be inserted (one can be improvised with a 19-gauge needle and the finger from a rubber glove in which a small perforation has been made); hypoventilation or respiratory arrest clearly calls for mouth-to-mouth respiration or the use of a portable breathing apparatus. However, it must be borne in mind that very forceful respiratory assistance or maintenance has two risks: first, that an unrelieved pneumothorax will be made worse; secondly, that particularly if the neck is not kept well extended air may be forced in considerable quantities into the stomach. The latter is more likely if an airway has been inserted over-enthusiastically, and the stomach can be ruptured in this way. This man-made disaster apart, a blown-up stomach can cause respiratory and circulatory difficulty later. Its presence should be sought in every casualty and it is one of the few indications for pre-operative nasogastric intubation.

Cerebral compression

The recognition of advancing cerebral compression is an indication for rapid evacuation or on occasion, it must be admitted, for the decision that nothing useful can be done and that other casualties if they are present may merit more attention—a form of crude triage (see below) that most of those at multiple incidents have had forced upon them. Speedy transport to a place where a burr hole can be made is more likely to save lives if advance warning can be given, and here again an efficient radio network is invaluable.

Haemorrhage

Finally, massive bleeding may have exsanguinated the patient. External haemorrhage from a single source can nearly always be controlled by local compression. Very occasionally an artery forceps may need to be applied to arrest a major arterial bleed. A tourniquet is justified if, and only if, the distal damage is such that the limb is subsequently to be amputated. When bleeding is internal the situation is comparable to a closed head injury; rapid evacuation is mandatory.

Two other questions to be asked when major bleeding has taken place are: should intravenous therapy be started, and should pain be relieved? While not to decry the value of the first, and while recognizing its place if a patient is trapped or evacuation is to be long delayed, it must also be admitted that most infusions set up under adverse circumstances fail to do their job; time can be wasted and if an infusion is successfully begun a false sense of security may be introduced. So, in general, efforts should be concentrated on getting the victim to a place where definitive treatment and volume replacement can go hand in hand. It is pertinent, if self-evident, to comment that for many casualties survival is possible without intravenous therapy, which often tends to be rather blindly thrust at them.

Pain

As to pain relief, there are two useful techniques. Nitrous oxide inhalers are carried by most ambulance crews for obstetric use and they are equally valuable and safe for the casualty. Alternatively, a very small dose of opiate given by the intravenous route is also quite safe and, in spite of all that is written in the textbooks, will not interfere with subsequent assessment. The technique for this situation (as in the relief of acute pain of other causes) is to dilute a 'standard' dose (say 15 mg morphine sulphate) in 10 ml of saline and inject 1 ml every 30 sec until relief is obtained. Less than 5 ml is often adequate.

Transport to hospital

The time has now come to move the patient. Again, first-aid maxims apply: the airway must be protected, skeletal injuries should be adequately immobilized and the possibility of spinal injury borne in mind. A neutral position with good support is the watchword for both limbs and trunk, and is usually more compatible with preventing additional problems than elaborate techniques designed to deal with particular injuries.

Methods of movement have already been briefly mentioned. The increase in speed of evacuation, and particularly the use of the helicopter, has revolutionized the management of the military casualty in the last two decades, although it has inevitably generated additional problems by presenting to the surgeon individuals who would otherwise have died at the point of injury or along the evacuation route. In civilian life the cost and complexity of airborne movement have made it difficult to deploy this technique, though at the Maryland Center for Trauma the greatest proportion (in excess of 75 per cent) of patients arrive by this method. Certainly, where 'three-dimensional' evacuation is thought to have an undoubted advantage in speed and smoothness, and particularly from difficult situations, it should be used if at all possible; medical practitioners have not pressed hard enough for it. Objective information on the unpleasantness of high-speed surface journeys is difficult to come by, but there is more than anecdotal evidence that being swung around in an ambulance is undesirable.

Whatever the technique, every endeavour should be made to see that there is one move and one move only. To shift a casualty in and out of different vehicles, move him from stretcher to couch and back again is deleterious, particularly if fractured bones have not been adequately immobilized.

Ideally, once on a stretcher he should proceed right to definitive treatment in the operating room. Modern accident departments and the organization for military casualties are designed with this in mind. In particular, delay in places such as the X-ray department must be avoided. Finally, in despatching a casualty some attention may have to be directed towards choosing the place he is to go according to his needs—for example, a neurosurgical centre, a thoracic or maxillofacial centre. Of overriding importance is the need to send him to a place geared to the reception of trauma, for there the expertise for the initial and life-saving management is most likely to be found.

In hospital

Assessment

Our injured man has now reached with all deliberate speed the casualty reception area. Here his formal and complete assessment can take place. Attention should initially be directed towards the following: hypoxia, hypovolaemia, gross anatomical problems (skeletal or vascular), cerebral compression, the possibility of visceral rupture, the presence of an expanding haematoma or of a constricting limb burn. Some of these may be self-evident on history or physical examination; some may require additional information for either diagnosis or confirmation; and some must be sought for with diligence if they are not to be missed. Details will not be entered into here, but some special points are worthy of emphasis. First, hypoxia may be suspected from the nature of the injuries, but should always, if possible, be looked for by blood gas tension analysis. Especially in long bone fractures, but also in extensive soft tissue injury, this will also establish a base line against which subsequent values can be assessed, should the suspicion of fat embolus arise. Secondly, it must be remembered that a normal blood pressure and pulse are not an assurance of normovolaemia; the history of the injury and its physical extent are a better guide to the amount of blood lost and therefore to transfusion requirements. Thirdly, the same observations (the damage profile in particular) and a little intelligent thought can often suggest, for example in motor car accidents, the possibility of closed injury to chest or abdomen. If the latter is thought at all possible then diagnostic peritoneal lavage should be undertaken without hesitation. This manœuvre has been recommended routinely in multiple injury (Gill et al., 1975), but unless resources are very large it adds a technical burden which few would wish to shoulder.

Priorities

From these general points an order of priorities and a plan of action will begin to emerge. As this is being developed, practical matters common to any major casualty should be being dealt with over and above those already considered. An adequate intravenous line must be established—if necessary by a cut-down in the arm—and, in addition, if the circumstances are complex and the team is skilled a further line may be inserted to measure central venous pressure. This apart, multiple intravenous infusions should be avoided: they add to the problems of management and usually only mean that a big enough single cannula has not been inserted. Administrative details of documentation, contacting relatives and obtaining permission are all important and tend to be overlooked. Finally, arrangements will have to be made for the patient to be fitted into an operating theatre schedule according to his need.

The details of early fluid therapy which follow when an intravenous pathway has been established, can be found in standard texts (e.g. Kyle, 1969; McNair, 1972), and will not be gone into here.

Planning of the timing and nature of surgery when more than one casualty is present is based on the classical precepts of triage—division into three classes: those too damaged to benefit from treatment (rare now in both civilian and military trauma); those who can wait because their injuries are minor or unlikely to progress; and those whose lives are threatened but who should respond to adequate management. It is with the last group that we are now concerned. The plan that emerges is based on an order of priorities as follows (McNair, 1972):

Immediate/urgent

 Relief of cerebral compression by burr holes.
 Correction of problems with respiration and intubation, including the use
  of intermittent positive pressure respiration. Arrest of continued large
  vessel bleeding, including the need for laparotomy and thoracotomy.

These need little comment. The last is a vexatious situation when internal bleeding into thorax or chest is so catastrophic that until it is arrested resuscitation cannot be achieved. Bold surgery may be necessary on an unanaesthetized or barely conscious patient to achieve control.

High priority

> Evident body cavity injury, including penetrating wounds.
> Expanding haematoma and/or long bone fractures with neurovascular involvement.
> Constricting limb burns.

Again little elaboration is necessary. Emphasis must be laid on the speed with which an arterial haematoma can expand and the exsanguination that can thus be produced. Further, as the lesion progresses, the technical side of control becomes ever more difficult.

Middle priority

> Long bone fractures, simple or compound but without neurovascular involvement.
> Extensive soft tissue injuries.
> Consultation and action on eye and ear injuries.

Low priority

> Removal of superficial foreign bodies.
> Small lacerations and burns.

Whatever the priorities established for an individual patient or for a group, two matters must be made clear. First, an order of priorities is not permission for neglect and as soon as possible all injuries should be formally and definitively dealt with. This is of particular importance in relation to damage that, if not properly treated, can later lead to cosmetic or functional defects which may thereafter cause the patient more prolonged distress than the major injuries that were life-threatening. Secondly, with an order established every effort should be made to treat all the injuries in the appropriate order and with despatch *at the one time*. Though it is impossible to prove that this is in the patient's interests, it is undoubtedly rational that where possible the total correction of his disorders must leave him best equipped to face the rigours of convalescence. Also, the interaction of injuries on his care may be of significance—a patient with an abdominal injury and a fracture of the shaft of the femur presents a more difficult nursing problem for the first later if the other has not been properly immobilized; good nursing care of a head injury may be rendered difficult if repeated trips to the operating theatre are needed or if a long bone fracture is not satisfactorily fixed.

This account of the principles of early management can conveniently end at the point where the well organized plan is put into action and the patient is about to enter the operating theatre, with all those necessary for his definitive treatment in attendance and clear as to their individual and joint roles. Obviously, unless they bring surgical skill to their work all initial planning will have been in vain. But without thought on principles the chances of a successful and uncomplicated outcome are seriously reduced.

References

GILL W., CHAMPION H. R., LONG W. B., JAMARIS J. and COWLEY R. A. (1975) Abdominal lavage in blunt trauma. *Br. J. Surg.* **62,** 121–124.

GRAY R. C. and COPPEL D. L. (1975) Intensive care of patients with bomb blast and gunshot injuries. *Br. Med. J.* **1,** 502–504, and subsequent issues.

KYLE J. (ed.) (1969) *Pye's Surgical Handicraft,* 19th edn. Bristol, John Wright & Sons.

MCNAIR T. J. (ed.) (1972) *Hamilton Bailey's Emergency Surgery,* 9th edn. Bristol, John Wright & Sons.

SNOOK R. (1974) *Medical Aid at Accidents.* London, Update Publications.

4

Swellings Around the Angle of the Lower Jaw

H. P. Cook, FDSRCS

Swellings located in the submandibular and lower jaw angle area are frequently caused by disorders affecting the teeth and alveolar bone. Such conditions may be relatively unfamiliar to general surgeons, who, having a wider spread of interests, may find these swellings somewhat of a diagnostic puzzle. The object of this paper is to try to offer simple clues to those who would like to unravel a not very dense mystery.

Bone dysplasias

Children as a group often present diagnostic problems which, in the lower jaw situation, can prove very difficult to diagnose. There are a number of congenital and familial disorders affecting the mandible which come into this category and are really in the nature of bony dysplasias. The condition of cherubism (Jones, 1933, 1938; Seward and Hankey, 1957) is such an example, and takes its name from the cherubic appearance caused by bilateral swellings affecting the lower part of the face and the rather bulging and upturned eyes. The enlargement, which affects both sides of the mandible, is uniform and usually painless. The child is usually brought for advice because of the observed swellings, or sometimes on account of delayed eruption of teeth. Radiographs of the mandible demonstrate bilateral expanding lesions of the bone, involving both ramus and body portions. The rarefied areas are often divided by well defined bony septa and may be related to unerupted teeth delayed beyond the average age of eruption. The values of serum calcium, phosphorus and alkaline phosphatase are within limits of normality.

Diagnosis of this condition may depend upon histological examination of biopsy material, as the typical cherubic appearance is not always present. This shows a well organized fibrous stroma in which are scattered aggregations of multinucleated giant cells. Once this information is obtained, other members of the same family may be found to have the condition in a 'burnt out' form. It may also be possible to trace the inherited defect with distortion of normal anatomy and unerupted teeth back for some distance in the family tree. Treatment is usually limited to bone trimming operations and curettage of the abnormal tissue, especially if tooth eruption needs to be encouraged.

Another unusual condition found in young individuals which seems at least to be a clinical entity is the localized monostotic fibrous dysplasia reported by Obwegeser et al. (1973) as a variation of fibrous dysplasia of the jaws.

This appears in children up to and including the late teens and is characterized by gross distortion and enlargement of the maxilla or mandible in the absence of involvement of other bones. The serum values for calcium, phosphorus and alkaline phosphatase are usually within normal limits, but a raised alkaline phosphatase has been reported. Radiographic examination of the jaws (Fig. 4.1) demonstrates enlargement of the bone and distortion of the normal anatomy. The normal bone trabeculae are lost and replaced by well defined rarefied areas.

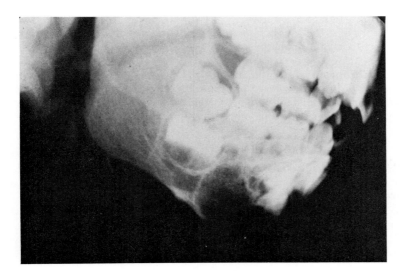

Fig. 4.1 Radiograph of mandible of child 2½ years of age. Lateral view shows area of enlargement and bone resorption affecting anterior part of body.

Histological examination of material from these areas may show soft tissue consisting of fibrous connective tissue, including osteoid and scattered giant cells consistent with fibrous dysplasia. Sometimes the areas turn out to be multiple pseudocystic cavities without epithelial lining and contain only clear fluid.

It is impossible to give a definite aetiology for these lesions at the present time as their pathology is not clearly understood. Both trauma and haemorrhage into the tissues have been suggested as factors, but both of these suggestions seem unlikely. Management consists of surgical trimming of the distorted bone when required for function or appearance. It seems likely that enlargement of these lesions may gradually become less after the age of 20 years, but Obwegeser et al. (1973) mentioned 2 of their patients in whom activity continued after this age.

Giant cell reparative granuloma of bone, first distinguished by Jaffe (1953), must also be considered in the situation where enlargement of the jaws is found. It is considered to occur most frequently in the age group below 25 years as described in Jaffe's original criteria for diagnosis. He defined it as a non-neoplastic benign giant cell lesion of bone, probably arising in response to some injury the nature of which is not always easy to establish. The histological appearances often reveal attempts at new bone formation so that the term 'reparative' seems justified. The giant cells seen often contain fat droplets and haemosiderin and are probably exerting a scavenging action. Sometimes the causation of the anomaly can fairly certainly be attributed to the teeth, as in a case described by this author (Cook, 1965). In that instance dental radiographs of the involved area taken seven years previously were available. These demonstrated the presence of carious teeth and related periapical chronic infection in the area subsequently involved by giant cell granuloma, It is therefore possible that chronic inflammation does have an aetiological effect.

The radiographs of such cases in general show expansion of the alveolar bone with well defined areas of rarefaction separated by fine bony septa. This configuration may suggest a pseudo-cystic appearance.

The blood biochemical investigations are usually normal, although some cases have been reported in which the acid phosphatase level has been elevated. The lesions can be quite vascular and on occasion may bleed freely when surgically curetted, which is the usual form of treatment (Cook, 1959).

Other benign causes

Trauma from compressed air

An occasional and unusual cause of swelling around the lower jaw may result from the presence of air in the tissues, causing surgical emphysema. This gains entrance through the tooth root in cases where a compressed air syringe is used to dry the tooth during root canal therapy. The blast of compressed air is forced into the tissues if the syringe nozzle is tightly inserted into the root canal entrance so that they are almost literally inflated as with a pump. The typical 'crackling' sensation felt when the tissues are palpated gives the diagnosis, but the cause may not at first be obvious.

Recurrent submandibular sialoadenitis

Calculi completely obstructing the main submandibular salivary duct will cause enlargement of the gland, but the history relating this phenomenon to mealtimes is usually enough to give the clue to the diagnosis. Radiographic examination confirms the presence of single or multiple stones which are usually opaque.

Acute infections

Acute pyogenic infection involving the soft tissues of the face occurs most commonly in relation to the ubiquitous lower wisdom tooth. Intraoral examination, if trismus permits this, should disclose the localized infection around the affected tooth. If inadequately treated such cases, even with the sophisticated antibiotics available today, can give rise to severe soft tissue infection which requires exten-

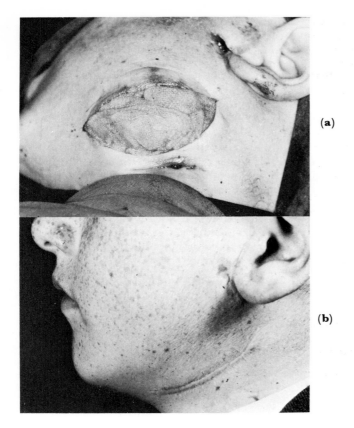

Fig. 4.2 Clinical photographs of boy aged 7 years suffering from acute osteomyelitis of mandible.
(**a**) After decortication of mandible—wound packed with paraffin gauze.
(**b**) Scar one year later.

sive drainage incisions to prevent extension of oedema to the glottis and airway obstruction. On occasion it may prove necessary to resort to wound packing with Vaseline gauze packs.

Acute osteomyelitis of the mandible can give rise to massive facial swelling and is usually the result of periapical infection around the roots of teeth. Often a chronic periapical infection which has been established for some months giving rise to very little in the way of symptoms suddenly becomes acute, resulting in the rapid onset of swelling. A good diagnostic sign with reference to mandibular disease is the presence of impaired sensation in the lower lip on the affected side. The patient will refer to this as being 'like pins and needles' or the effect of a dental injection. The area should be tested with a sharp point to demonstrate diminished pain response.

Radiographic evidence of sequestrum formation will certainly not be present unless the disease has been established for 4–6 weeks. Radiographic signs of periosteal activity may be found much earlier and should always be sought. Fine linear calcified shadows can be seen running concentric with the main mandibular outline and indicate progressive lifting and irritation of the periosteal membrane. Radical surgical decortication of the mandible may be needed to clear up such infections (Fig. 4.2).

Chronic infection

Of the chronic inflammatory granulomata, tuberculous and syphilitic disease appear infrequently to involve the mandible. When seen in the mouth the lesions of these diseases usually involve mucous membrane by ulceration. Occasionally, tuberculous involvement of a tooth socket occurs in a patient with an infected sputum.

Actinomycosis presents at the angle of the jaw, not infrequently in modern urban communities although the classical textbook appearance of patients with severe cicatrization and multiple discharging sinus is not usually seen. The facial form encountered is usually not very florid.

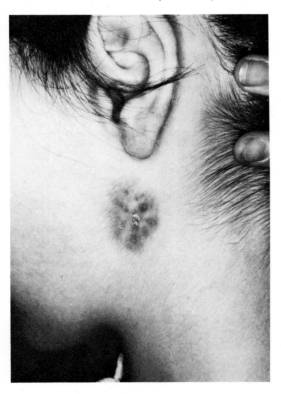

Fig. 4.3 Clinical photograph of girl aged 13 years suffering with actinomycosis—swelling at angle of jaw.

The patient usually presents with a fairly well defined swelling just below the angle of the jaw. This is dusky or plum coloured with defined margins and frequently fluctuant, accompanied by some surrounding soft tissue induration (Fig. 4.3). There is usually a history of a dental extraction or of jaw injury some time previously, which interval may be as long as 3 months.

If the swelling is fluctuant it should be aspirated through a wide-bore needle as the liquid can be quite viscid, and the pus sent for examination. When the diagnosis is established, a prolonged course of antibiotic is given which should result in resolution of the condition. Usually some localized scarring of the skin in the area occurs, which appears rather like a fine-textured primary vaccination scar.

Occasionally actinomycosis presents as an acute inflammatory episode in relation to a partly erupted wisdom tooth. Any such episode which fails to resolve with adequate treatment, especially where subcutaneous induration develops, should be suspected of being other than simple pyogenic infection.

Lymph node enlargement affecting the submandibular and upper deep cervical groups may occur from a virus or other inflammatory agent unrelated directly to the teeth and jaws. Glandular fever (infectious mononucleosis) is by far the most common cause in this group. Adenovirus may also be responsible for cervical lymph node enlargement. In recent years a number of cases have appeared caused by *Toxoplasma gondii* and these may initially be easily confused clinically with Hodgkin's disease. This finding probably represents a change in the pattern of disease so far as the UK is concerned.

Cysts and odontomes

The group comprising cysts and odontomes of dental origin are apt to cause much confusion in the minds of general surgeons. A general understanding of their developmental origin makes the situation less obscure.

Odontomes

Odontomes composed of calcified tissues occur as buried masses in the alveolus, which result in an enlargement of the alveolar size. They are usually painless unless they become infected, and it is often this latter event which calls attention to their presence. They are usually discovered in children and young adults, and associated with buried or missing normal teeth.

These odontomes are development aberrations derived from the tooth germs and are composed of a disordered mixture of the hard dental tissues, enamel, dentine and cementum. There is a wide range of shapes and sizes and a great variation in the degree of formal pattern. The commonest sites of occurrence are in the incisor areas, and the molar and premolar areas.

The two varieties which are formed to any size are the compound composite odontome and the complex composite odontome. The former consists of a fibrous tissue bag which contains a varying number of denticles of many different sizes. These are composed of dentine, enamel and cementum, and there are often as many as 20 or 30 individual denticles present. The latter consists of a misshapen mass of enamel dentine and cementum irregularly arranged together. These malformations are very hard in consistency and may prove difficult to remove because of their size, shape and position.

Both these examples of odontomes are of great theoretical and academic interest. Although they do not endanger life, they cause considerable disruption to the dentition and occlusion by their situation. They often present a difficult technical problem in removal, when at the same time the minimal damage to normal structures is required.

Cysts

Dental cyst

The most common cyst of the alveolus is the dental cyst, or root cyst. This occurs mainly in adults and may slowly and painlessly enlarge over a long period. It is benign and non-invasive. Very rare cases of malignant propensity have been recorded.

The cyst is found in relation to a dead tooth or root—although the latter may have been extracted, in which case the cyst is called 'residual'. The chronic inflammation associated with such a tooth stimulates epithelial developmental remnants (epithelial debris of Malassez) in the periodontal membrane to become active so that growth occurs which results in the formation of a simple cyst lined by stratified squamous epithelium. Once established, further growth is probably stimulated by osmotic pressure changes across the lining cyst membrane, as shown by Toller (1948). Recent work by Harris (1974) suggests that prostaglandins may also be involved in their growth. These cysts can grow to a considerable size, giving rise to smooth bony enlargement, but once the bone covering has been resorbed the physical sign of fluctuation is observed. Sometimes secondary infection of the cyst occurs with attendant physical signs. Nerve trunks are displaced by the enlarging lesions so that loss of sensation in the lower lip is not usually observed.

It is usually possible to excise these cysts completely by carefully dissecting them free. Sometimes in the upper jaw the maxillary sinus may be involved. As the cyst enlarges the volume of the antral cavity becomes reduced, which may present problems with nasal drainage.

Dentigerous cyst

Probably the next most common cyst of dental origin is the dentigerous cyst (follicular odontome) which occurs in children and young adults. This is because it is of developmental origin and grows without the requirement of stimulation by chronic inflammation. Typically there is an unerupted tooth in close relation to the cyst, often the crown portion of which lies in the cavity of the lesion. Such an appearance supports the theory that this cyst is derived from the remains of the enamel organ of the tooth germ which fails to involute and continues to grow in an abnormal manner, thus involving the tooth which it has lately formed.

The teeth most commonly affected are the upper and lower third molars, upper canines and, less frequently, the premolar teeth.

These cysts can grow to a considerable size if untreated, causing a hard swelling

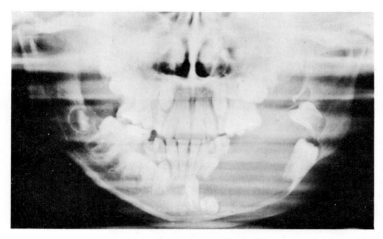

Fig. 4.4 Radiograph of mandible of boy aged 10 years, showing large dentigerous cyst of mandible. Note displacement of inferior dental nerve and first and second molar teeth.

of the jaw at the sites mentioned. The radiographic appearance is of a radiolucent area in the bone which possesses clearly defined margins. The related tooth will be observed at some point in its outline. Structures such as the inferior dental canal containing the neurovascular bundle will be displaced and not invaded by the enlarging lesion (Fig. 4.4). When removed, these cysts do not tend to recur and their histological examination reveals a simple stratified epithelium.

Odontokeratocyst

The non-recurring propensity of the previous group is certainly not found in odontokeratocysts (primordial cysts). This lesion has been defined more accurately in recent years and investigated in some detail because of its consistent tendency to recur. Because of the more active nature of their component epithelial cells, they are probably derived from remnants of the dental lamina which retain their activity after most of their number differentiate into the enamel organ of the tooth germ. Sometimes it is likely that this differentiation fails to occur at all so that, instead of the formation of a tooth in the normal series, all the formative activity goes into the production of an odontokeratocyst. In such cases a tooth (or teeth, if the lesion is bilateral) will be absent from the series.

These cysts are usually found in the lower third molar area where they are sometimes bilateral, and also in the lower incisor tooth area. They may reach a very large size before the patient attends for treatment, and cases with a 20-year history are known. The patient usually presents with a large painless swelling in the mandibular ramus area. Radiographic examination reveals massive bone loss caused by a multiloculated type of cyst containing many bony septa. These may or may not be related to a buried tooth (Fig. 4.5).

Such a massive lesion will present a difficult technical problem in its removal, but it is not this fact alone which accounts for the almost invariable recurrence

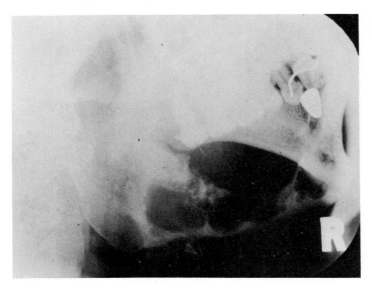

Fig. 4.5 Radiograph of mandible of male aged 35 years, showing large odontokeratocyst. Known history of 9 years.

as was at one time believed. Even in cases where it has been possible to remove every portion of abnormal epithelium, recurrence of the cyst has been observed some years later. Radiographic follow-up can also be deceptive and unreliable in this situation. Post-operative radiographic follow-up may demonstrate complete healing of the affected area, with complete filling in of a cavity by new bone, only to revert several years later to cystic cavity formation.

The nature of these cysts has been investigated by Toller (1971), who has shown by labelling their epithelial cells with tritiated (radioactive) thymidine that they are capable of undergoing considerable mitosis. This can be demonstrated by autoradiography and comparison with the results obtained by the same method in clinically less active cysts.

In view of the very active behaviour of these cells it seems likely that the high recurrence rate of odontokeratocysts can be explained by unavoidable spillage of cells into the bone cavity which occurs during their operative removal. This view is supported by recurrence of such cysts in bone grafts which have been inserted to replace resected portions of involved mandible (Schofield, 1971; Attenborough, 1974). Following such reports it has become the practice to wash out bone cavities caused by odontokeratocysts with an aqueous solution of 1 : 500 mercury perchloride. This acts as a protein coagulant capable of killing residual cells which could otherwise remain and continue to proliferate by implantation. A similar procedure was described by Lloyd-Davies and Naunton Morgan (Lloyd-Davies, 1948; Lloyd-Davies and Naunton Morgan, 1950); they successfully reduced the development of tumour recurrences at the sight of the anastomosis following resection of carcinoma of the colon, by washing out the lumen of the bowel with mercury perchloride solution. It is to be hoped that the recurrence rate of odontokeratocysts will be reduced in the same manner.

It was also shown in a separate piece of investigation by Toller (1966) that the fluid content of these cysts was different from that of dental and dentigerous cysts. Aspiration specimens of odontokeratocysts frequently contained flakes of keratin material. Also, the albumin content of the cyst fluid is relatively low compared with the patient's own serum or other cyst fluids. This is easy to demonstrate by electrophoresis and can sometimes be used diagnostically.

These cysts must always be treated with care. Although not a danger to life they can be a great nuisance to a patient, requiring multiple operations to eradicate. They should always be considered in diagnosis and distinguished from ameloblastoma (adamantinoma) which they can closely mimic.

Malignant swellings

Ameloblastoma

Ameloblastoma (adamantinoma) has been well known and well described for many years. It is often illustrated in textbooks as a tumour of enormous size affecting the lower jaw of patients in less developed communities. It is in fact not a very common tumour in Europeans. In the vast majority of cases it is the mandible which is affected, but a few instances have been reported in which the maxilla was involved (Fox and Dyson, 1975).

There has been a good deal of speculation concerning the origin of this lesion, but nobody to date has produced a better suggestion than Willis (1968), who considers it to be a carcinoma of dental basal cell remnants. The tumour can occur at any point in the mandible. Examples have been seen in the midline and, more commonly, involving the ramus and the angle area. They enlarge fairly slowly, producing destruction and enlargement of the mandible locally. Eventually ulceration occurs, and if this involves the intraoral mucous membrane it is possible for fragments of tumour to be detached and inhaled into the bronchial tree. The occasional known cases of secondary pulmonary tumours are thought to arise in this way, as ameloblastomas do not give rise to lymph node or blood-borne metastases.

The radiographic appearances show gross expansion and distortion of the bone outline. The tumour area contains large radiolucent portions which are bounded by bony septa of varying size. In such cases a biopsy is required to confirm the diagnosis.

Surgical treatment of these tumours is necessarily radical if they are to be completely removed. Reconstruction of the mandible is usually required by means of a metal prosthesis or a bone graft in order to restore appearance and function. More conservative forms of surgery have their advocates in special circumstances; for example, in elderly or otherwise unfit patients. These localized procedures can keep the tumour under control for quite long periods.

A number of excellent results have also been seen following high-energy irradiation treatments.

Other malignant tumours

The mandible may be the site of primary, metastatic or multicentric tumours

(Fig. 4.6). These may cause swelling in the bone or give rise to lymph node involvement which itself produces swelling in the submandibular or upper cervical sites. The salivary glands, because of their anatomical situation, impinge on the area so that an adenoidcystic carcinoma of the parotid gland or an anaplastic

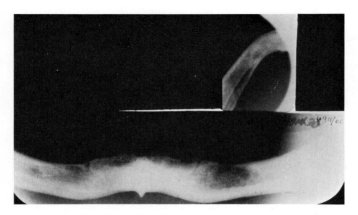

Fig. 4.6 Radiograph of mandible of male aged 54 years. Panoral and occlusal views showing deposit of multiple myeloma. Skull and left and right humerus also affected.

carcinoma of the submandibular salivary gland can present as a swelling near the jaw angle.

Squamous cell carcinoma and adenocarcinoma occurring in the oral cavity give rise to mandibular involvement from several sites, such as the tongue, floor of the mouth, alveolus, tonsil and buccal mucous membrane.

Metastatic tumours involving the mandible are derived from any of the primary tumours which commonly metastasize to bone; for example, breast, prostate, kidney, thyroid, bronchus and melanoma. All of these may present diagnostic as well as therapeutic problems. The same might also be said of multicentric tumours, such as multiple myeloma and reticulum cell sarcoma.

Fibrosarcoma, chondrosarcoma and osteosarcoma can all occur in the lower jaw and usually require combined treatment from surgeon, oncologist and radiotherapist to obtain the best possible control of the disease.

References

ATTENBOROUGH N. R. (1974) Recurrence of an odontogenic keratocyst in a bone graft: report of a case. *Br. J. Oral Surg.* **12**, 33–39.
COOK H. P. (1959) Giant cell reparative granuloma. *Proc. R. Soc. Med.* **52**, 745–747.
COOK H. P. (1965) Giant-cell granuloma. *Brit. J. Oral Surg.* **3**, 97–100.
FOX J. E. and DYSON D. P. (1975) Ameloblastoma of the maxilla; a report of two cases. *Br. Dent. J.* **138**, 61–64.
HARRIS M. (1974) Review of recent experimental work on the dental cyst. *Proc. R. Soc. Med.* **67**, 1259–1262.

JAFFE H. L. (1953) Giant cell reparative granuloma, traumatic bone cyst, and fibrous (fibro-osseous) dysplasia of the jaw bones. *Oral Surg.* **6,** 159–175.

JONES W. A. (1933) Familial multilocular cystic disease of the jaws. *Am. J. Cancer* **17,** 946–950.

JONES W. A. (1938) Further observations regarding familial multilocular cystic disease of the jaws. *Br. J. Radiol.* **11,** 227–241.

LLOYD-DAVIES O. V. (1948) Radical excision in carcinoma of rectum. *Proc. R. Soc. Med.* **41,** 822–827.

LLOYD-DAVIES O. V. and NAUNTON MORGAN C. (1950) Conservative resection in carcinoma of the rectum. *Proc. R. Soc. Med.* **43,** 701–710.

OBWEGESER H. L., FREIHOFER H. P. M. and HOREJS J. (1973) Variations of fibrous dysplasia in the jaws. *J. Maxillofac. Surg.* **1,** 161–171.

SCHOFIELD J. J. (1971) Unusual recurrence of an odontogenic keratocyst. *Br. Dent. J.* **130,** 487–489.

SEWARD G. R. and HANKEY G. T. (1957) Cherubism. *Oral Surg.* **10,** 952–974.

TOLLER P. A. (1948) Experimental investigation into factors concerning growth of cysts of the jaws. *Proc. R. Soc. Med.* **41,** 681–687.

TOLLER P. A. (1966) Permeability of cyst walls in vivo: investigations with radioactive tracers. *Proc. R. Soc. Med.* **59,** 724–729.

TOLLER P. A. (1971) Autoradiography of explants from odontogenic cysts. *Br. Dent. J.* **131,** 57–61.

WILLIS R. A. (1968) *Pathology of Tumours*, 4th edn. London, Butterworths.

5

Surgery in the Haemorrhagic Diatheses

A. J. Gunning, MA, FRCS, DLO

The importance attached to blood throughout the ages is recalled in sacrifice, hunting and warfare.

Blood, this juice 'of rarest quality', is common to the surgery of all tissues and organs. In the surgery of the brain, the lung or the intestine we accept the blood

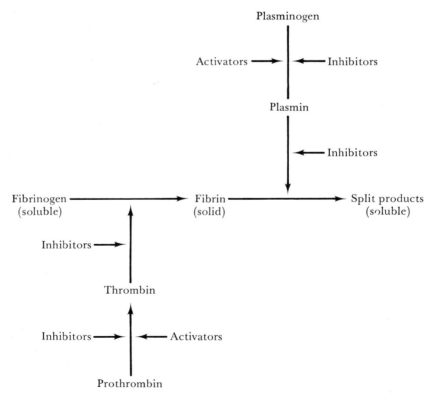

Fig. 5.1 The haemostatic balance.

as an intruder that must be properly controlled lest it mar the efficiency of technique.

Surgeons make incisions, clamp, cauterize or ligature a few dozen of the larger vessels they have cut and feel they have made a major contribution towards haemostasis whereas in reality thousands upon thousands of small cut vessels have been sealed by a natural process, the failure of which would be catastrophic. Artificial haemostatic measures are relatively useless without the natural mechanism and many patients with haemostatic defects have bled to death from apparently trivial injuries despite every effort to stop the bleeding by conventional surgical means. A surgeon trying to stop bleeding during an operation on a patient with a haemostatic defect would be like trying to stop water going through a shirt by suturing the buttonholes!

Normal haemostasis

During the last 20 years considerable advance has been made in the understanding of the haemostatic mechanism, its defects and the development of effective methods for treatment. However, the process of clotting outside the vascular system and in certain circumstances when blood is still retained in the vessels appears to become more complicated each year as more and more factors are concerned in its regulation, but it has become more intelligible as a biological phenomenon.

The normal fluidity of the blood is maintained by a balance between substances that tend to make it clot and other substances which prevent this (Fig. 5.1). Most of the confusion concerning the clotting mechanism has been eliminated by the acceptance of an international code of roman numerals instead of names for the various clotting factors and the acceptance of the 'cascade theory' of MacFarlane (1964) of Oxford to describe the clotting sequence (Fig. 5.2).

Haemostasis in a wound is achieved by the interlocking operation of three different mechanisms which are dependent upon one another. These are: (1) changes in the vessels; (2) platelet effects; and (3) the coagulation factors (Fig. 5.3).

Changes in vessels

Trauma causes a vascular response which is manifest as active constriction in all vessels except the capillaries. This constriction is an important haemostatic mechanism in large vessels, but is less obvious in smaller vessels though it can be seen in damaged arterioles and venules and also in undamaged vessels in their vicinity. The vascular endothelium becomes sticky and permeable to fluid, resulting in a rise in extravascular pressure which causes the capillary endothelial walls to stick together. Fluid loss leads to packing of the red cells, with a consequent rise in viscosity which slows the rate of flow of blood through the capillary. The mechanism for these vascular effects is obscure. In the large vessels it is probably neurogenic in origin. The reaction in the smaller vessels is probably due to vasoactive substances released in the area of the injury, particularly by the platelets which secrete serotonin and catecholamines. Other substances produced as a result of trauma are derived from the activation of the kinin system, including bradykinin which causes local pain and increases vascular permeability.

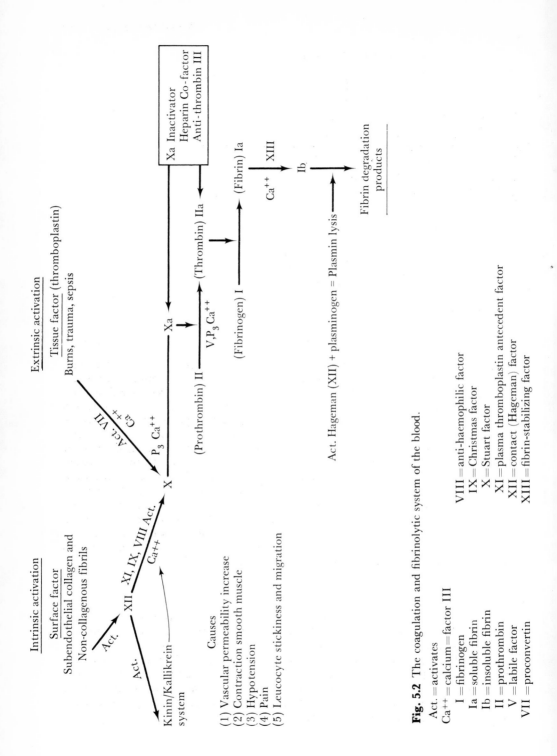

Fig. 5.2 The coagulation and fibrinolytic system of the blood.

Act. = activates
Ca++ = calcium = factor III
I = fibrinogen
Ia = soluble fibrin
Ib = insoluble fibrin
II = prothrombin
V = labile factor
VII = proconvertin

VIII = anti-haemophilic factor
IX = Christmas factor
X = Stuart factor
XI = plasma thromboplastin antecedent factor
XII = contact (Hageman) factor
XIII = fibrin-stabilizing factor

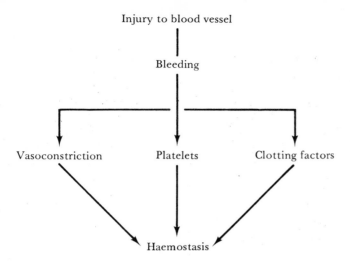

Fig. 5.3 Mechanism of haemostasis.

Role of platelets

The vascular endothelium constitutes the first line of defence against bleeding or clotting. Injury to the intimal layer results in the following sequence of events:

The platelets adhere to the subendothelial collagen or to recently described non-collagenous microfibrils. Adenosine diphosphate (ADP) is then released from the vessel wall, damaged red cells and the adhered platelets, causing other platelets in the blood stream to adhere to the site of injury and to each other to form a haemostatic plug. Simultaneously there is activation of Hageman factor (XII) by exposed collagen and platelets. This activates the intrinsic clotting mechanism, leading to the generation of small amounts of thrombin. Thrombin then causes an irreversible aggregation and fusion of platelets with release of the intraplatelet pool of serotonin and catecholamines which produce further platelet aggregation. Minutes later, as additional thrombin is formed, fibrin is laid down which strengthens and stabilizes the haemostatic plug. Activated platelets, in addition to forming haemostatic plugs, accelerate the coagulation mechanism by making available platelet factor 3, a surface phospholipid.

Clotting mechanism

The steps leading to the formation of a fibrin gel from its precursor, fibrinogen, are complicated. Blood coagulation involves a sequential reaction of a number of plasma proteins or clotting factors which act in a step-wise or 'cascade' fashion. Each proteolytic enzyme converts its protein substrate to an active form which acts as an enzyme for the next reaction in the series. The result is the formation of thrombin from prothrombin, which leads to the conversion of fibrinogen to an insoluble fibrin gel. Calcium and phospholipids (platelet factor III) from the platelets are also necessary for the reaction.

Prothrombin activation occurs by two processes: the extrinsic system, which requires the interaction of tissue factor or thromboplastin with plasma factors VII, X and V and with calcium (factor III); or the intrinsic system, whereby contact of the plasma with foreign surfaces leads to a series of reactions involving only blood constituents such as factors XII, XI, IX, VIII, X and V together with the platelets. At least one additional plasma factor (factor XIII) is necessary to effect the polymerization of fibrin (see Fig. 5.2) by promoting cross-linkage.

Built into this cascade system is a feature of amplification—for the minute quantity of factor XII present in plasma, staggeringly large amounts of factor I become available.

Our vascular system is constantly being traumatized by the hurly-burly of everyday activities. It is suggested that clotting is a prerequisite for vascular integrity. If this is so and it is occurring continuously, then mechanisms must be available in the system to eliminate fibrin as fast as it is formed. Without them the vascular system would become obliterated.

Three mechanisms are available to prevent this. First, the reticuloendothelial system clears active coagulation products from the blood as it passes through liver, spleen and lungs. Secondly, natural anticoagulants occur, particularly those that actively neutralize thrombin, for example anti-thrombin III, or interfere with fibrin formation. Thirdly, the fibrinolytic enzyme system constitutes a mechanism capable of breaking down large quantities of fibrin (Fig. 5.2).

Abnormal haemostasis

A haemostatic abnormality may be congenital or acquired. A careful history and physical examination and a few simple coagulation tests will usually reveal the true nature of a pre-existing coagulation disorder. Most patients with a congenital haemostatic abnormality will give a voluntary history of excessive bleeding: therefore, never dismiss a patient's claim of excessive bleeding. The best and commonest lesion to question any patient about, if there is a suggestion of a bleeding tendency, is the open wound bed following a tooth extraction. This is a severe test for the haemostatic mechanism. Beware of the young patient with spontaneous ecchymoses and petechiae. Many women and old people bruise easily and do not, as a rule, have a bleeding disorder.

The majority of clinically important coagulation defects will be detected by routine tests available in all haematological laboratories.

Abnormal haemostasis, either as an increased bleeding tendency or extensive thrombosis, results from; (1) vascular defects; (2) platelet dysfunction and defects; and (3) coagulation disorders.

Vascular defects

The majority of causes of bleeding from vascular defects rarely confront the surgeon but may prove troublesome if present in patients requiring surgery. They may be classified as:

(a) Defects in the supporting tissue of vessels, e.g.
   (i) purpura of old age; (ii) Cushing's syndrome and steroid therapy;
   (iii) haemorrhagic telangiectasis.

(b) Defects in the vessel wall, e.g. Marfan's syndrome and Ehler–Danlos syndrome.
(c) Infections, e.g. mycotic aneurysms.
(d) Metabolic, e.g. sprue.

Platelet defects and dysfunction

Platelet defects, which may be qualitative or quantitative, account for a considerable number of clinical problems. The main manifestation is bleeding because platelet abnormalities may affect not only the vascular endothelium but also the coagulation of blood. Thrombocytopenia is well tolerated, but below 15,000–20,000 platelets/mm³ bleeding may occur spontaneously and haemorrhage can occur anywhere, but especially into the subcutaneous tissues, intestine, urinary tract and central nervous system. Patients with thrombocytopenia for which a cause is not readily apparent need a bone marrow examination or a lymph node biopsy to rule out such diseases as leukaemia, lymphoma or multiple myelomatosis.

The commonest form of platelet deficiency, thrombocytopenic purpura, is due to the action of chemical poisons; drugs are probably the most important to the surgeon because so many drugs in common use, for example sedatives, antibiotics, etc., can cause a thrombocytopenic purpura. Other causes are radiation and viral infections. Surgery on these patients is made possible only by stopping the

Table 5.1 Haematological disorders amenable to splenectomy

1. *Haemolytic anaemias:*
   Hereditary spherocytosis
   Hereditary elliptocytosis
   Hereditary non-spherocytic haemolytic anaemia
   Thalassaemia
   Sickle cell disease
   Idiopathic autoimmune haemolytic anaemia
   Idiopathic thrombocytopenic purpura
   Thrombotic thrombocytopenic purpura

2. Primary hypersplenism
   Secondary hypersplenism

3. Myeloid metaplasia
   Hodgkin's disease, lymphosarcoma, leukaemia and reticulum cell sarcoma

4. *Miscellaneous disorders:*
   Felty's syndrome
   Sarcoidosis
   Gaucher's disease
   Niemann–Pick's disease
   Fanconi's syndrome
   Porphyria erythropoietica
   Spontaneous rupture, e.g. glandular fever, malaria

offending drug and by using platelet transfusions; steroids and fresh blood before, during and after operation.

The condition known as idiopathic thrombocytopenic purpura is similar to the above condition and is now accepted as being a manifestation of temporary or long-term autoimmunity. The condition is important to recognize as it can, with other bleeding diatheses, be cured by removing the spleen. Steroids and fresh blood transfusion may be necessary to get patients fit for surgery. Immunotherapy may be necessary in some patients. Table 5.1 shows a list of bleeding conditions which are treated by splenectomy. In secondary hypersplenism the operation of anastomosing the portal vein to the inferior vena cava will relieve the bleeding tendency. The influx of a coloured population has necessitated extra care and tests to rule out red cell sickling before administering an anaesthetic and so avoiding a bleeding crisis during an operation on coloured patients.

Defects of coagulation

Theoretically, absence of any one of the factors concerned in blood coagulation could cause bleeding. In practice, however, absence of factors VIII, IX, V and XIII are the most likely to cause bleeding. Congenital absence of factors VIII and IX, i.e. haemophilia and Christmas disease respectively, are by far the most frequent and, to the surgeon, the most difficult and frustrating to deal with.

Haemophilia

Haemophilia is a disease caused by a genetic defect. An individual who suffers from it bleeds too freely because he cannot activate a factor in the blood which causes the plasma to coagulate. It is a sex-linked recessive defect originally resulting from the mutation of the gene on the X chromosome of the germ cell, either the sperm of the father or the ovum of the mother. If a child is a male he will be a haemophilic; if a female she will be a carrier of the disease although she will rarely suffer from it and the chances are 1 in 2 that her sons will be haemophilic and her daughters carriers. The sons of a haemophilic father will carry no trace of the hereditary defect because they receive his Y and not his X chromosomes. All his daughters, however, will be carriers. The disease has gained a certain notoriety because it plagued European royalty for three generations.

Haemophilia (or factor VIII deficiency) is the most important, most common and one of the most serious of the bleeding diatheses. Approximately 1 in every 10,000 persons in England is affected by the disease. There are therefore about 3,000 haemophilics in England. Table 5.2 shows the degree of bleeding which can be expected in patients with varying percentages of factor VIII in the blood.

The commonest lesion in the haemophilic is haemarthrosis, either from spontaneous bleeding or from trivial trauma, and especially bleeding into and around the knee-joint. The joint may become very large and very painful, and repeated bleeds lead to crippling arthritis, joint dysfunction and deformity. Splinting, aspiration, administration of the necessary blood factor and analgesics are required in treatment. Major orthopaedic procedures such as arthrodesis, hip replacement and tendon transplantation are now accepted procedures in a patient suffering from haemophilia.

Table 5.2 The relationship between observed natural blood levels of factor VIII and the occurrence of haemorrhagic symptoms

Blood level of factor VIII(%)	Level of haemostatic efficiency
100	Normal
25–50	Liability to abnormal bleeding after major trauma. Often not diagnosed
10–25	Severe bleeding after minor trauma or surgical operations
5–10	Gross bleeding after minor injuries. Some haemarthroses and 'spontaneous' bleeding
<5	Severe haemophilia. Haemarthroses and muscle haemorrhages, with crippling

Table 5.3 The level of factor VIII required in patient's blood and the therapeutic materials used for the treatment of different lesions

Lesion	Level of factor VIII desired in patient's blood immediately after transfusion (percentage normal)*	Therapeutic material
Uncomplicated spontaneous bleeding into joints and muscles	5–20 (0–5)	Cryoprecipitate. Human freeze-dried concentrate AHG
Haematoma in dangerous situation	20–40 (5–10)	
Dental extractions		Pre-extraction: epsilon-aminocaproic acid (EACA: Epsikaprin); aminomethyl cyclohexane carboxylic acid (AMCA: Cyklokapron); cryoprecipitate. *Then* EACA 0.1 g/kg for 6–10 days orally
Major surgery and accidents	100–150 (25–40)	Human freeze-dried concentrate AHG
Any source of bleeding with AHG Inhibitors	Requires maintained high levels	Animal AHG or Freeze-dried human concentrate

*The figures in parentheses are the approximate levels to which the factor VIII level will have fallen 24 hours after transfusion.
†AHG = Anti-haemophilic globulin.

Peculiar to the haemophilic are the huge haemophilic pseudo-tumours or cysts caused by bleeding into muscles, especially in the lower half of the body. They erode through and deform underlying bone. If they erode through the skin or are inadvertently aspirated or biopsied they become infected. The organized thick cyst wall has extensive ramifications. Small tumours resolve well with factor VIII administration and immobilization. Wide radical excision, however, may be necessary, and even amputation to free the patient of the cyst (Gunning, 1966). Major surgery in the haemophilic has become safer with the development of effective plasma concentrates in the last few years; however, treatment is still not simple because of expense, recurrent bleeding, especially if infection supervenes and healing is prolonged, and the development of natural or acquired inhibitors of factor VIII by the patient. Indeed, no patient with haemophilia should ever be submitted to surgery without testing for inhibitors. Their presence may well preclude any surgical treatment. Table 5.3 shows the preparations used for treating haemophilia and the amounts of factor VIII necessary to achieve haemostasis. The level of factor VIII must be maintained at a steady level of 80–100 per cent for at least 7 days, and preferably 10 days, to allow for primary healing. This is difficult to achieve because factor VIII is only effective for 12 hours. The use of factor VIII concentrates which necessitate only small volumes of fluid—20–50 ml—being administered at any one time have revolutionized the treatment of haemophilia. An important aspect of the surgical treatment of a haemophilic patient once the diagnosis of haemophilia has been made is to make quite sure that the hospital you are working in is capable of dealing with these patients. If the hospital has not enough concentrate or the necessary personnel experienced in determining the factor levels two to three times daily, the patient should be transferred to a centre where such treatment and management is available.

Factor IX deficiency (Christmas disease)

Factor IX deficiency (or Christmas disease) is clinically indistinguishable from haemophilia. It is only one-tenth as common as haemophilia. Concentrates for the treatment of factor IX deficiency are also available.

Patients with haemophilia and Christmas disease require surgery not only for the lesions of the bleeding defects but also for those surgical conditions from which ordinary people are liable to suffer.

Patients with haemorrhagic disorders are subject to unique intra-abdominal emergencies. Abdominal pain presents a clinical problem calling for careful assessment and observation because of the dangers of surgical treatment in haemophilics. The commonest cause of intra-abdominal pain in haemophilics is bleeding into the psoas muscle, or the intraperitoneal tissues. Bleeding may also occur into the mesentery and this may cause gangrene or intussusception of the involved portion of bowel. Bleeding into the intestinal wall is not uncommon and may result in partial or complete obstruction of the bowel. Bleeding into the urinary tract causes renal colic and haematuria. Because bleeding is the commonest cause of pain, it is always advisable to administer anti-haemophilic concentrate, which will effect a cure, and to observe the patient over 8–24 hours or until such time as symptoms and signs indicate that surgical treatment is necessary.

The diagnosis of acute appendicitis may be very difficult, but it is probably fair to say that more haemophilics have died from unnecessary surgical treatment than from neglected appendicitis. It should be remembered that haemorrhage alone may be associated with pyrexia, tachycardia, leucocytosis, nausea and vomiting. When in doubt it is best to give anti-haemophilic concentrate to ensure haemostatic competence, and antibiotics; to restrict oral intake; and, most important, to make careful repeated observation.

Gastric bleeding is a serious problem in the haemophilic. If haematemesis and malaena are shown by barium meal and gastroscopy to be due to a gastric or duodenal ulcer, it is best to operate under anti-haemophilic cover. The operation of choice should be one which gives the least chance of recurrence, and in my

Table 5.4 Surgery on haemophilic patients from January 1968 to May 1974. (From the Oxford Unit)

Type of operation	Total
Removal of haemophilic cyst	1
Hernia repair	7
Cholecystectomy	2
Laparotomy	3
Vagotomy and pyloroplasty	2
Circumcision	4
Haemorrhoidectomy	5
Gastrectomy	1
Abdominoperineal resection	2
Aortic valve replacement	1
Appendicectomy	2
Vagotomy and antrectomy	3
Excision of pilonidal sinus	1
Total	34

experience this has been a vagotomy and antrectomy, restoring intestinal continuity with a Billroth I procedure.

With the efficient fibrinogen-free, small volume, human anti-haemophilic concentrates commercially available today it is possible to do any major operation, as can be seen from Table 5.4, which shows the range of surgical operations personally performed from the haemophilic unit in Oxford.

Factor XIII deficiency

Factor XIII deficiency is rare, but important to surgeons because it results in secondary post-operative wound bleeding and poor wound healing. Pre-operative or intra-operative blood or plasma will prevent bleeding.

Von Willebrand's disease

Von Willebrand's disease is a haemorrhagic state inherited as a simple autosomal dominant in which all three components of the haemostatic mechanism appear to be involved. Clinically it presents, in males and females, with repeated episodes of bleeding from mucous membrane surfaces. The laboratory findings suggest three components at fault in von Willebrand's disease, one or all of which may cause bleeding:

1. Vascular   —prolonged bleeding time
2. Platelets   —reduced adhesiveness and a failure to aggregate with the anti-biotic, ristocetin
3. Coagulation—a low level of factor VIII

An interesting and curious factor in von Willebrand's disease is that when patients with the disease are transfused with normal blood or fractions of plasma rich in anti-haemophilic factor the concentration of this factor rises immediately to a level one would anticipate. But within 6–8 hours, the concentration of anti-haemophilic factor rises still higher, as if the synthesis of factor VIII had been induced, and thereafter its titre falls at a much slower rate than it does in patients with classic haemophilia. Even more remarkable is the fact that the transfusion of haemophilic plasma into patients with von Willebrand's disease stimulates the appearance of anti-haemophilic-factor-like activity. This phenomenon only occurs in vivo. Indeed, it is now thought that von Willebrand's disease, rather than haemophilia, is associated with a true deficiency of factor VIII antigen. In other words, von Willebrand's disease patients require a factor in haemophilic or normal plasma to stimulate the formation of functional anti-haemophilic factor, and the haemophilic patient has the antigen but lacks a factor which must combine with the antigen to make the coagulation factor.

The condition is clinically mild except in unusual instances, especially when factor VIII level is below 20 per cent. Bleeding is rapidly controlled by blood transfusions or plasma factor VIII concentrates.

Medical diseases associated with bleeding tendency

There are patients with certain medical conditions who, if they require surgery, may bleed excessively during or after the operation. The surgeon operating, especially in emergency situations on patients with these conditions, should be aware of this possibility and enlist the help of a haematologist.

1. Polycythaemia vera. The incidence of complications in these patients is as high as 80 per cent in uncontrolled cases, 30 per cent in controlled. The mortality is 15–20 per cent; 65 per cent bleed, 25 per cent develop thrombosis and 20 per cent become infected. Causes of bleeding include a deficiency of clotting factors, poor organization of the clot, deficiency of platelet factor 3, low platelet concentration, deficiency of anti-plasmin, and fibrinolysis. Treatment includes phlebotomy, giving fresh blood and myelosuppressive drugs.

2. Patients with myelofibrosis, leukaemia or lymphoma have the same complications as item 1, above. Avoid surgical procedures if possible.

3. Obstructive jaundice, cirrhosis of the liver, prolonged antibiotics, sprue and intestinal fistula all lead to prothrombin and vitamin K deficiency. Vitamin K is necessary for the synthesis of factors II, VII, IX and X. Treatment is to administer vitamin K. For urgent cases give fresh frozen plasma containing prothrombin.

4. Uraemia—renal failure results in a variable degree of disturbance of the normal haemostatic mechanism. This occurs in two ways. First, some degree of depression of vitamin-K-dependent factors may occur, e.g. prothrombin and factors VII and X. Secondly, and possibly more significant, there may be a disturbance of platelet function. The platelet release reaction is variably depressed and collagen aggregation may be deficient.

5. Mismatched blood causes a thrombocytopenia and hypofibrinogenaemia.

The treatment is a combination of heparin and mannitol to combat the fibrinolysis, and the transfusion of fresh blood as a source of platelets.

6. Cyanotic congenital heart disease—these patients develop a polycythaemia secondary to their anoxaemias, but they also have a shortage of most of the clotting factors and a tendency to increased fibrinolysis for reasons not well understood.

7. Shock from gram-negative organisms leads to intravascular clotting with consumption of clotting factors, which leads to a fall in platelets, fibrinogen, factor VIII and factor V. Fibrinogen degradation products rise from lysis and promote bleeding.

8. Patients on anticoagulant therapy. Watch out for the odd patient who is secretly taking anticoagulants to induce bleeding to gain admission to hospital.

9. Acquired anticoagulants may occur—spontaneously, in middle-aged

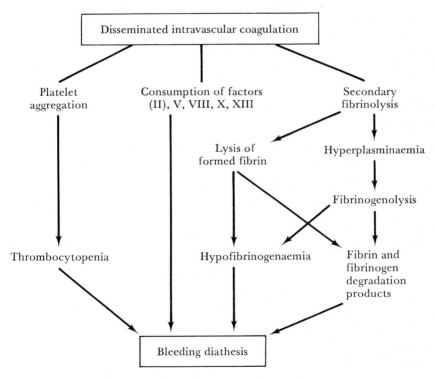

Fig. 5.4 Activation of clotting in circulation.

people and in patients with systemic lupus erythematosus and rheumatoid arthritis—and lead to bleeding. The anticoagulant usually destroys anti-haemophilic factor in these patients. The situation usually resolves spontaneously.

Bleeding during an operation may be expected in open-heart surgery, transplant surgery (especially liver transplants), and after massive homologous blood transfusions of stored blood. After the administration of 8–10 units of stored blood one should, if possible, go on to fresh blood until the bleeding is controlled. If fresh blood is not easily available then 1–2 units of fresh frozen plasma should be given. To this may be added cryoprecipitate. If all else fails to stop bleeding, the author has on one occasion tried the effect of a direct blood transfusion from donor to recipient with cessation of bleeding.

Extensive surgical resections for carcinoma, especially of the prostate, lung and pancreas, can lead to the rapid development of clotting abnormalities and bleeding. Diffuse intravascular coagulation and fibrinolysis have been blamed for bleeding in these conditions.

Fibrinolysis and intravascular clotting is too complex a subject to discuss here. Briefly, a number of agents—physical, chemical or bacterial—after entering the blood stream can cause platelet aggregation without vascular injury. These aggregations block the capillaries of organs and limbs. The platelets lyse and coagulation proceeds intravascularly, leading to fibrin formation. The fibrin is lysed to fibrin degradation products, causing severe bleeding. It is thought that this is the most frequently acquired haemostatic defect occurring in medical patients requiring surgery (Fig. 5.4).

It is often considered by surgeons that a bleeding tendency is rare and it certainly is if you consider haemophilia and Christmas disease only. It should be remembered as shown above that other medical conditions have the ability to convert a simple straightforward surgical procedure into a surgical nightmare!

References

GUNNING A. J. (1966) The Surgery of Haemophilic Cysts. In: BIGGS R. and MCFARLANE R. G. (ed.) *Treatment of Haemophilia and other Coagulation Disorders*. Oxford, Blackwells, p. 262.

MACFARLANE R. G. (1964) An enzyme cascade in the blood clotting mechanism, and its function as a biochemical amplifier. *Nature* **202,** 498–499.

Further Reading

RATNOFF O. D. (1974) Some recent advances in the study of hemostasis. *Circ. Res.* **35,** 1–14.

6

The Pathogenesis and Management of Embolism in the Vascular Tree

H. H. G. Eastcott, MS, FRCS

Embolism means the movement of any abnormal material or object in macroscopic amounts from one part of the circulation to another. In most instances, it is blood thrombus that migrates. Other objects have been described as behaving in the same way: fat globules, air bubbles, tumour masses, hydatid daughtercysts, small bullets or missile fragments, plastic tubing in various lengths, fragments of guide-wire and even mercury that has gained access from an arterial manometer, and many others. Thrombus, however, heads the list: in fact the processes of its formation and migration are now often considered together under the title 'thromboembolism', the two processes being inseparable in both their causes and treatment. There have been striking advances in recent years in our understanding of the processes of thromboembolism and the treatment of its various forms. None of this new knowledge, however, has in any way altered Virchow's classic concept of a threefold disease process depending upon the presence of stasis, injury to the vessel wall and hypercoagulability. In the past these three great principles existed, it seemed, to be learned and largely forgotten, perhaps because further advances in knowledge were so slow in developing. The past few years have brought advances on all three fronts. It is now believed that hypercoagulability is the dominant factor in venous thromboembolism; that damage in the endothelium with consequent platelet adherence is the prime factor in arterial occlusive disease; and that stasis is equally important on both sides of the circulation. The study of blood viscosity at both high and low rates of shear, for blood is a non-Newtonian fluid, and of the processes of fibrin deposition and removal, all closely related to one another, have opened up the way for real advances in the understanding of thromboembolic disease and its management. Until recently, almost all such studies were qualitative. Now that the normal and abnormal can be measured, further advances are certain to follow (Dormandy, 1970).

There are some risk factors that are common to both arterial and venous thrombosis. Tobacco smoking, diabetes, congestive heart failure, shock and polycythaemia vera all tend to increase blood viscosity, which in turn is augmented by stasis, either locally or of the body as a whole. Injury, likewise, has both local and general damaging effects on vascular flow. Cancer, leukaemia and an unfavourable reaction to the contraceptive pill can also bring about occlusion of any part of the vascular tree.

Venous thromboembolism

Limited thrombi can be detected in the veins of the calf in 25 per cent of patients recovering from surgical operation (Kakkar et al., 1969). Improved modern methods of detection of lower limb thrombi (radioiodine-labelled fibrinogen for the calf (Fig. 6.1) and popliteal regions; Doppler ultrasound for the femoral (Fig.

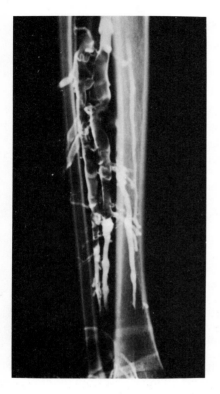

Fig. 6.1 Calf vein thrombosis in a girl of 22 years who was taking the contraceptive pill.

6.2) and iliac veins) have shown that in 50 per cent or more of patients with deep venous thrombosis there may be no detectable clinical evidence of this (Nicolaides et al., 1975). It is common for massive pulmonary embolism to transform a quiet recovery into a desperate illness within the hour. The post-operative care of surgical patients should now properly include the most rigorous methods of prevention and detection that are now becoming practicable. The value of post-operative physiotherapy, leg bandaging and elevation and early ambulation cannot be proven nor can these measures withstand the scrutiny of modern methods of thrombus detection. This is hardly surprising when these new methods have established that in the majority of cases thrombosis begins during the actual operation itself. To be effective, therefore, prevention must begin in the operating

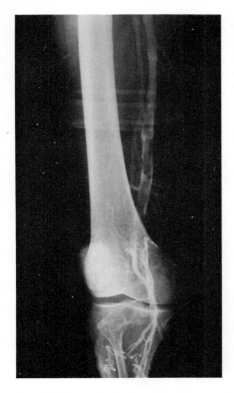

Fig. 6.2 Femoral vein thrombosis in a surgical patient, detected with Doppler ultrasound, from failure to elicit a previously normal flux signal at the groin on calf squeezing. (From *Thromboembolism*, edited by Nicolaides, Meadway and Irving, 1975, by kind permission of the authors and the publishers, Medical and Technical Publishing Ltd.)

theatre or even beforehand. Time spent in hospital awaiting operation should be reduced to the minimum. This has been shown to be more effective than the various post-operative measures already mentioned. During operation, mechanical calf compression, sporadic stimulation of calf contractions and the low dosage subcutaneous heparin regimen are known to be useful in this order of increasing effectiveness. The early results of large-scale trials of 8-hourly subcutaneous injections of heparin 5,000 units are showing a significant decrease in fatal post-operative pulmonary embolism (*Lancet*, 1975). Difficulties still remain, however. There is a slight but definite tendency to increased operative and post-operative blood loss and drainage.

Preventive femoral vein ligation has never been much used in Britain, nor have various methods of incomplete obstruction of the inferior vena cava become accepted. Apart from some doubt about the effectiveness of these surgical methods of prevention, they also carry a real risk of obstructive and gravitational difficulties in the lower limb which can develop as early as the convalescent period. Nevertheless, the low dosage heparin method has still fully to establish its usefulness in the special high-risk situations in which effective prevention is so much needed. Though it can be fully accepted that proximally extending calf vein thrombosis can be almost eliminated by low dosage heparin, there remains some uncertainty as to whether it may work equally well for the large and dangerous iliac vein thromboses that so often complicate major hip reconstruction (Fig. 6.3),

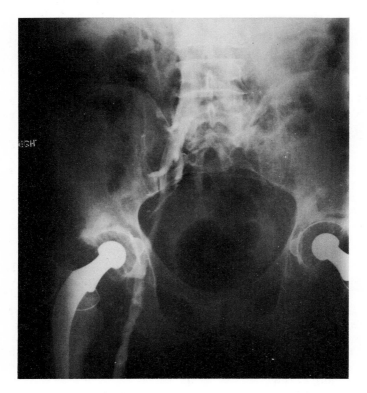

Fig. 6.3 Localized iliofemoral venous thrombosis as an early complication of hip reconstruction. High risk of embolism.

pelvic cancer operations and some otherwise successful cases of renal transplantation (Kakkar and Jouhar, 1973).

Other drugs, known to be effective against some components of the mechanism of thrombosis, have been subjected to carefully controlled trials against venous thromboembolism. These include aspirin, low molecular weight dextran and dipyridamole. None of these could be shown conclusively to reduce the incidence of thromboembolism after operation.

Prevention by surgical means

For practical purposes, this is considered only after pulmonary embolism has already occurred, particularly if the patient is already having anticoagulant

treatment. Vein ligation with or without removal of the thrombus, or thrombectomy with reconstruction of the vein, have all been advocated during the past
decade (Mavor and Galloway, 1969). Though thrombectomy cannot be said to
have contributed significantly to the prevention of pulmonary embolism, nor perhaps either to the reduction of post-thrombotic stasis, it does have a real place
as the only potential cure for developing venous gangrene. While ligation of the
femoral vein below the profunda entry is not often followed by stasis effects, iliac
or caval ligation usually is. Because of this, it has been the more recent practice
amongst those who believe in interruption of the venous pathway to the lungs
to narrow the inferior vena cava by sutures, by coarsely serrated clips or by the
insertion of an umbrella filter (Mobin-Uddin et al., 1971) introduced from the
neck, down through the right atrium, to a point below the renal veins.

Objections to these operations include the risk of late stasis effects in the lower
limbs, the fact that they largely exclude effective anticoagulant treatment at a
time when it is most needed and, above all, that they may not be effective in
achieving their object. Thrombus has often been demonstrated beyond a clip
or ligature at post mortem in patients who have succumbed from secondary
embolism. Late post-operative venography seldom shows a patent channel after
reconstructive thrombectomy.

The most effective preventive measure against secondary embolism is heparin
in full therapeutic dosage, up to 60,000 units in 24 hours, preferably given by
regulated drip or infusion but otherwise by intermittent 6-hourly injections via
an indwelling cannula. Most British surgeons believe that this regimen continued
for 7–10 days will largely exlude the problem, though it is conceded that there
may be a place for operation in resistant or chronic cases of small repeated embolism resulting in pulmonary hypertension. A natural extension of the heparin concept (which may permit or possibly even promote natural fibrinolytic activity)
is the induction of active thrombolysis by the patient's own plasmin activated
by streptokinase. This method, which has been under examination for almost
as long as surgical interruption, is proving under controlled trial to be most effective, not only in clearing thrombus but in preserving valvular function. As with
heparin, there is the risk of haemorrhage. Also, it is more difficult to control and
levels of the various components in the blood reaction should be monitored; this
may not everywhere be possible. Sensitivity to the bacteria of origin is necessarily
set up at the first course, which should therefore be long enough not to require
repetition.

Pulmonary embolism

Like the venous thrombosis that precedes it, pulmonary embolism can produce
clinical pictures of widely differing degrees of severity, depending most probably
on the size of the occluding thrombus and the efficiency of the collateral circulation around it. Nevertheless, the factors responsible for its initiation are probably
the same in both the minor and the major types of case. Obviously, there will
be more risk of loosening of thrombus at the upper limit of a long femoroiliac
occlusion, where both the force of the venous flow from the re-entering venous
collaterals and also the turbulence will be greater. One can picture the free end
of the thrombus loosely moving about in this stream, ready to become detached

either from these forces alone or as a result of additional aggravating factors such as straining, the resumption of ambulation by the patient, and further loosening of the thrombus in its more distal, occluding portion where its contact with the venous intima generates fibrinolysis which tends to loosen the slight adherence between the two. The process can be likened to the slipping of a large accumulation of snow from a roof during a fall. The analogy may be pursued further. The fibrinolytic thaw, under other circumstances, will dissolve the accumulation without dislodging it. On a matter of degree, therefore, may depend which of the two actions takes place. Certainly, it cannot be seriously suggested that therapeutic fibrinolysis dislodges emboli, yet its success in reducing massive thrombosis is undisputed.

Pulmonary embolism may range in severity from a minor pleurisy with chest pain and haemoptysis, where a small embolus has lodged in a peripheral bronchus near the pleural surface, to a massive fatal occlusion of the main pulmonary arterial trunk causing immediate cardiac arrest. Between these two extremes lies a large, common group of cases characterized by the collapse of a previously recovering patient, with dyspnoea, cold extremities with collapsed veins, a small, rapid pulse, and central venous congestion. Diagnosis (Oakley, 1970) may be difficult. There may be no obvious signs in the chest or heart, and chest x-rays may be normal. However, a normal-looking chest x-ray may on more careful scrutiny show diminished vascular shadows in the zone of the lung fields affected by the embolism. The main pulmonary artery shadow may be enlarged in the more severe cases. Later on, secondary changes in the lung and pleura are more obvious. Electrocardiography should show right ventricular strain at some stage. Once a strong suspicion of pulmonary embolism has formed, investigations of a more invasive kind are justified. Pulmonary arteriography via an upper limb vein not only shows the arterial filling defect, but allows pressure measurements to confirm a rise in pulmonary and right heart pressures. The catheter should be left in place, if the results are positive, for it offers the most convenient and direct route for the administration of streptokinase. Later on, lung scanning is useful for checking progress in a known case. In diagnosis this method, though sensitive, is less useful since other conditions give a similar image on scanning. A negative scan, however, goes a long way towards eliminating the diagnosis of pulmonary embolism, particularly when the results of other investigations agree with this.

The treatment of pulmonary embolism in the practice of today derives from long experience of the several available methods over many years, during which all of these methods met with a measure of success. What has changed and has helped to define more clearly the treatment of choice today is the refinement of diagnostic and progress studies such as those already mentioned. Now that the actual extent and effect of the pulmonary occlusion can be estimated so accurately, the indications for and the effectiveness of the various methods are much better understood.

Surgeons, of course, will naturally incline to a mechanical solution of an obstructive difficulty. As long ago as 1908, Trendelenburg developed the concept of direct pulmonary embolectomy through the chest. Before World War II there were at least four successful operations of this kind, and by the 1960s the number had grown considerably. Yet for such a common and lethal condition, successes were few and far between. The severity of the procedure in an emergency situation, often without the supporting facilities for cardiac bypass, and even with them, were real objections to its general use. After a phase of moderate success with emergency surgery, using the light disposable oxygenator primed with saline, opinion has more recently inclined towards what Murley (1970) has called a 'medical embolectomy'. This has the overwhelming advantage that the patient need not be moved to a special unit for it can be carried out in any well equipped general hospital.

After essential supportive treatment, such as the correction of metabolic acidosis by the infusion of sodium bicarbonate, and improvement of heart function by the use of inotropic drugs, the definitive medical treatment is begun. These are the same methods as have already been discussed when we considered the prevention of pulmonary embolism by anticoagulant and thrombolytic drugs. Heparin, being the simpler and more readily available agent, will always be used first. Not only will it prevent the spread of stasis thrombus in the occluded zone, but it may, by preventing any further intravascular thrombosis, allow the beginning of spontaneous recovery through the normal fibrinolytic mechanisms, always present in health and exacerbated by stress. This latter effect was clearly recognized by John Hunter nearly 200 years ago.

The success of heparin in the treatment of pulmonary embolism of intermediate severity, and above all in the prevention of so-called secondary embolism, has been surprisingly overlooked, especially outside Europe. The tendency, as in the treatment of major deep vein thrombosis, has been to give heparin but for too short a time and to rely on oral anticoagulants as soon as possible, even as early as the second day. This may account for the popularity of caval ligation and for the wave of acceptance of pulmonary embolectomy during the past ten years. It is now becoming more generally realized, however, that heparin should be given for at least 1 week and often longer in major thromboembolism affecting the right side of the circulation. In most cases of moderate severity this will be enough, though it should be followed by oral anticoagulants before and after the patient's discharge from hospital for 3–6 months or even longer.

It is the massive, life-threatening pulmonary embolism that has proved so amenable to thrombolytic treatment. Streptokinase is infused through the pulmonary arteriogram cannula in an initial dose of up to 600,000 units, followed by 100,000 units hourly for up to 3 days* (Miller, 1972). It is important to maintain the treatment for a sufficient length of time. The pulmonary arteriogram can be repeated to check the progress of the condition and pressure readings should also improve.

The place remaining for pulmonary embolectomy is now a small one. It is probably confined to those few patients who, having survived a massive pulmonary embolism, are yet unable to maintain a circulation without cardiac massage and whose blood pressure will not respond to vasopressor drugs. It would also be used in the event of failure of thrombolytic treatment (Paneth, 1970). The mortality remains very high, even in experienced units.

Chronic pulmonary embolism is a much less common condition that develops over a long period in response to repeated embolism, or it may be the end-result

*In some cases a smaller dose is indicated or the substrate, plasminogen, may be exhausted. The partial thromboplastin time is a guide to this.

of a single, massive embolism which has only partly resolved. Anticoagulant treatment is usually given in the hope of preventing repeated embolism. A few cases of surgical relief of the obstruction have been reported. Vena caval clipping, while theoretically suited to a preventive role, is probably open to the same objections as in the acute condition.

Arterial embolism

Whereas we may visualize the process of venous to pulmonary embolism as something of a drifting process, the events of arterial embolism will naturally be rather quicker. The Greek word *embolus* means 'something thrown in', and that, no doubt, is a good description of the way in which partly organized and fairly solid thrombus from the heart or an arterial aneurysm comes loose and is whipped away on the fast-flowing arterial stream. No doubt, also, the pathway of the embolus through the arterial tree and its final resting place are determined by the forces of gravity as well as by the direction of the blood stream. This may well be why large carotid emboli are so rare and similarly why acute mesenteric ischaemia rarely arises from arterial embolism; the natural track for the embolus to follow would be downwards and backwards, rather than upwards or anteriorly. From this one would expect that the sites of final impaction of arterial emboli would be the lower limbs. Acute ischaemia of one or both lower limbs is indeed the most important clinical presentation.

There is, however, nothing specific in the local clinical symptoms and signs of arterial embolism that distinguishes it in any way from other causes of acute limb ischaemia (Lewis, 1946). Acute thrombosis, compression by a fracture or foreign body, or the application of an arterial clamp will produce exactly the same sequence of events, their severity depending on the position of the obstruction and the state of the collateral circulation. The most important factor here is the age of the patient. The capacity to develop an alternative circulation progressively diminishes with age. Along with this, there is the likelihood of a declining cardiac efficiency which will also lessen the prospects of limb survival (Eastcott, 1973).

The best way to distinguish between arterial embolism and other causes of acute limb ischaemia is to examine the rest of the patient. Valvular heart disease (Fig. 6.4) and recent myocardial ischaemia account for almost all cases. The clinical features of these cardiac causes are not difficult to discern. The presence of atrial fibrillation should always give rise to the suspicion of cardiogenic embolism. On the other hand, acute limb ischaemia in middle age and later, unassociated with cardiac disease, is most likely to be due to arteriosclerotic thrombosis.

The state of the heart, moreover, may be crucial not only to the diagnosis of arterial embolism but also to its treatment, and it should never be ignored. It may determine the outcome both as regards limb and life more surely than anything that transpires in the operating theatre.

It should not be too difficult to determine the site of impaction of an arterial embolism without having recourse to arteriography, with its inevitable delay and discomfort, of especial importance in the elderly subjects who are really too ill and distressed to undergo any but the most essential investigations. The best guide, as in chronic arterial occlusion, is the state of the peripheral pulses in the affected

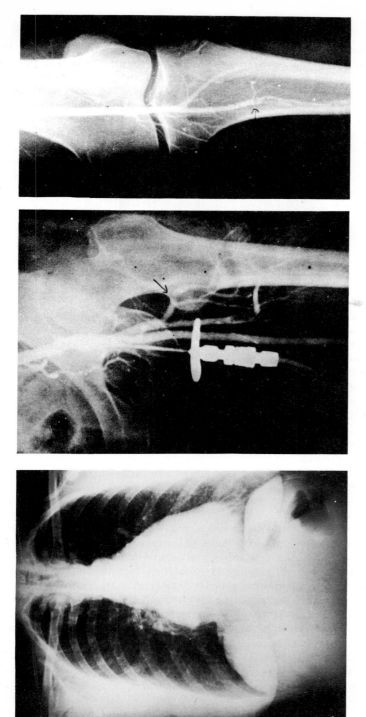

Fig. 6.4 Radiological appearances in embolism from mitral valve disease. (**a**) Chest radiograph of a patient with well compensated mitral stenosis, admitted with bilateral lower limb ischaemia. Note slight obstructive 'corrugation' appearance in superficial femoral. (**b**) Left femoral arteriogram showing fragments of embolus in profunda branches. This is transient and non-specific to any particular cause of the block beyond it. (**c**) Further embolic fragments in the posterior tibial artery, also associated with well marked corrugation in the proximal artery and the popliteal. (This patient's ischaemia on the left was mild and improved spontaneously. On the right side the common femoral was occluded and embolectomy was required, after which a transmetatarsal amputation healed well.)

limb. For practical purposes this means that if the common femoral pulse is absent the embolus is either lodged there, in which case the artery is firm and often tender, or higher up the main artery, most probably in the common iliac, in which case the femoral artery is soft and non-tender. Similarly, the popliteal pulse is absent and the artery tender when the embolism is within it. Sometimes the popliteal pulse is full and bounding, even stronger than that on the unaffected side. This happens when a small embolus impacts at the bifurcation of the artery below the level of the knee. The pulse can usually be traced down to the point where it meets the obstruction: here there is often a tender small swelling and the pulse is lost.

A special situation arises when the embolism arises from a proximal arterial aneurysm, such as the axillary beyond a compressing cervical rib (Eastcott, 1962), or the popliteal, usually arteriosclerotic or less often post-stenotic, from entrapment by the gastrocnemius muscle (Hall, 1964). In these circumstances the embolism is often repeated and small, with consequent loss of run-off and collateral branches. Serious ischaemia beyond that which would be expected with the occlusion of these arteries should therefore lead to the suspicion of a proximal aneurysm as the cause, when a careful local examination of the whole limb will usually show it if present.

Abdominal aortic aneurysm, surprisingly, seldom gives rise to major lower limb embolism. It does, however, sometimes discharge diffuse atheroembolic material widely throughout the lower limbs, producing the serious form of that normally innocuous condition, livedo reticularis. This is sometimes seen after resection and grafting of the aneurysm. Much more often the occlusion is more major, and this is the only common way for larger lower limb embolism to occur in these patients. No doubt stasis thrombus and loose fragments of mural thrombus from the lesion combine and migrate downwards at the moment of unclamping the aorta. Adequate heparinization during the operation and the establishment of a good back-flow from the iliac openings should prevent this serious complication. It is not always possible to pass the embolectomy catheter down these kinked and irregular iliacs. In this event, if embolism is suspected from a slowness of the return of the skin circulation to the foot, a formal embolectomy from the common femoral should be undertaken. It will usually succeed if the distal artery was previously patent.

Acute ischaemia of severe degree presents itself with a waxy pallor of the extremity, extending up the limb to a degree proportional to the severity of the arterial block. This means that not only is the occlusion likely to be high up in the course of the artery, but also that the extent of the consecutive stasis thrombus beyond it in the main trunk and its branches is more massive, and that the untreated prognosis is bad. When pallor definitely improves—usually from above downwards, often with the advance of cyanosis at first, and then later a pink colour—this all means that some recovery of the arterial circulation is taking place. In the conscious patient this may be accompanied by the return of skin sensation down the extremity. If this fails to show itself within 2 hours of the occlusion occurring or being first recognized, some death of tissue is certain to ensue, unless the circulation can be re-established and, with it, the sensation (Jacobs, 1959).

More serious physical signs of massive ischaemia, short of actual limb death, include ischaemic muscle contracture, more familiar in the upper limb yet commoner in the lower, because its cause occurs more often. Like simple paralytic foot drop, for which it is sometimes mistaken, it is very often missed during the clinical examination. Attempted dorsiflexion of the foot is painful to the patient, and the calf muscles are exquisitely tender at first, particularly the tibialis anterior which, in its tight and relatively isolated compartment, experiences the changes of acute ischaemia often at the same time as the toes. There may well be a purple-stained patch of skin at the centre of the muscle area where underlying necrosis is far advanced. This tightness of the muscles within the fascial sheath of the whole limb is an important contributory cause of the ischaemia, and may need to be relieved by a fasciotomy even though the arterial flow appears to have been restored. Some special dangers of the revascularization of partly infarcted muscle will be referred to later.

The operation of arterial embolectomy has become one of the easiest in general surgery, thanks to the invention of the Fogarty balloon catheter (Thompson et al., 1970; Fogarty et al., 1971). A totally inexcusable tendency to conservatism in the management of acute embolic limb ischaemia still persists, as indeed it does in the treatment of suspected major arterial injury. It is almost never justifiable to leave such a patient for later review. Only when good pulsations can be felt in mid-limb and the patient is definitely improving by the criteria mentioned already can delay be allowed. Nowadays, to these clinical signs may be added the direct and measured evidence of Doppler ultrasound flow testing over the tibial pulse points with estimation of the pressure at the cuff region of the calf or ankle. Still, most patients will need operation.

Usually, local anaesthesia is preferable. Particularly in the patient with recent myocardial infarction, the stress and the vasodilatation of general anaesthesia may prove fatal. Now that with the Fogarty catheter almost all recent emboli can be removed from any point between the umbilicus and the ankle through a short incision in the groin, the local method is always to be preferred. Only when the patient is clinically well and the anaesthetist or cardiologist gives his approval should a general anaesthetic be considered. An exception may also have to be made in the case of a restless or confused patient who cannot co-operate.

With the lower limb fully prepared and towelled as for a varicose vein operation, a longitudinal incision is made over the common femoral artery. There is no place for cosmetically pleasing skin-crease incisions in this work. Access and extendability are the only considerations. The femoral vascular sheath is opened and more local anaesthetic may be needed. The common femoral artery is gently freed from its bed using a curved artery forceps such as Moynihan's cholecystectomy forceps, and a tape is passed beneath it and used to lift the artery up while the rest of its length is cleared. Using a dissecting pledget, and if necessary further sharp dissection, the first 2·5 cm or so of the superficial femoral and the origin of the profunda femoris are cleared sufficiently to permit the application of a bulldog arterial clip. No clamps or clips must yet be applied, however. Systemic heparin should already have been given. If it has been omitted, or if some hours have elapsed since it was given, 5,000 units should be injected either into the intravenous drip line or preferably into the pulsating proximal part of the femoral if this is patent. With the arterial sling tape held up and no clamps applied, a short cut is made over the middle of the common femoral artery to reveal the embolus or consecutive thrombus beneath. This can often then be allowed to deliver itself through the arteriotomy by the force of the arterial pulse above it. If it does this, and is followed by a brisk spurt of arterial blood, the proximal clamp is applied, usually a curved Craafoord coarctation clamp. Toothed or other hard-acting clamps should be avoided. A short curved soft intestinal clamp will serve well. The distal thrombus is then removed with the Fogarty balloon catheter. Usually a No. 5 or 6 will serve well. The stilette is removed and the balloon gently tested with the correct amount of saline injected, from as small a syringe as possible, for better accuracy and control of the tension in the balloon. With the balloon deflated, the lubricated catheter is passed as far as possible down the main artery; the balloon is gently inflated till resistance is felt in the syringe, and then the catheter is gently withdrawn, adding slightly more saline to the balloon as the artery size increases proximally. A long coiled black thrombus with paler pieces of embolus will then emerge from the arteriotomy. Several passes may be needed to remove all possible thrombus, and to achieve a back-bleed of arterial blood. The same manœuvre is then repeated down the profunda (see Fig. 6.4). Each artery is clipped with a soft bulldog clamp as soon as it is cleared.

The procedure for a larger, proximal embolus is very similar. The taped common femoral artery is incised as before, when often a spurt of non-pulsatile arterial blood will come out instead of thrombus. The distal femoral is clipped and the sling held up to check the blood loss, while the Fogarty catheter is inserted upwards through the occluding sling which is partly released for a moment to allow the catheter to enter the iliac artery. It is then passed upwards for at least 25 cm, inflated and pulled gently down into the wound. A gush of arterial blood under full pressure and portions of the embolus then usually emerge. Pieces of the embolus are retrieved for both histological and bacteriological examination. More than one pass may be necessary, and distal fragments or stasis thrombus should be searched for in the femorals as already described.

The repair of the artery is by a continuous atraumatic round-bodied needle carrying a 5/0 arterial suture of silk, or now preferably polypropylene (Prolene). The distal clamps are removed first, and any leaks secured with further interrupted sutures. It is preferable whenever possible not to reverse the action of the heparin at this point, but to allow it to continue with the useful work of reducing stasis thrombus, and perhaps to aid its removal from the smaller, still occluded branches, for as we saw in considering venous thromboembolism, the patient's own fibrinolytic activity may be helped in this way. A vacuum drain is advisable.

In some complicated or late cases, not all of the thrombus can be removed via the common femoral. This is why the leg was fully prepared for more extensive exposure of the lower course of the vessels. A medial approach to the popliteal, below the knee, and sometimes the posterior tibial at the ankle, will often permit a fuller clearance of extensive or adherent thrombus from these areas. The balloon catheter in smaller sizes can be usefully employed from these sites also. Irrigation upwards is also a most valuable method of clearing obstinate obstructions without the use of too much force. Vollmar's non-cutting arterial ring strippers can be gently used, but with great care for it is quite easy to damage these small, softened arteries, and a false aneurysm or arteriovenous fistula has often resulted from such instrumentation and even from the softer Fogarty catheter itself (Mavor et al., 1972).

In late cases of severe ischaemia, e.g. after the first day, with doubtful limb viability and established muscle contracture, the revascularization of the limb may bring with it a profound and sudden metabolic acidosis from the obstructed area. It is well to offset this effect by the infusion of sodium bicarbonate solution systemically, 100 mmol or more if the area of ischaemia is very large, otherwise a cardiac arrest may occur in such a case.

As with all severe ischaemia, there is the risk of anaerobic infection from the

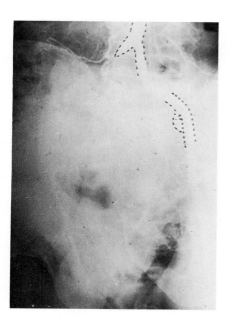 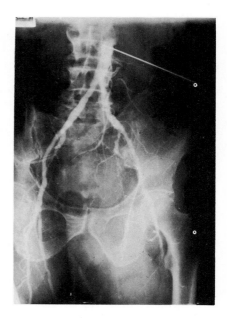

Fig. 6.5 Late embolectomy. (**a**) Early lumbar aortogram in an elderly man with acute right lower limb ischaemia after a myocardial infarct. With cardiac recovery the limb survived, but claudication was severe and he was referred for arterial surgery. (**b**) Post operative lumbar aortogram following removal of right common ilac embolus via the common femoral, using balloon catheters and loop strippers. Full recovery.

patient's own bowel organisms, so it is advisable to give a preventive course of penicillin.

Embolism to the peripheral arteries remains a serious condition. The introduction of the balloon catheter has reduced limb loss to 20 per cent or less. Nevertheless, the associated cardiac and other mortality is high (Haimovici et al., 1975). It might be said that some survive with their affected limb intact, only later to succumb to their heart disease. Even so, the alternative to embolectomy being in most cases a major amputation with much higher risks, the arterial operation should always be undertaken if possible.

It sometimes happens that limb recovery follows general improvement after a myocardial infarct with arterial embolism. Intermittent claudication is then a serious further obstacle to general convalescence. In such patients a late embolectomy may succeed in restoring ambulation (Fig. 6.5).

References

DORMANDY J. A. (1970) Clinical significance of blood viscosity. *Ann. R. Coll. Surg. Engl.* **47,** 211–228.

EASTCOTT H. H. G. (1962) Reconstruction of the subclavian artery for complications of cervical-rib and thoracic-outlet syndrome. *Lancet* **2,** 1243.

EASTCOTT H. H. G. (1973) *Arterial Surgery,* 2nd edn. Tunbridge Wells, Pitman Medical, p. 264.

FOGARTY T. J., DAILY P. O., SHUMWAY N. E. and KRIPPAEHNE W. (1971) Experience with balloon catheter technique for arterial embolectomy. *Am. J. Surg.* **122,** 123–237.

HAIMOVICI H., MOSS C. M. and VEITH F. J. (1975) Arterial embolectomy revisited. *Surgery* **78,** 409–410.

HALL K. V. (1964) Intervascular gastrocnemic insertion. *Acta Chir. Scand.* **128,** 193–196.

JACOBS A. L. (1959) *Acute Arterial Embolism in the Limbs.* Edinburgh and London, Churchill-Livingstone, p. 28.

KAKKAR V. V., HOWE C. T., FLANC C. and CLARKE M. B. (1969) Natural history of deep-vein thrombosis. *Lancet* **2,** 230–232.

KAKKAR V. V. and JOUHAR A. J. (ed.) (1973) *Thromboembolism: Diagnosis and Treatment.* Edinburgh and London, Churchill-Livingstone.

LANCET (1975) Prevention of fatal postoperative pulmonary embolism by low doses of heparin. An international multicentre trial. *Lancet* **2,** 45–51.

LEWIS T. (1964) *Vascular Disorders of the Limbs.* London, Macmillan, p. 27.

MAVOR G. E. and GALLOWAY J. M. D. (1969) Iliofemoral venous thrombosis: pathological considerations and surgical management. *Br. J. Surg.* **56,** 45–59.

MAVOR G. E., WALKER M. G., DAHL D. P. and PEGG C. A. S. (1972) Damage from the Fogarty balloon catheter. *Br. J. Surg.* **59,** 389–391.

MAVOR G. E., DAHL D. P., DAWSON A. A., DUTHIE J. S., WALKER M. G., MAHAFFY R. G. and ALLARDYCE A. (1973) Streptokinase therapy and deep vein thrombosis. *Br. J. Surg.* **60,** 468–474.

MILLER G. A. H. (1972) The diagnosis and management of massive pulmonary embolism. *Br. J. Surg.* **59,** 837–839.

MOBIN-UDDIN K., TRINKLE J. K. and BRYANT L. R. (1971) Present status of the inferior vena cava umbrella filter. *Surgery* **70,** 914–919.

MURLEY R. S. (1970) Massive pulmonary embolism: what can be done to encourage survival? *Br. J. Surg.* **57,** 771–775.

NICOLAIDES A. N., MEADWAY J. and IRVING D. (1975) The value of clinical signs in the diagnosis of deep venous thrombosis. In: NICOLAIDES A. N. (ed.), *Thromboembolism.* Lancaster, Medical and Technical Publishing.

OAKLEY C. M. (1970) Diagnosis of pulmonary embolism. *Br. Med. J.* **2,** 773–777.

PANETH M. (1970) Surgical management of massive pulmonary embolism. *Br. Med. J.* **2,** 778–779.

THOMPSON J. E., SIGLER L., RAUT P. S., AUSTIN D. J. and PATMAN R. D. (1970) Arterial embolectomy: a 20 year experience with 163 cases. *Surgery* **67,** 212–220.

7

Occlusion of the Mesenteric Vessels

A. G. Horsburgh, FRCS

Occlusion of the vessels of the mesentery is one of the most serious intra-abdominal conditions which can occur. It is accompanied by a high mortality and recurrent attacks are frequent. The classical clinical picture of acute obstruction to the superior mesenteric artery by embolus or by thrombus has been well recognized for many years. Nevertheless, despite modern methods of treatment, its mortality remains high at 70–80 per cent. In more recent years chronic narrowing of the arteries, without occlusion, producing the picture of mesenteric angina, has been clearly described.

Success in treatment depends, amongst other things, on early diagnosis and early laparotomy with resection of the affected bowel and end-to-end anastomosis. With the development of vascular surgery, attention has been paid to direct surgical intervention at the site of obstruction in the vessel in the hope of re-establishing circulation and avoiding or reducing the amount of resected bowel.

Thrombosis in the mesenteric veins has received less attention. It is sometimes a less dramatic event and carries a lower, but still considerable, mortality of 40–50 per cent. It often presents with symptoms which are distinguishable from arterial occlusion and not infrequently appears as an intestinal obstruction. It is important that, at laparotomy, mesenteric venous thrombosis is recognized clearly from mesenteric arterial occlusion, as in recent years different forms of treatment have been applied to these two conditions.

Mesenteric arterial occlusion

Occlusion of the mesenteric arteries can be classified into two main types. First and most commonly, there is obstruction due to atherosclerosis, often with superimposed thrombosis. Secondly, there is obstruction due to embolus, usually associated with a cardiac arrhythmia or mural thrombus secondary to myocardial infarction.

Atherosclerosis most commonly occurs in the superior mesenteric artery, but the coeliac axis is often affected as well. The main trunk of the artery near its origin is the site of maximum damage, and the more distal trunk and branches are seldom affected. Occlusion of the main trunk of the inferior mesenteric artery is much less common. When it does occur the results may be less dramatic, due to a better collateral circulation.

Atherosclerosis is a disease which increases with age, particularly in men. Most subjects with mesenteric occlusion, therefore, tend to be elderly males. This must, in part, account for the high mortality associated with treatment of mesenteric occlusion.

In mesenteric embolus the subjects may well be younger. The embolus commonly arises in a heart with a disturbance of rhythm. The site of the obstruction will, of course, depend upon the size of the embolus. Commonly it is well beyond the origin of the superior mesenteric artery and may be in one or other of the more distal branches. Consequently, the length of infarcted bowel is likely to be less than in the atherosclerotic obstruction. It is in these subjects that most success has been obtained in surgical treatment, whether by resection of affected bowel or by direct surgery on the artery.

Pathological effects of mesenteric artery occlusion

The superior mesenteric artery terminates in end-arteries and therefore the collateral circulation is not usually good enough to compensate for occlusion of the main trunk. Following occlusion, clot forms at the site of obstruction and propagates distally. At the moment of occlusion the affected bowel goes into intense spasm. This probably accounts for the severe pain which occurs in the classical description of the acute condition. Oedema then occurs, first in the mucosa and then spreading outwards to the serosa. The submucous layer becomes filled with blood. The mucosa becomes ulcerated and necrotic, and changes extend outwards. The muscularis propria (deep muscle layer) is more resistant to deprivation of blood than the mucosa and submucosa (Morson, 1971) and may survive for longer. Ultimately, complete necrosis takes place. In non-occlusive ischaemia of the bowel or when only a very small segment is affected by occlusive ischaemia, the condition may not proceed to complete necrosis. Ulceration of mucosa can heal by granulation tissue. This is followed by fibrosis, cicatrization and formation of a stricture.

Following the initial intense spasm, the bowel relaxes and dilates. The segment no longer transmits peristalsis. There is a vast outpouring of fluid into the bowel, which may result in a depletion of circulating blood volume. A peritoneal exudate occurs. This is, at first, clear and yellowish, but later becomes blood-stained. Later still, as bacteria flourish in the stagnant bowel content and migrate through the wall, the exudate becomes offensive. Bacterial peritonitis is now present and perforation of the bowel can occur.

Clinical types

Acute occlusion

Acute occlusion can occur without any previous symptoms, as in embolus or occasionally in atherosclerosis, or can follow a period of chronic ischaemia. The main symptom is pain and, although this is sometimes the acute, severe, classical picture with signs of an intra-abdominal catastrophe, it is by no means always so and the onset may be quite insidious (Mavor, 1961). Vomiting occurs often later and there may be the passage of a bloody stool. It may be several hours before the classical picture, with circulatory collapse due to intra-abdominal fluid collection and absorption of toxin, occurs. The object of treatment should be to carry out laparotomy before this state develops. There are not many aids to diagnosis here. A raised leucocyte count is perhaps the most useful and, in these circumstances, it is as well to regard such a rise as due to ischaemia unless proved otherwise. Occasionally a bruit may be heard in the right iliac fossa.

X-ray of the abdomen shows distended small bowel loops with fluid levels, but is not specific to this condition. Angiography has been used to help demonstrate the occlusion (Williams et al., 1967). However, it is not often readily available in emergencies and, if normal, will not avoid a laparotomy as the abdominal picture will still demand surgery.

The most useful aid to diagnosis is to bear the condition in mind, particularly in the atherosclerotic or in the patient with cardiac arrythmia.

Chronic ischaemia

This occurs in the atherosclerotic patient with gross reduction in blood flow due to mesenteric stenosis. It can go on for many months or even years and may or may not culminate in an episode of acute occlusion. Again, the main symptom is abdominal pain, which Mikkelsen (1957) describes as 'intestinal angina' and is also referred to as mesenteric angina. The pain is often cramp-like and postprandial. Food intake is reduced in an effort to overcome this. There is often diarrhoea and weight loss with the presence of occult blood in the stools. Steatorrhea may be present and malabsorption.

Again, it is not easy to make a correct diagnosis here unless the condition is borne in mind. The symptoms are most often diagnosed as one or other form of intra-abdominal malignancy. Quite often an abdominal bruit may be heard. In these chronic occlusive cases, angiography is a much more worthwhile investigation and several writers have described its use (Stoney and Wylie, 1966; Bergan, 1967). An aortogram with lateral views is most useful and may demonstrate stenosis of the main trunk of the superior mesenteric artery and sometimes the coeliac axis as well.

Treatment

Despite improvements in resuscitation and in diagnostic aids, there has been very little change in the mortality from this condition in the last quarter of a century. Up until 1957, when Shaw and Rutledge first carried out a successful mesenteric embolectomy without resection of bowel, surgical treatment of the acute occlusion was entirely dependent on resection of ischaemic bowel. This is still by far the commonest operation.

Acute occlusion

In early cases, before general circulatory changes have occurred, laparotomy should be carried out as soon as the diagnosis is suspected and as a matter of urgency. In later cases, delay should only be for fluid and electrolyte correction. This can be done quite quickly even though large volumes may be needed. Here, a central venous line is useful. At laparotomy, the extent of intestinal involvement is noted and the mesentery inspected closely to differentiate arterial from venous occlusion. In the latter, pulsation will be seen or felt right up to the bowel wall, while in arterial occlusion there is no pulsation beyond the point of obstruction.

Although the history of cardiac irregularity may help in differentiating embolic from atherosclerotic obstruction, at laparotomy it may be difficult to establish the precise cause of the obstruction. This is specially so if a fairly large embolus has lodged near the origin of the artery, as this is the main site for atherosclerosis.

Dissection of the origin of the superior mesenteric artery is difficult, particularly in an obese subject. The patient is often not a suitable subject for such a lengthy procedure. Probably the best step to take is to expose the ileocolic artery at a place distally in its course, where it is of sufficient size to admit a size 4F Fogarty embolectomy catheter (Marston, 1971). This is then passed up the artery and the clot or embolus withdrawn. It is recommended that the common iliac arteries should first be clamped with soft clamps to prevent any thrombus passing into the legs. If this manœuvre is successful in restoring circulation as seen by mesenteric pulsation and improvement in bowel colour, then the ileocolic artery is ligated at the point of catheterization. If it is not successful in restoring circulation, then retrograde revascularization may be attempted. This, in its simplest form, involves a side-to-side anastomosis between the ileocolic artery and the right common iliac artery. Other methods include bypass using autogenous vein graft or artificial tube between the ileocolic artery and the right common iliac artery or aorta (Morris et al., 1962).

Direct exploration of the origin of the superior mesenteric artery, in order to carry out end-arterectomy with or without patch graft, is most suitable in the chronic case (De Bakey, 1969) and has only occasionally been successful in acute occlusion.

Whatever method of restoration of circulation is used, a review of the affected bowel is now necessary. Any portion still not viable is resected. A definite opinion on viability is not always easy. After restoration of blood flow there is a good deal of bleeding into the lumen and also considerable oedema of the bowel wall. If, after a period of careful observation, there is still some doubt, it is reasonable to close the abdomen and re-explore on the following day to assess the situation. It has been suggested that this should be done as a routine procedure anyway in all cases (Glotzer and Glotzer, 1966).

Problems following restoration of blood flow

The successful restoration of blood flow in an acutely obstructed superior mesenteric artery with avoidance of resection is a considerable surgical achievement. Regrettably, it is only rarely that one reaches this satisfactory state. Even when this is achieved, serious problems can occur when blood flow is restored.

First, there is active loss of a large quantity of blood and fluid into the lumen of the damaged bowel. This, in itself, may produce a profound fall in blood pressure. Possibly the hypotension is also due to a sudden increase in the arterial vascular bed (Mavor et al., 1963). In addition, toxic substances from the damaged bowel may pass into the portal and systemic circulations. Certainly, there appears to be a rise, first in the portal and later in the systemic potassium levels. A number of patients have succumbed from one or more of these effects, after initially successful surgery. The hypovolaemia is best combated by adequate transfusion with blood and plasma. The 'toxaemia' and rise in potassium are more difficult to deal with. Mavor et al. (1963) have experimented with perfusion of the mid-gut loop in dogs using oxygenated blood, and found that this will prevent a rise in portal potassium levels. It is doubtful, however, whether this will become of widespread practical use in man. Apart from the circulatory problems, renal and pulmonary complications are frequent.

Long-term effects of bowel resection

Most patients will tolerate resection of short segments of bowel without disturbance. However, when segments 2 metres or more have to be resected for infarction, symptoms do develop. Even so, there is remarkable individual variation here. The nature and severity of the symptoms will be governed, to some extent, by the exact site of the resected bowel and whether or not the remainder is affected by chronic vascular insufficiency. For those few patients who survive massive resection of half or more of the small bowel, the condition known as the 'short bowel syndrome' develops. In this, there is diarrhoea—often very severe—with malabsorption, weight loss, metabolic acidosis, vitamin deficiencies and megaloblastic anaemia. Severe cases can waste away at a most alarming rate.

Treatment in patients with less severe symptoms consists of dietary adjustments, replacement of deficiencies and the use of drugs to reduce intestinal motility. In patients with severe short bowel syndrome, these measures are insufficient and the mortality is high. A few of these patients have been helped by one or other variety of the anti-peristaltic reversed segment operation. In its simplest form, this consists of reversing a short segment of small bowel, near its end, and re-anastomosing it in continuity, in an anti-peristaltic position. This slows down the passage of intestinal content and allows improved absorption. The exact length of the reversed segment appears to be critical. Somewhere about 8–10 cm seems to be optimum. Too short a segment may not achieve sufficient result and too long a segment has been known to produce obstruction.

Chronic ischaemia

The indications for surgery are less clear-cut here than in the acute case. The patient is usually an elderly man with extensive arteriosclerosis and often cardiac insufficiency. In reaching a decision regarding surgery, this general state must be considered in conjunction with the severity of the symptoms and the appearance of the aortogram, particularly in its lateral view. Complete obstruction of the origin of the superior mesenteric artery does not necessarily produce severe symptoms, particularly if the collateral circulation is better than usual. The disease seldom affects more than the origin of the main trunk of the artery.

Symptoms, however, can be very severe in this condition, with post-prandial pain, loss of weight, diarrhoea and malabsorption. Also, at any moment and particularly if an episode of cardiac insufficiency produces a reduction in circulation, thrombosis may occur with acute bowel infarction.

If the aortogram shows obstruction limited to the origin of the superior mesenteric artery and good filling beyond this, and if a decision to operate is made, one of two procedures is available. A direct attack can be made on the site of obstruction at the origin of the artery. The exposure is not easy, due mainly to the close proximity of the origin of the portal vein and its tributaries around the neck of the pancreas. However, end-arterectomy with closure and enlargement of the vessel with a Dacron patch graft has been successful in some cases (De Bakey et al., 1969).

A more frequently used operation is the bypass procedure. A number of different techniques are described. If the coeliac axis is not involved in the obstructive disease, the splenic artery may be used to re-vascularize the superior mesenteric distal to the obstruction. Unfortunately, the coeliac axis is often at least partly obstructed by atherosclerosis, which will have been seen on the lateral aortogram, and the splenic artery will therefore not be suitable. A bypass from the aorta, below the renal arteries, to the superior mesenteric artery and, if necessary, to the coeliac artery as well, can be made using Dacron (Morris et al., 1962) or an autogenous vein graft.

It appears that these bypass procedures carry a rather better success rate than direct surgery at the site of the obstruction.

Something over 100 patients have been treated in this fashion. A mortality rate of around 5 per cent is quoted. Most patients get relief of pain from this procedure. Rather fewer are cured of malabsorption. The longer-term results are yet to appear.

Mesenteric venous occlusion

This is a far less well recognized entity than is mesenteric artery occlusion. Relatively little has appeared on it in the British literature, although rather more in North America. Nevertheless, mesenteric venous thrombosis was recognized as a separate condition from the arteries as long ago as Trotter's description in 1913. It is probably much commoner than is generally realized. At laparotomy, it is not always easy to differentiate arterial from venous obstruction in a fat-laden mesentery, unless a particular effort is made to do so. Resected specimens are sometimes reported simply as 'infarcted bowel', unless particular attention has been paid to the state of the small vessels of the mesenteric border.

Aetiology

The reported age incidence of patients suffering from mesenteric venous thrombosis varies widely from 20 to 80 years. The majority appear to occur in the sixth and seventh decades. Unlike arterial occlusion, where men predominate, in venous thrombosis men and women are affected equally. Cases may be broadly classified into those in which a predisposing cause can be detected and those in which one cannot. In the former group, Warren and Eberhard (1935) have described venous thrombosis in association with pelvic and abdominal infective conditions, with portal stasis, with tumours, volvulus and adhesions and with blood dyscrasias, such as splenic anaemia and polycythaemia. It has also been described in association with thrombophlebitis migrans. Reed and Coon (1963) described a case occurring in association with the contraceptive pill, and since then other cases have been reported (Civetta and Kolodny, 1970).

In all these cases the occurrence of mesenteric venous thrombosis, secondary to some other intra-abdominal condition or to a disturbance of blood coagulation, would not seem surprising. However, it is with the other group of cases, in which no predisposing cause can be found, that the greater problems of diagnosis occur.

Pathological appearances

Thrombosis in the veins results in a cessation of circulation. It is not surprising, therefore, that the affected bowel shows the same oedema, haemorrhage and mucosal disintegration that occurs in arterial occlusion. Microscopic examination shows the most striking features in the vessels of the mesentery, adjacent to the bowel. Here the arteries are seen to be quite patent. The veins, on the other hand, are filled with clot and, in some cases, clot of differing ages can be recognized (Fig. 7.1). The occurrence of earlier and lesser episodes of clotting may

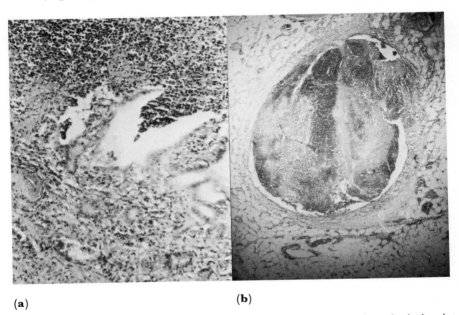

(a)   **(b)**

Fig. 7.1 (a) Section of ileum from a case of superior mesenteric venous thrombosis showing disruption of the wall with haemorrhage. **(b)** Section of the adjacent mesentery showing a small vein full of blood clot. Clot of differing age can be recognized.

account for the long prodromal symptoms sometimes seen. The idiopathic cases characteristically show the thrombus confined to these small mesenteric veins. In the group, however, where the thrombus is secondary to other abdominal conditions or to abnormalities of the blood, the larger tributaries and main trunk of the superior mesenteric vein undergo thrombosis, and spread to the vena cava may be rapid.

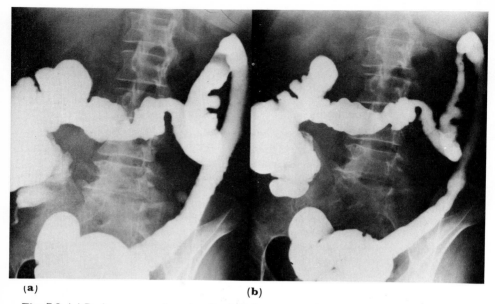

(a)   **(b)**

Fig. 7.2 (a) Barium enema 3 weeks after inferior mesenteric venous thrombosis, showing mucosal oedema and ulceration. **(b)** Barium enema 6 weeks later, showing stricture formation.

Because the thrombosis is often confined to the small veins, short segments of bowel may be affected. The collateral circulation may be sufficient to maintain viability and spontaneous recovery can occur. The bowel wall heals with the laying down of fibrous tissue. This may undergo cicatrization to form a stricture, an event that can sometimes take place within a few weeks (Fig. 7.2). When the thrombosis has occurred in the tributaries of the inferior mesenteric vein, the features are remarkably similar to the ischaemic colitis described by Marston et al. (1966). In ischaemic colitis, usually no predisposing cause is found and no arterial obstruction seen. It may be that some of these cases are due to small vein thrombosis. Murley (1971) reported such a case. The specimen there showed, on section, features of ischaemic colitis and thrombosis of small veins in the adjacent mesentery.

Even after successful treatment or spontaneous resolution of an episode of mesenteric thrombosis, further episodes are common and may occur within a few days or sometimes months later. The over-all mortality of the condition is stated to be around 40–50 per cent.

Clinical types

In general, the over-all picture in venous thrombosis tends to be slower and less severe than in arterial occlusion. Two clinical types can be recognized. First, those cases secondary to some other intra-abdominal condition or to blood coagulation disturbances. Here, because the larger mesenteric veins are often affected, wider segments of bowel are damaged. The onset of symptoms is more acute and deterioration rapid. It is usually impossible to differentiate this from arterial occlusion. Secondly, the idiopathic group, in which a slower onset is characteristic. Donaldson and Stout (1935) first drew clear attention to a definite clinical difference between venous thrombosis and arterial obstruction. The clinical picture typically includes a prodromal phase, which may vary from 2 to 21 days or possibly be several weeks in length. During this time there is vague abdominal discomfort, sometimes with colicky pain. The bowel action is normal or occasionally loose and, at this stage, symptoms may be attributed to a dietary indiscretion or an enteritis. The pain then increases in frequency and there is usually some

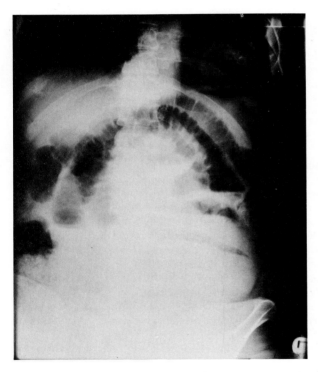

Fig. 7.3 Abdominal x-ray in a case of superior mesenteric venous thrombosis presenting as an intestinal obstruction.

abdominal distension and vomiting, although this latter symptom is not often copious. Constipation now occurs and it may be at this stage that the patient is first referred for a surgical opinion. Examination then shows a patient with a relatively low pulse rate at around 80–90 per minute and slight to moderate dehydration. The abdomen is a little distended and bowel sounds are active. There is tenderness in all areas with, at times, a little guarding, but no rigidity. Rectal examination is usually negative, although occasionally stale blood may be found on the examining finger. This is particularly so if the thrombosis affects the inferior mesenteric vein with resultant damage to the colon. Abdominal x-ray commonly shows distended loops of bowel with fluid levels (Fig. 7.3). The condition is often mistaken for one of partial or complete intestinal obstruction and, indeed, it may be difficult to tell them apart. Usually, however, the vomiting and abdominal distension are much less in thrombosis. The only useful laboratory investigation to help with diagnosis is the white cell count. This is moderately raised to around 13,000–20,000/mm³, a feature one would not expect in an obstruction. Later on, the patient's condition will deteriorate; the pulse rate rises, the abdomen becomes distended and the white cell count rises to 25,000/mm³ or above. Gangrene of the bowel has now occurred and, in the absence of surgery, death will follow.

Treatment

Early surgery with wide resection of the affected segment of bowel is the usual recommended treatment. A precise diagnosis of mesenteric venous thrombosis can be extremely difficult, as is often the case in arterial occlusion. It must be constantly borne in mind. The suspicion of its presence is sufficient indication for laparotomy, especially in a patient with symptoms of obstruction, and an elevated white cell count. Delay should only be for rapid resuscitation if this is required.

On opening the abdomen, free fluid is present. In the early stages, this is clear and moderate in amount. Later, it is copious and blood-stained. The affected segment of the bowel shows oedema, reddening and the omentum may be lightly adherent. The adjacent mesentery is oedematous, but this seldom extends down to the root and is usually confined to a centimetre or two from the bowel wall. The mesenteric arteries are seen to be pulsating well, right up to the bowel wall. In later cases, however, there may be frank gangrene of the bowel.

In cases of gangrene, the standard treatment of resection is required. However, the anastomoses do not heal well and anastomotic breakdown accounts for some part of the high mortality in this condition. Trinkle et al. (1969) pointed out the high rate of anastomotic breakdown following resection and anastomosis, and indeed, because of this, recommended exteriorization of the bowel ends after resection, rather than anastomosis.

Because of the very unsatisfactory results seen with resection and anastomosis, it is suggested that a more conservative approach may be made to these cases of early mesenteric venous thrombosis, in which, at laparotomy, the gut is still viable. The laparotomy is, of course, still essential, both to confirm the diagnosis and to check the viability of the bowel. If it is thought likely that the bowel is viable, the abdomen is closed. The patient is then maintained with intravenous fluids, and intravenous heparin and low molecular weight dextran are given. A very close watch must be kept on the situation, particularly with regard to the pulse rate, the reappearance of bowel sounds and the white cell count, with a view to re-opening the abdomen on the slightest suggestion of deterioration.

The use of anticoagulants in mesenteric venous thrombosis and also in mesenteric arterial occlusion has been a debatable point. It would seem important to try to prevent any extension of the thrombotic process, particularly in a bowel which is only just viable. On the other hand, there is a risk that an anticoagulant will produce further blood and fluid loss into the lumen of the bowel and also into the peritoneum. This has been seen in one case of thrombosis affecting the small tributaries of the inferior mesenteric vein. This patient was first treated with heparin. After a few days, warfarin was started. One 30-mg dose produced a rise in prothrombin time to 50 seconds, and a sharp haemorrhage from the colon necessitated reversal with vitamin K. Because of this, it is probably best to keep these patients on intravenous heparin until the condition is well settled. In general, patients have done better on this regimen than with resection and anastomosis.

With regard to the low molecular weight dextran, there is certain animal experimental evidence for its value in bowel infarction due to mesenteric obstruction. Whether its property of improving blood flow in small vessels is of practical use in mesenteric venous thrombosis in man is not established. It appears to be free from any disadvantages.

Once the thrombotic condition has settled and gastrointestinal function been established, anticoagulation is maintained orally to avoid the common complication of early recurrent thrombosis. How long these drugs should be continued is, of course, open to discussion. An arbitrary period of 3 months is advised. That thrombosis can occur after this is certain and we have had a case appearing with a second episode 7 months later. However, the prolonged use of anticoagulants in the elderly is not free from problems of its own.

The management of mesenteric venous thrombosis, like mesenteric arterial occlusion, is an extremely difficult clinical problem. The frankly gangrenous bowel must, of course, be resected. There does, however, seem to be a place for a more conservative approach in the early case with still viable bowel, and so far results have been better than those achieved with a resection and anastomosis.

References

BERGAN J. J. (1967) Recognition and treatment of intestinal ischemia. *Surg. Clin. North Am.* **47,** 109–126.

CIVETTA J. M. and KOLODNY M. (1970) Mesenteric venous thrombosis associated with oral contraceptives. *Gastroenterology* **58,** 713–716.

DE BAKEY M. E., MORRIS G. C. and DIETHRICH E. B. (1969) Abdominal vascular surgery. In: MAINGOT R. (ed.), *Abdominal Operations*, 5th edn. New York, Meredith.

DONALDSON J. K. and STOUT B. F. (1935) Mesenteric thrombosis. *Am. J. Surg.* **29,** 208.

GLOTZER D. J. and GLOTZER P. (1966) Superior mesenteric embolectomy. Report of two successful cases using the Fogarty catheter. *Arch. Surg.* **93,** 421–424.

MARSTON A. (1971) Acute mesenteric vascular occlusion. In: BOLEY S. J. et al. (ed.), *Vascular Disorders of the Intestine*. London, Butterworths.

MARSTON A., PHEILS M. T., THOMAS M. L. and MORSON B. C. (1966) Ischaemic colitis. *Gut* **7,** 1–15.

MAVOR G. E. (1961) Superior mesenteric artery occlusion. *Proc. R. Soc. Med.* **54,** 356–359.

MAVOR G. E., LYALL A. D., CRYSTAL K. M. R. and PROCTOR D. M. (1963) Observations on experimental occlusion of the superior mesenteric artery. *Br. J. Surg.* **50,** 536–541.

MIKKELSON W. P. (1957) Intestinal angina: its surgical significance. *Am. J. Surg.* **94,** 262–267.

MORRIS G. C., CRAWFORD E. S., COOLEY D. A. and DE BAKEY M. E. (1962) Revascularization of the celiac and superior mesenteric arteries. *Arch. Surg.* **84,** 95–107.

MORSON B. C. (1971) Histopathology of intestinal ischaemia. In: BOLEY S. J. et al. (ed.), *Vascular Disorders of the Intestine.* London, Butterworths.

MURLEY R. (1971) Comment on a paper read to the Society. *Proc. R. Soc. Med.* **64,** 1083.

REED D. L. and COON W. W. (1963) Thromboembolism in patients receiving progestational drugs. *N. Engl. J. Med.* **269,** 622–624.

SHAW R. S. and RUTLEDGE R. (1957) Superior-mesenteric-artery embolectomy in the treatment of massive mesenteric infarction. *N. Engl. J. Med.* **257,** 595–598.

STONEY R. J. and WYLIE E. J. (1966) Recognition and surgical management of visceral ischemic syndromes. *Ann. Surg.* **164,** 714–722.

TRINKLE J. K., BENJAMIN F. R., FULLER M. A., BRYANT L. R. and RAMS J. (1969) The operative management of idiopathic mesenteric venous thrombosis with intestinal infarction. *Am. Surg.* **35,** 338–341.

TROTTER L. B. C. (1913) *Embolism and Thrombosis of the Mesenteric Vessels.* Cambridge, Cambridge University Press.

WARREN S. and EBERHARD T. P. (1935) Mesenteric venous thrombosis. *Surg. Gynecol. Obstet.* **61,** 102–121.

WILLIAMS L. F., ANATASIA L. F. and HASIOTIS C. A. (1967) Non-occlusive mesenteric infarction. *Am. J. Surg.* **114,** 376–381.

8

Modern Surgical Attitudes to Peptic Ulceration

D. Johnston, MD, ChM, FRCSEd, FRCSGlas

'If the pylorus does not relax, it is evident that a wave approaching it pushes the food into a blind elastic pouch, the only exit from which is through the advancing constricted ring. The constrictions are deeper near the end of the antrum, and the rings are small; consequently the food is squirted back through them with considerable violence. As has been noted, the pylorus opens less frequently for a while after a solid piece of food comes to it. In such a case the slow driving waves squeeze the hard morsel and the soft food about it up to the sphincter, only to have the whole mass shoot back, sometimes half way along the antrum. Over and over again the process is repeated till the sphincter at last opens and allows the more fluid parts to pass.'

W. B. Cannon (1898)

For the surgeon dealing with peptic ulcer, the most important discoveries of the last 10 years have been that vagal release of gastrin in man is relatively unimportant and that truncal vagotomy is followed by a significant *increase* in serum gastrin levels. These findings imply that vagal denervation of the antrum is unnecessary and that the use of drainage procedures can be discarded. The sphincteric mechanism at the exit of the stomach can thus be preserved.

The stomach as a reservoir: control of gastric emptying

It should never be forgotten that the stomach's principal function is to act as a reservoir. The stomach is a muscular bag, equipped with sphincters at either end. The cardiac sphincter stops acid and pepsin regurgitating into the oesophagus and so protects us against heartburn and all the pathological consequences of acid-pepsin reflux. At the other end of the stomach the sphincteric mechanism controlling gastric emptying is in two parts, the terminal antrum and the pyloric sphincter. Gastric emptying of solids is controlled in large measure by the vigorous contraction of the distal 4 cm of antrum, which has the effect of retropelling particulate matter into the body of the stomach (Cannon, 1898; Carlson et al., 1966). The resulting 'to and fro' movement of solid food in the stomach has been demonstrated beautifully by means of cine-radiography in dogs by C. F. Code, whose film of these events is a remarkable record of the 'antral mill' in action.

Beyond the terminal antrum lies the pyloric sphincter proper. For many years it was unfashionable to speak of the pylorus as a sphincter. However, the pylorus is now acknowledged to be a true sphincter (Fisher and Cohen, 1973) encompassing a zone of high intraluminal pressure. Its musculature is sensitive to hormones such as secretin and cholecystokinin which are released when acid chyme reaches the duodenum (Isenberg and Csendes, 1972; Fisher and Cohen, 1973), and its functions are not only to assist in the regulation of gastric emptying but also, and perhaps more important, to prevent reflux of potentially injurious bile salts into the stomach during contraction of the duodenal bulb. Gastric emptying is thus controlled to a large extent by the antrum, pylorus and proximal duodenum, which act in a co-ordinated manner under the influence of nerves and hormones. Such controlled gastric emptying is a pre-requisite for normal digestion and absorption and thus for good health.

Destruction of gastric reservoir by standard operations

All the standard operations for duodenal ulcer destroy or at least severely impair this normal control of gastric emptying. In both Polya gastrectomy and vagotomy with antrectomy, the antro-pyloro-duodenal segment is removed entirely, with the result that both solids and liquids leave the stomach in an unregulated fashion. Vagotomy with a drainage procedure $(V+D)$ also produces dramatic changes in the pattern of gastric emptying. After $V+D$, the stomach has been shown to be 'incontinent' of liquids (McKelvey et al., 1969; McKelvey, 1970; Cobb et al., 1971; Clarke and Alexander-Williams, 1973) and emptying of solids may also be precipitate during the first 15 minutes or so after a meal (Colmer et al., 1973). Hence, it is incorrect to say that $V+D$ 'preserves the gastric reservoir'. Thus, all the standard operations for duodenal ulcer greatly impair the principal functions of the stomach, as the 'hopper' and the 'mill' of the alimentary tract. The uncontrolled gastric emptying which they produce, and the rapid intestinal transit which follows, produce in susceptible individuals such well known symptoms as early dumping and diarrhoea, while the ready access of bile salts to gastric mucosa which these procedures afford may produce nausea, epigastric discomfort, bilious vomiting and even gastric ulceration (Capper, 1967; Rhodes et al., 1969; Bushkin et al., 1974).

Clinical results after the standard operations for duodenal ulcer

Since the currently popular operations of truncal vagotomy (TV) or selective vagotomy (SV) with a drainage procedure $(TV/SV+D)$ possess many of the physiological defects of partial gastrectomy, it is perhaps not surprising that in the long run they have been found to yield clinical results which are little if any better than those of gastric resection, and they are by no means free from long-term sequelae such as anaemia and loss of weight. For example, in the late 1950s Professor Goligher and his colleagues in Leeds and York instituted a prospective randomized controlled trial of TV plus gastroenterostomy (GJ), TV plus antrectomy (A) and two-thirds Polya partial gastrectomy (PG) in the elective surgical treatment of duodenal ulcer (Goligher et al., 1968a). Patients were reviewed 'blindly' at yearly intervals at a special gastric follow-up clinic. At the end of 5–8 years it was found (Table 8.1) that only 70 per cent of patients had achieved a good clinical result (Visick grades 1 and 2) after TV+GJ, whereas about 78 per cent of patients had good results after TV+A and PG. Mean weight loss, however, was significantly greater (5 kg) after TV+A and PG than after TV+ GJ (1·8 kg). There was no operative mortality in any of the three groups of

Table 8.1 Visick grading of functional results 5–8 years after operation in Leeds/York trial*

Category	V+GJ (% of 119 cases)	V+A (% of 116 cases)	Subtotal G (% of 107 cases)
1	44 ⎫ 70	50 ⎫ 78	49 ⎫ 77
2	26 ⎭	28 ⎭	28 ⎭
3	19	14	17
4	11	8	6

*Data from Goligher et al. (1968a).

patients. In a similar trial which had been initiated in Glasgow by Sir Charles Illingworth and his colleagues to compare TV+GJ and PG, no significant difference between the results of the two procedures was found (Cox, 1968). More recently, prospective trials by Jordan and Condon (1970), Jordan (1974) and Postlethwait (1973) have confirmed that the over-all clinical results after V+ D are no better than those of V+A or PG. Indeed, Jordan (1974) recommends TV+A as the standard operation for duodenal ulcer, on the basis of an ulcer-recurrence rate of 1 per cent, compared with 9 per cent after V+D, an operative risk which is little greater than that of V+D provided that the surgeon is experienced, and side-effects which are little worse than those of V+D. Jordan advises, however, that V+D be used in poor-risk patients and in situations where technical difficulty in closing the duodenal stump can be anticipated. On a more optimistic note, a recent prospective random trial of TV+P versus TV+GJ by F. Kennedy et al. (1973) in Glasgow showed that both procedures were yielding excellent clinical results 4 years after operation. Why TV+D should yield better results in Glasgow than in Leeds/York or in Houston is difficult to explain. The vagotomies were not better done, according to the results of the insulin tests, and the drainage procedures in all four cities were of standard type. My personal opinion is that the criteria used for judging the results may have been different, because the operations were the same and their physiological sequelae must presumably have been the same. Perhaps our criteria in Leeds are too stringent. Certainly many patients who have a Visick grade 3 ('moderate' or 'fair') result are reasonably satisfied with the outcome.

Prospective random trials cannot, however, provide a complete assessment of an operation for ulcer. They do not 'measure' the relative operative risks of two or more operations, because the numbers of patients involved are not large enough: nor do they provide a measure of long-term sequelae, because they come to an end after 5 or 10 years, whereas it may be 25 years or more before long-term sequelae such as cancer of the gastric stump appear. In a recent report on 255 patients who were followed up for 15–20 years after TV+GJ (Wheldon et al., 1970), 33 per cent of the men and 60 per cent of the women were found to have lost more than 6 kg in weight, iron-deficiency anaemia had been diagnosed in 44 per cent of men and 84 per cent of women, and no fewer than 7 per cent had contracted pulmonary tuberculosis. Thus, nutritional problems after gastric surgery are by no means confined to patients who have undergone gastrectomy. Perhaps in the long run the apparently minor degree of malabsorption of fat and other nutrients after TV+D takes its toll, though diminished intake of food and other factors are probably also involved.

Truncal vagotomy with a drainage procedure thus yields clinical results which are neither very good nor very bad. Recurrent ulceration is found in from 3 to 20 per cent of patients (Herrington, 1972), depending upon the individual surgeon's ability to achieve a complete vagotomy (Johnston et al., 1967; Johnston and Goligher, 1971; F. Kennedy et al., 1973). The incidence of episodic diarrhoea is 25 per cent, and of severe diarrhoea is from 2 to 5 per cent. Approximately 30 per cent of patients have to limit the size of their meals because of an unpleasant sensation of post-prandial fullness, 10–15 per cent 'dump', and an equal number experience bilious vomiting. There is little evidence that truncal vagotomy with a drainage procedure yields better clinical results than does partial gastrectomy or vagotomy with antrectomy. Its main advantage compared with gastrectomy is that it is much safer in the hands of relatively inexperienced surgeons.

Choice of drainage procedure: Pyloroplasty versus gastroenterostomy

Both in the Leeds/York and in the Glasgow trials, which commenced in the 1950s, GJ was used as the drainage procedure with truncal vagotomy. During the 1960s, pyloroplasty (P) gained in popularity because the creation of a blind loop was avoided and it was felt that release of secretin and cholecystokinin-pancreozymin (CCK-PZ) might be closer to normal, chyme would mix better with bile and pancreatic juice, and problems at the stoma such as retrograde intussusception or kinking would be avoided. In addition, pyloroplasty was not expected to have much effect on the control of gastric emptying or to produce dumping, because the pylorus was not thought to be a sphincter. The honeymoon period with pyloroplasty did not last long. By 1968, Goligher et al. (1968b) were reporting that after a 2-year period of follow-up, TV+P gave worse clinical results than TV+GJ, V+A or PG! Only 64 per cent of patients had achieved a really good (Visick grades 1 and 2) result. Goligher et al. (1972) later reported that 5–8 years after TV+P, the over-all results were little better than at 2 years: only 68 per cent of patients had good-to-excellent results, 7 per cent had proved recurrent ulceration and a further 7 per cent were suspected of having recurrence. Side-effects were as frequent after TV+P as after TV+GJ.

The long-term metabolic effects of TV+P and TV+GJ were reviewed by

Wastell (1974). The increase in faecal fat output was found to be as great after TV + P as after TV + GJ. Weight loss and anaemia were less common after TV + P than after TV + GJ.

The respective merits of pyloroplasty and gastrojejunostomy have now been evaluated by means of prospective random trials, of TV + P versus TV + GJ in Glasgow (F. Kennedy et al., 1973) and SV + P versus SV + GJ in Belfast (T. Kennedy et al., 1973a, 1974). No significant difference was found in either trial between P and GJ, with respect either to side-effects or to recurrent ulceration. Recurrence was slightly more common after P, bilious vomiting more common after GJ. Hence, when the duodenal cap is badly scarred or very inflamed, GJ should be preferred to P on the grounds of safety. T. Kennedy also makes the interesting suggestion that, since V + GJ gives as good results as V + P, GJ should usually be preferred to P because a GJ can be undone whereas a P in general cannot. Thus if a patient suffers from intolerable and persistent side-effects such as bilious vomiting, diarrhoea, early dumping or 'late' dumping after V + GJ, the GJ can simply be dismantled. When this is done some years after the initial operation, Kennedy finds that the vagotomized stomach will usually empty satisfactorily without the addition of a drainage procedure, presumably because of recovery of muscular tone and perhaps also because of some degree of vagal reinnervation of the stomach.

Selective vagotomy

In SV the stomach is denervated from cardia to pylorus, the nerves of Latarjet to the antrum are cut, but the hepatic and coeliac vagal fibres are preserved. For many years, H. Burge in Britain and C. A. Griffith in the United States advocated the use of selective vagotomy (SV) rather than truncal vagotomy (TV). In theory, TV was always an irrational procedure, because cutting the parasympathetic nerve supply to the liver, gall bladder, bile ducts, pancreas, small intestine and half the large intestine could not be expected to assist the healing of a duodenal ulcer. Dragstedt had advocated TV as a means of reducing the inappropriate secretion of acid and pepsin by the stomach (Dragstedt and Owens, 1943), but had feared to use or advocate SV because he thought that a high incidence of incomplete vagotomy and hence of recurrent ulceration would follow. Burge (1964) and Griffith (1969), on the other hand, maintained that SV would actually lead to a lower incidence of incomplete vagotomy than did TV. They also pointed out that vagal denervation of the extragastric viscera (in animals) led to alterations in their function which, in man, could prove harmful. Secretion of bile and pancreatic juice, for example, was diminished after TV (see below) and since these secretions were alkaline, neutralization of hydrochloric acid (HCl) in the duodenum after TV might be impaired. Moreover, the extragastric vagal fibres had been shown to inhibit gastric acid secretion in the dog, probably through the agency of some humoral substance, and if they were cut, as in TV, acid secretion increased (Kelly et al., 1964; Landor, 1964; Middleton et al., 1965; Stening and Grossman, 1970; Klempa et al., 1971).

In the realm of clinical practice, Burge and Griffith made two important claims for SV. First, they said that, compared with TV, it lowered the incidence of postvagotomy diarrhoea and, secondly, that it produced a more complete vagal denervation of the stomach. These claims were greeted with some scepticism, but they have both been vindicated by the results of prospective random trials of SV + D versus TV + D (T. Kennedy et al., 1973b; T. Kennedy, 1973, 1974; Sawyers et al., 1968) (Table 8.2). However, although T. Kennedy et al. (1973b) recorded significantly less diarrhoea and incomplete vagotomy and many fewer recurrent ulcers after SV + GJ than after TV + GJ, the *over-all* clinical results which they obtained after SV were little better than the clinical results after TV.

Table 8.2 Comparison of results of truncal and selective vagotomy, each with a drainage procedure

Procedure	No. of patients	Diarrhoea (%)	Recurrent ulcer		Hollander positive (%)
			Proven	Suspected	
TV + D[1]	46	28	3	1	19
SV + D[1]	49	8	0	1	4
TV + D[2]	90	21	1	–	11
SV + D[2]	53	11	0	–	2

[1]Kennedy et al. (1973b); Kennedy (1974).
[2]Sawyers et al. (1968).

Similarly, the clinical results achieved by the patients of Sawyers et al. (1968) after SV + D were little better than those of patients after TV + D. Although diarrhoea is less common after SV + D than after TV + D, early dumping may be more common (T. Kennedy and Connell, 1969; Kraft et al., 1967; Tovey, 1969). Clinical experience, admittedly uncontrolled, with SV + D in Leeds has been far from encouraging (Mason et al., 1968). The incidence of positive Hollander tests 1 week after SV was 19 per cent, no lower than after TV, and 5–8 years after operation the incidence of recurrent ulceration was 10 per cent and only about 66 per cent of patients had achieved good-to-excellent clinical results (Goligher et al., unpublished data). Thus while T. Kennedy (1974) achieved a significantly better vagal denervation of the stomach with SV than with TV in his prospective random trial, this does not mean that *every* surgeon would achieve similar results: indeed, some might achieve a significantly better vagal denervation of the stomach with TV than with SV! We showed previously that some surgeons have no positive Hollander tests 1 week after TV, others have 50 per cent positive (Fig. 8.1); some have no positive Hollander tests after SV, others have 30 per cent positive (Johnston and Goligher, 1971); and, as we shall see, some surgeons have almost no positive Hollander tests 1 week after HSV, while others have 60 per cent positive. The fault lies not in the vagotomy, but in ourselves.

To sum up, prospective random trials in Britain and North America have confirmed many of Burge's and Griffith's claims for SV, but there is still no convinc-

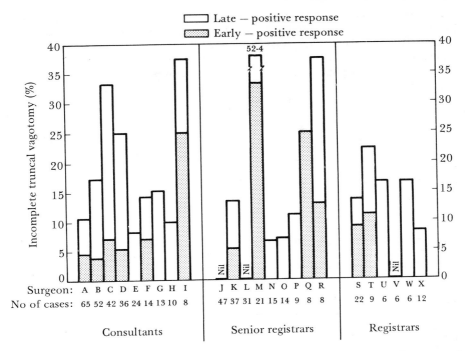

Fig. 8.1 The great inter-surgeon variation in the ability to achieve a complete truncal vagotomy is shown. Surgeons J and L did 47 and 31 vagotomies, respectively, all of which were complete, whereas several other surgeons left 25–50 per cent of their patients with the vagotomy still incomplete. Similar inter-surgeon variation is found on insulin testing after selective and highly selective vagotomy. These findings provide an explanation for the great variations in the quoted incidences of recurrent ulceration after each type of vagotomy. The above insulin tests were performed 5–10 days after operation. Note that consultants were not better vagotomists than registrars.

ing evidence that the over-all clinical results after SV with a drainage procedure are significantly better than the results of TV with a drainage procedure.

Selective vagotomy without a drainage procedure

By the late 1960s it was clear that many of the side-effects of vagotomy with drainage were attributable to the drainage procedure (at least in part), rather than to the vagotomy. For this reason, attempts were made to treat patients with duodenal ulcer by vagotomy without drainage. Bilateral selective vagotomy (SV) was used, because TV without drainage was known to produce gastric stasis. Burge and his colleagues (1969) treated more than 100 patients by SV without drainage, with favourable results in the short term. Burge's patients were carefully selected—in that they had no pyloroduodenal narrowing—and Burge himself stated that fewer than 50 per cent of all patients coming to operation for duodenal ulcer were suitable for SV without drainage. Less happy results than Burge's were recorded by Kirk (1970) who had to re-operate on 2 out of 25 patients to relieve gastric stasis, and by Clarke et al. (1972b) who, in a short-lived prospective random trial of SV alone versus SV with drainage, found that omission of the drainage procedure led to delayed gastric emptying in most patients (Clarke and Alexander-Williams, 1973) and to gastric ulceration in 3 out of a total of 15. In another study, severe gastric retention after SV without drainage was found in 3 out of 9 patients (T. Kennedy, 1973). These findings were in agreement with previous observations in dogs that vagal denervation of the antrum led to considerable impairment of antral motility (Wohlrabe and Kelly, 1959a, b; Stavney et al., 1963) and that SV without drainage produced gastric stasis (Shiina and Griffith, 1969; Clarke and Alexander-Williams, 1973). For these reasons, selective vagotomy without a drainage procedure 'should no longer be considered as a method of treatment for duodenal ulcer'.

Highly selective vagotomy (parietal cell vagotomy)

History and nomenclature

Because of my close acquaintance with the disappointing results of the Leeds/York trial (Goligher et al., 1968a) and also because of a long-continued interest in mechanisms which control and inhibit gastric secretion and emptying, I began in 1968 to think about how to keep the pylorus intact in the course of operations for duodenal ulcer. This had for long been a surgeon's dream (Ferguson et al., 1960; Flynn and Longmire, 1960; Friesen and Rieger, 1960; Killen and Symbas, 1962; Maki et al., 1967; Amdrup and Griffith, 1969a,b), because of the potential benefits to the patient in terms of better-controlled gastric emptying and fewer side-effects, but progress had been blocked by surgeons' distrust of the gastric antrum, derived from knowledge both of the disastrous clinical consequences of the antrum-exclusion operation (Von Eiselsberg, 1920; Devine, 1925; Kay, 1959) and of experiments in animals which showed that vagal stimulation released gastrin from the antrum (Pe Thein and Schofield, 1959; Nyhus et al, 1960). Hence many surgeons believed firmly that the antrum should nearly always be resected (Smithwick et al., 1961; Herrington, 1969), while the remainder agreed with Nyhus et al. (1960) that at least it should invariably be vagally denervated and 'drained'. Vagal denervation of the antrum, as explained earlier, weakens its propulsive power and leads to the need for a drainage procedure, which in turn either destroys or bypasses the sphincteric mechanism at the exit of the stomach.

It seemed to me that if the pyloric sphincter and the terminal antrum were to be preserved, it would be necessary to leave the antrum vagally innervated. Vagotomy would have to be confined to the acid- and pepsin-secreting part of the stomach, the parietal cell mass (PCM) (Fig. 8.2). This operation had first been used by Griffith and Harkins in dogs in 1957. They reported that gastric emptying was satisfactory, that insulin tests were either negative or weakly positive, and that clinical application seemed feasible. Amdrup and Griffith (1969a) subsequently confirmed these findings, but found a 47 per cent increase in acid output from Heidenhain pouches. They concluded that the operation would

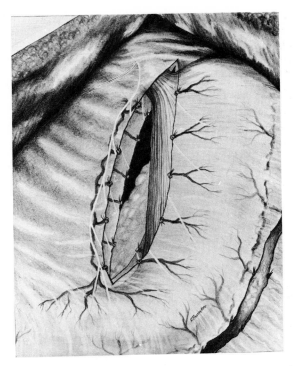

Fig. 8.2 HSV is half completed. The lesser curvature has been laid bare. Note anterior nerve of Latarjet in lesser omentum. Although the lower oesophagus has been laid bare, a further 5 cm of distal oesophagus must now be cleared of all blood vessels and nerve fibres.

eliminate dumping, but might be followed by a high incidence of recurrent ulceration because of excessive gastrin release from the innervated antrum. 'Selective proximal vagotomy' with pyloroplasty or antrectomy was first used in man by Holle and Hart (1967), their rationale being that the vagal nerves to the antrum mediated inhibition of gastric secretion (Hart, 1966, 1968). Vagotomy confined to the parietal cell mass without a drainage procedure was first used by Johnston and Wilkinson (1969, 1970) and by Amdrup and Jensen (1970) from the beginning of 1969. Viewing the new operation as a logical extension of selective vagotomy, we call it highly selective vagotomy (HSV), Amdrup terms it parietal cell vagotomy (PCV), while others prefer the term proximal gastric vagotomy. Amdrup and I, having developed this operation which preserves the sphincteric mechanisms at the exit of the stomach, hope that our colleagues will be generous enough to grant us the privilege of naming it. We are in agreement that if the extent of the antrum is 'mapped' at operation, the operation should be called PCV, while if anatomical landmarks are used, the operation should be called HSV (Amdrup and Johnston, 1975). Since HSV and PCV are so similar, and because to date they have yielded virtually identical results, they will be considered together here under the title of HSV.

Rationale

Highly selective vagotomy is based on the hypotheses that side-effects of gastric surgery will be minimized if controlled gastric emptying can be preserved through an intact pylorus, and that if this is to happen the vagal nerve supply to the gastric antrum must be preserved.

The truth of the first hypothesis is self-evident. Vagal denervation of the antrum had previously been regarded as essential because it was thought that gastrin release was thereby reduced (Forrest, 1956; Oberhelman et al., 1957; Nyhus et al., 1960). It was certainly true that vagal release of gastrin was easy to demonstrate in dogs equipped with separated or transplanted antral pouches which were shielded from the inhibitory influence of endogenous acid (Pe Thein and Schofield, 1959). Similarly, in man, profuse release of gastrin had been responsible for the prohibitive incidence of recurrent ulceration after the antral exclusion operation (Von Eiselsberg, 1920; Devine, 1925; Kay, 1958). However, when the antrum was either left in continuity with the 'acid stream' from the body of the stomach or bathed with HCl (in dogs), vagal release of gastrin was much more difficult to demonstrate (Oberhelman et al., 1952; Burstall and Schofield, 1953, 1954) than when the antrum was 'excluded', because acid in contact with the mucosa of the antrum inhibits gastrin release (Oberhelman et al., 1952; Gillespie, 1959). Moreover, vagal denervation of an antral pouch which had been transplanted to the alkaline milieu of the duodenum failed to reduce the profuse acid output from the stomach (Woodward et al., 1954) and vagal denervation of an isolated antral pouch did not alter gastrin release elicited by meat broth (Wohlrabe and Kelly, 1959b). Of course, there was plenty of evidence to support the orthodox view, so that the literature on the effect of vagal denervation of the antrum on gastrin release is thoroughly contradictory. Besides, most of it pertains not to man but to the dog. Thus, the idea that the gastric antrum must always be vagally denervated and 'drained' in the course of vagotomy operations for ulcer in man seemed open to question. When the antrum was 'in situ', vagal release of gastrin might not be excessive, particularly because any gastrin that was released would have to act on vagally denervated, and hence less sensitive, parietal cells (Uvnäs, 1942; Payne and Kay, 1962).

Finally, we suggested that protective and inhibitory mechanisms mediated by the nerves of Latarjet (Hart, 1966, 1968), the hepatic and coeliac vagal fibres (Kelly et al., 1964; Landor, 1964) and by the alkaline secretions of the antrum, Brunner's glands, liver and pancreas would remain unchanged after HSV, whereas they might be impaired after any of the standard operations.

Comparison of the effects of truncal, selective and highly selective vagotomy on the physiology of the alimentary tract

In Leeds, we studied gastric secretion, serum gastrin, gastric emptying, the provocation of dumping and diarrhoea, gall bladder function, pancreatic function, glucose–insulin metabolism and faecal fat excretion in matched groups of healthy patients, more than 1 year after each of the three types of vagotomy. Each patient had been shown to have a complete vagotomy (of the PCM) by the Hollander insulin test soon after operation. The comparisons made between these groups of patients are felt to be relatively free from bias.

Serum gastrin

Measurement of serum gastrin by radioimmunoassay has shown that vagotomy of any type leads to an *increase* in serum gastrin (Hansky et al., 1972; Stadil, 1972; Hansky and Korman, 1973; Jaffe et al., 1974; Korman et al., 1973a, b; Kronborg et al., 1973; Stern and Walsh, 1973). This is true both of gastrin levels in fasting patients and of gastrin levels after a meal. There is no evidence that either fasting or post-prandial gastrin levels are higher after HSV than after truncal vagotomy (Jaffe et al., 1974; Stadil and Rehfeld, 1974); indeed, Hansky and Korman's (1973) data suggest that gastrin levels are significantly higher after TV than after HSV. These results suggest that the main determinant of the concentration of serum gastrin is the pH of the contents of the antrum rather than the integrity or otherwise of the vagal nerve supply to the antrum. When the vagus nerves are stimulated by insulin-induced hypoglycaemia, gastrin release is demonstrable both in patients with intact vagi and in patients after HSV (Hansky et al., 1971, 1972; Hansky and Korman, 1973; Korman et al., 1973a, b). After truncal or selective vagotomy, no increase in gastrin levels after insulin was found by Korman et al (1973a, b), but Stadil and his colleagues found that gastrin levels still increased in response to insulin (Stadil, 1972; Kronborg et al., 1973; Stadil and Rehfeld, 1974). The finding that TV increases rather than decreases serum gastrin in man is of great clinical importance because it suggests that vagal denervation of the gastric antrum is unnecessary. If vagal denervation of the antrum is unnecessary, drainage procedures are probably unnecessary also.

Gastric secretion

Basal acid output (BAO)

HSV reduces BAO by 80 per cent (Johnston et al., 1973a; Greenall et al., 1975) for up to 5 years after operation. This reduction is at least as great as that produced by TV or SV+D.

Maximal acid output (MAO)

Maximal acid output is reduced by 50 per cent in the long term (Johnston et al., 1973b, Greenall et al., 1975), which again is as large as the reductions in MAO after TV or SV (Jepson et al., 1973).

Insulin response

Only 3 of the first 100 patients had positive insulin tests 1 week after HSV in Leeds (Fig. 8.3; Johnston et al., 1973b), but 3–5 years later 90 per cent of the tests had become positive. However, even then, the peak acid response to insulin (PAO[I]) (minus BAO) was only about 3 mEq/hour, compared with 33 mEq/hour

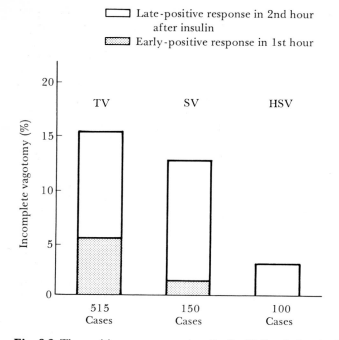

Fig. 8.3 The positive responses to insulin (by Hollander's criteria) 1 week after TV, SV and HSV. Note that only 3 of 100 patients were Hollander-positive after HSV. The apparent superiority of HSV over TV and SV is probably spurious (see text), but the 3 per cent positive incidence after HSV indicates that there is no need for the high incidences of incomplete vagotomy which are sometimes quoted. Patients who are insulin-positive at this time are much more likely to develop recurrent ulceration than are patients who are insulin-negative (F. Kennedy et al., 1973).

before operation (Lyndon et al., 1975). That is, most of the acid responses to insulin are very small and the mean reduction in PAO[1] in the long term after HSV is approximately 90 per cent. Since very few (2 out of 250) of our patients have so far developed recurrent ulceration after HSV, the finding of a positive response to insulin more than 1 year after HSV is unlikely to have prognostic significance.

The finding of a Hollander-positive response to insulin 1 week after HSV is quite a different matter. At this time, there is great inter-surgeon variation in the ability to achieve a complete vagotomy of the PCM, just as we showed previously in patients who had undergone TV and SV (Fig. 8.1) (Johnston and Goligher, 1971). The use of HSV certainly carries no guarantee that the PCM will be completely denervated, and we know of surgeons who have, respectively, 0, 10, 28 and 58 per cent incidences of positive insulin tests 1 week after HSV. Patients with positive insulin tests 7–10 days after TV (particularly those with large, early-positive responses) have been shown to be more likely to develop recurrent ulceration than are patients who have negative insulin tests (Johnston et al., 1967; F. Kennedy et al., 1973), and there is some evidence that a similar correlation exists between 'insulin-positivity' soon after HSV and recurrent ulceration (Wastell et al., 1972; Kronborg and Madsen, 1975). Thus, in our own series, 97 of the first 100 patients had negative insulin tests after HSV. None of the 97 has so far developed recurrent ulceration in a 3–6-year follow-up, but 1 of the 3 with positive tests developed a recurrent ulcer. Amdrup and Jensen's patients who underwent PCV in Copenhagen had virtually identical patterns of acid secretion to those of our patients after HSV in Leeds (Johnston et al., 1973a, b) and none of their patients has developed recurrent duodenal ulceration (Amdrup et al., 1974). In contrast, 28 per cent of Wastell et al.'s (1972) 16 patients had positive insulin tests 1 week after HSV, and 2 of them (13 per cent) quickly developed recurrent ulceration. Of Kronborg and Madsen's (1975) patients, 58 per cent had positive insulin tests 1 week after HSV and no fewer than 22 per cent of them developed recurrent ulceration. Thus it seems likely that the incidence of recurrent duodenal ulceration is determined not so much by the variety of vagotomy which is employed as by its degree of completeness, as determined by the insulin test 5–10 days after operation.

Acid response to a test meal

Acid response to a test meal was found to be no greater after HSV (mean, 10 mEq/hour) than after TV + P (mean, 14 mEq/hour) or SV + P (10 mEq/hour) (Johnston, 1972).

Pepsin output

Pepsin output is reduced as much by HSV as by TV or SV in man (our unpublished observations) and dog (Kaynan et al., 1973).

Gastric motility and receptive relaxation

Both TV and SV without drainage lead to disorganized myoelectrical activity in the stomach of man and dogs (Nelsen et al., 1967; Kelly and Code, 1969; Stoddard et al., 1973; Wilbur and Kelly, 1973), impair gastric motility, and produce gastric stasis (Wohlrabe and Kelly, 1959a; Stavney et al., 1963; Shiina and Griffith, 1969; Kirk, 1970; Amdrup et al., 1971; Clarke et al., 1972). Compared with TV and SV, HSV has been shown to produce less disturbance in myoelectrical activity, motility and emptying (Stoddard et al., 1973; Wilbur and Kelly, 1973). Although the vagotomized stomach is often thought of as 'flaccid', in fact gastric vagotomy has been shown to impair receptive relaxation (hence the symptom of epigastric fullness after meals), increase intragastric pressure, accelerate the emptying of liquids and produce dumping in susceptible individuals (Jansson, 1969; Stadaas and Aune, 1970; Kolster and Madsen, 1970; Wilbur and Kelly, 1973). These changes are more marked after vagotomy with a drainage procedure than after HSV.

The observations of Wilbur and Kelly (1973) identified the key role of the vagally innervated proximal stomach in regulating gastric emptying of liquids by controlling intragastric pressure and the key role of the vagally innervated antrum in regulating gastric emptying of solids by controlling the terminal antral contraction.

Gastric emptying

Stasis

HSV does not produce gastric stasis. If patients with clinical evidence of pyloric stenosis are excluded, fewer than 1 per cent of patients who underwent HSV for duodenal ulcer have required re-operation for the relief of gastric stasis (Amdrup et al., 1974). At the gastric follow-up clinic, symptoms suggestive of gastric retention, such as vomiting and flatulence, have been found to be less common after HSV than after TV or SV with a drainage procedure. Finally, studies of gastric emptying of fluids (Interone et al., 1971; Humphrey and Wilkinson, 1972; Moberg et al., 1972) and of food-and-barium (Pedersen and Amdrup, 1970; Madsen et al., 1973; Wilkinson and Johnston, 1973) have revealed no evidence of gastric stasis in man after HSV, whereas complete gastric vagotomy without drainage frequently produces gastric stasis both in man (Kirk, 1970; Clarke et al., 1972b) and in experimental animals (Shiina and Griffith, 1969; Amdrup et al., 1971).

Regulation of gastric emptying

Granted that HSV rarely produces gastric stasis, is the pattern of gastric emptying normal after HSV? The answer is that gastric emptying is not normal after HSV, but that it is closer to the normal than is gastric emptying after vagotomy with a drainage procedure. After HSV in man, gastric emptying of fluids is significantly faster than before operation, presumably because of impaired receptive relaxation by the denervated body of the stomach (Humphrey and Wilkinson, 1972; Moberg et al., 1972; Clarke and Alexander-Williams, 1973). It is significantly *slower* than gastric emptying after truncal or selective vagotomy with a drainage procedure, both of which render the stomach 'incontinent' of liquids (McKelvey, 1970; Cobb et al., 1971; Clarke and Alexander-Williams, 1973). Such gastric incontinence after vagotomy with drainage may be an important cause of so-called post-vagotomy diarrhoea (McKelvey et al., 1969). Thus, when a hypertonic test meal is given orally to patients who have undergone either HSV or vagotomy with pyloroplasty (V+P), significantly more dumping, diarrhoea and hypotension ensue in the patients who have undergone V+P than in the patients who have undergone HSV (Humphrey and Wilkinson, 1972; Humphrey et al., 1972; Johnston et al., 1972a; Madsen et al., 1973). Radiological studies of the gastric emptying and intestinal transit of a thick mixture of food and barium after HSV showed that the pattern of emptying was similar to that of pre-operative patients with duodenal ulcer, and significantly slower than that of patients who had undergone truncal or selective vagotomy with pyloroplasty (Wilkinson and Johnston, 1973). Both Pederson and Amdrup (1970) and Madsen et al. (1973) found that gastric emptying of a 'nutritional contrast medium' was significantly faster after selective vagotomy and pyloroplasty than after HSV. A preliminary report has suggested that gastric emptying of solid food is within normal limits after HSV in man (Alexander-Williams et al., 1973).

Biliary tract

The 'resting' gall bladder has been shown to dilate significantly after TV in man (Johnson and Boyden, 1952; Rudick and Hutchison, 1964). After both SV (Rudick and Hutchison, 1964) and HSV (Parkin et al., 1973), it does not dilate. Contraction of the gall bladder in response to a meal is relatively unimpaired after each of the three types of vagotomy (Glanville and Duthie, 1964; Parkin et al., 1973).

Vagal nerve stimulation leads to an increase in bile flow and in the output of bile acids (Tanturi and Ivy, 1938; Fritz and Brooks, 1963; Baldwin et al., 1966; McKelvey et al., 1973). Truncal vagotomy in man abolishes this response (McKelvey et al., 1973), while in the dog bile flow diminishes and the bile becomes more lithogenic in composition (Fritz and Brooks, 1963; Fletcher and Clark, 1969; Schein et al., 1969; Cowie and Clark, 1972; Tompkins et al., 1972).

The clinical significance of these observations is not clear. Several reports have suggested that TV leads to an increased risk of gallstone formation (Nielsen, 1964; Nobles, 1966; Miller, 1968; Clave and Gaspar, 1969; Tompkins et al., 1972), which could be due to stasis of bile in the dilated gall bladder, to changes in the composition of the bile or to both factors. Clave and Gaspar (1969) found evidence of gall bladder disease in 23 per cent of 92 patients after TV + P: gallstones were found in 13 of 55 patients in whom both pre-operative cholecystograms had been normal and the gall bladder had been felt to be normal at operation. In the study of Tompkins et al. (1972), 16 per cent of 50 patients who had undergone TV 1–5 years previously, and who had normal gall bladders at operation, were found to have developed gallstones: this was four times the expected incidence in the general population. Thus there is strong, although still inconclusive, evidence that TV increases the risk of gallstone formation. Whether gallstones will develop less frequently after SV or HSV than after TV remains to be seen.

Pancreas and small intestine

Pancreatic secretion is under neurohumoral control. A cephalic phase of pancreatic secretion has been demonstrated in man (Sarles et al., 1968; Novis et al., 1971). Truncal vagotomy in man abolishes or greatly impairs the pancreatic exocrine response to vagal stimulation by insulin hypoglycaemia (Dreiling et al., 1952; Pfeffer et al., 1952; Gamble, 1970), whereas after both SV and HSV in man, such stimulation elicits a significant increase in enzyme output (McKelvey et al., 1973; Smith et al., 1973). The clinical importance of vagal stimulation of the pancreas, compared with that of humoral stimulation by endogenous secretion and CCK-PZ, is not clear. Certainly the effect of TV on pancreatic secretion is disputed, and there is little evidence that absorption of fat in man is better after SV than after TV (Kraft et al., 1965; Wastell and Ellis, 1966; Williams and Irvine, 1966).

Bicarbonate output in response to a meal of meat has been shown to be greatly diminished after TV in the dog (Davis et al., 1973). Truncal vagotomy may thus damage an important defence against the corrosive action of acid and pepsin in the duodenum.

There is also evidence that endogenous stimulation of pancreatic exocrine and endocrine secretion may be impaired after TV, because release of secretin (Moreland and Johnson, 1971), CCK-PZ (Malagelada et al., 1974) and perhaps of insulin-stimulating hormones (Humphrey et al., 1975) has been found to be diminished after TV.

Faecal fat excretion

Both TV+D and SV+D increase faecal fat output in man significantly, from about 2·5 g/day to a mean of 6–8 g/day (Wastell and Ellis, 1966; Williams and Irvine, 1966). About 40 per cent of patients have steatorrhoea after TV+GJ (Cox et al., 1964). Much of the increase in fat output may be due to the drainage procedure rather than to the vagotomy (Wastell, 1966). After HSV, faecal fat output in man does not change significantly (Edwards et al., 1974).

The clinical importance of these increases in faecal fat after vagotomy lies not so much in the malabsorption of fat itself as in the associated malabsorption of protein, minerals and vitamins. Patients who have not lost weight before operation tend to lose weight after TV+D (Cox et al., 1964), which suggests that TV+D does have an adverse effect on nutrition. Weight loss, iron-deficiency anaemia and even tuberculosis are not uncommon in the long term after TV+GJ (Wheldon et al., 1970), and while one cause is certainly inadequate intake of nutriments, impaired absorption is no doubt important also.

Comparison of operations for duodenal ulcer

HSV has now been in use for $6\frac{1}{2}$ years. Prospective trials of HSV against V+D are now in progress and preliminary results are available from two of them. The combined Leeds/Copenhagen series of 400 patients is both the largest series and also the one with the longest period of follow-up. The results achieved in these patients will be described and compared with the results obtained after vagotomy with drainage (V+D) in the same centres. It is emphasized that while the series of patients in both cities were virtually consecutive (for example, 98 per cent of the author's elective cases were treated by HSV), a prospective random trial of HSV versus V+D was not undertaken and hence the comparisons presented may not be free from bias. So far as we are aware, however, the criteria for selection of patients for operation did not change. In Leeds, patients after TV, SV and HSV attended a special gastric follow-up clinic in company with patients who had undergone a wide variety of gastric operations, ranging from simple suture of perforation to total gastrectomy for carcinoma. They were assessed in 'blind' manner by a panel of three doctors, who recorded the answers to a standard set of questions and wrote down their collective verdict according to a modified Visick system of grading before being permitted to learn which type of operation had been performed.

Selection of patients

Four hundred patients were operated upon electively for duodenal ulcer from 1969 to 1974 inclusive. Patients with *clinically manifest* pyloric stenosis (until 1972 in Leeds), acute haemorrhage or perforation were excluded. All obese patients and those with considerable pyloroduodenal scarring without *clinical* pyloric stenosis were included. Thus HSV was not merely a 'minimal operation for minimal disease'. The series included a high proportion of patients with severe, active ulceration.

Operative technique

Parietal cell vagotomy (PCV) in Denmark involved routine mapping of the antrum, the proximal boundary of which was found to lie 8–10 cm from the pylorus (Amdrup and Jensen, 1970). In Leeds, the main nerves of Latarjet were spared, which meant that 5–8 cm of distal stomach were left innervated (Fig. 8.2). The clinical results after HSV and PCV were very similar and their effects on gastric secretion were almost identical (Johnston et al., 1973a, b; Amdrup et al., 1974).

The success or failure of an operation for peptic ulcer is determined by four principal factors. These are: (1) the operative mortality (and post-operative complications), (2) the side-effects, (3) the incidence of recurrent ulceration, and (4) the long-term sequelae. The clinical results of the various operations for duodenal ulcer will therefore be discussed under these four main headings.

1(a). Operative mortality

The operative mortality in 400 HSV operations for duodenal ulcer in Leeds and Copenhagen was 0 per cent. In a recent world-wide survey of the operative mortality of elective HSV, 17 deaths were recorded after 5,257 operations, an operative mortality of 0·31 per cent (Johnston, 1975). Five of these deaths were due to necrosis of the lesser curvature of the stomach, which seems to be a rare but specific complication of HSV (Newcombe, 1973), occurring in about 1 in 500 cases and resulting perhaps from the relative paucity of anastomosing blood vessels in the submucosa along the lesser curve (Barlow et al., 1951; Womack, 1969).

For comparison, Cox et al. (1969) in a review of 6,500 elective V + D operations found that the operative mortality was 0·8 per cent. The mean operative mortality of elective vagotomy–antrectomy is approximately 1·2 per cent (Herrington, 1969) and of Polya partial gastrectomy is about 2 per cent (Fig. 8.4). Of course, these figures are inevitably biased, if only because published series are usually written by enthusiasts and by surgeons with greater-than-average experience. Hence the *over-all* operative mortality of most procedures is probably a good deal higher than the published data would suggest. It is also certainly true that experienced surgeons can, by a combination of good luck and good judgement, sometimes perform many hundreds of elective gastric resections without a death (Goligher et al., 1968a; Ochsner et al., 1970; McKeown, 1972).

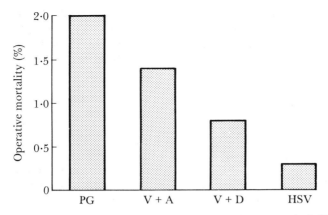

Fig. 8.4 Operative mortality of HSV was 0·3 per cent in 5,000 cases and that of V+D was 0·8 per cent in over 6,000 cases. These data refer not to the 'best' series, but to the world average. The difference between HSV and V+D is statistically significant. Data refer to *elective* operation for duodenal ulcer.

Despite their imperfections, however, the data from large collected series have to be used when the relative operative risks of different operations are calculated, because the numbers of patients included in prospective random trials—usually a few hundred at the most—are inadequate for the purpose, several thousands of patients being needed in each group to establish that a difference is of statistical significance, when the risk of death is, let us suppose, 1 in 100 in one group and 1 in 300 in another.

In conclusion, in patients treated electively for duodenal ulcer, the operative mortality of HSV is 0·3 per cent, of V+D is 0·8 per cent, of V+A is 1·2 per cent and of Polya PG is about 2 per cent. In other words, the risk that a patient will die soon after his operation is twice as great after V+D as after HSV; after gastric resection, it is four times as great as after HSV. These differences are both statistically significant ($P<0·01$) and clinically significant.

1(b). Post-operative complications

Complications specific to HSV have been very uncommon in our experience. Presumably this is because of the absence of any suture line or stoma. Patients are given 2 litres of intravenous fluid during the operation and after operation are nursed without either a nasogastric tube or an intravenous drip. This allows them to get out of bed and to move about relatively soon after operation. Gastric retention in the early post-operative period has been rare and a nasogastric tube has had to be passed in only 3 of my last 100 patients. Transient gastric stasis, manifested by the vomiting of food, occurred in 4 patients in Leeds within 2 months of HSV, but in none of Amdrup and Jensen's patients in Copenhagen. This gastric retention responded to conservative management in the form of a fluid diet and all these patients have now achieved good clinical results. Only 3 patients out of 400 (0·8 per cent in Leeds and Copenhagen) have subsequently required the addition of a drainage procedure for the relief of gastric stasis. These findings have been confirmed by many other surgeons, and in the survey of 5,257 elective HSV operations (Johnston, 1975), post-operative stasis was found to be uncommon and only 0·6 per cent of patients needed to have a drainage procedure added later.

2. Side-effects of gastric surgery

The clinical results which were achieved in 108 patients who had undergone HSV in Copenhagen and Leeds 2–4 years previously were published recently (Amdrup et al., 1974). While that report has the defect that there was no comparison with a randomized series of patients who had been allocated to one of the standard operations, the results obtained after HSV leave little doubt that the incidence of side-effects is significantly reduced compared with the incidence found after

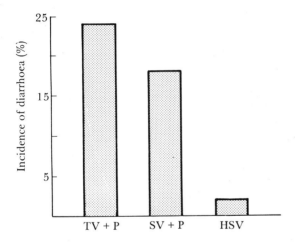

Fig. 8.5 Incidence of diarrhoea 1 year after vagotomy. Diarrhoea is defined as the passage of liquid stools, with urgency. It is usually episodic. HSV virtually abolishes so-called post-vagotomy diarrhoea. The incidence after HSV was no higher than the incidence in 50 control subjects who had undergone herniorrhaphy or operation for varicose veins. Incidences of diarrhoea 2 years and >5 years after TV, SV and HSV in Leeds are similar to the incidences recorded 1 year after operation.

any of the standard operations. Episodic diarrhoea, for example, was recorded in only 5 per cent of patients after HSV, compared with 15 per cent of patients after SV + P and 25 per cent of patients after TV + P. Severe diarrhoea was noted in none of the patients after HSV, 2 per cent after SV + P and 5 per cent after TV + P. These findings confirmed our earlier report that diarrhoea was much less common after HSV than after TV + P or SV + P (Johnston et al., 1972b) (Fig. 8.5). Similar findings have been reported by De Miguel (1972). Early dumping was noted in 6 per cent of patients after HSV, in 32 per cent after SV + P and in 11 per cent after TV + D. This, too, confirmed our previous report

(Humphrey et al., 1972). In Leeds, there has been no clinically troublesome dumping after HSV. Mild dumping after HSV is no doubt attributable to the accelerated emptying of liquids which has been described by Humphrey and Wilkinson (1972), Clarke and Alexander-Williams (1973) and Wilbur and Kelly (1973). Bilious vomiting was recorded in 2 per cent of patients after HSV, in 8 per cent after SV + P, in 11 per cent after TV + P and in 16 per cent of patients after TV with gastroenterostomy. Other side-effects of gastric surgery, such as dysphagia, flatulence and heartburn, were no more common after HSV than after vagotomy with a drainage procedure. These results suggest that preservation of an innervated antrum and intact pylorus virtually eliminates dumping, diarrhoea and bilious vomiting as clinical problems, while the incidence of other side-effects is not increased. The experience of other authors has been similar. For example, De Miguel (1972), Hedenstedt et al. (1972), Grassi et al. (1973), Liedberg and Oscarson (1973), Liavag and Roland (1973) and Madsen and Kronborg (1973) have all reported that the incidence of dumping and diarrhoea was low after HSV. Preliminary reports of prospective random trials from Belfast and Copenhagen confirm that there are significantly fewer side-effects after HSV than after complete gastric vagotomy with a drainage procedure (T. Kennedy, 1975, personal communication; Kronborg and Madsen, 1975). Since side-effects after V + A or PG are at least as severe as after V + D (Cox, 1968; Goligher et al., 1968a; Jordan and Condon, 1970; Postlethwait, 1973), it may be concluded that HSV produces significantly fewer side-effects than any of the standard operations for duodenal ulcer.

3. Recurrent ulceration

Side-effects are often at their worst during the first year or two after operation. In contrast, a long period of follow-up—ideally 10 years or more—is needed before the true incidence of recurrent ulceration can be estimated. However, recurrent ulceration after both V + D and HSV is characteristically early, often occurring within 2 years of operation (Fawcett et al., 1969; Wastell et al., 1972; Small, 1973). Hence, although the figures for recurrence after HSV must be regarded as provisional, by 5 years after operation the worst is probably over. In Leeds, 70 patients have now been followed up for a mean period of 5 years after HSV, and only 1 of them (1·4 per cent) has developed recurrent duodenal ulceration and none has developed gastric ulceration. The patient with recurrence had a late-positive insulin test 1 week after operation and developed recurrent pain 4 years later. Of the total of 250 patients who have undergone elective HSV in Leeds in the past 6½ years, only 2 have proven recurrent ulceration. These patients are followed up at yearly intervals and follow-up is 94 per cent complete. When Amdrup et al. (1974) reviewed the clinical results of 108 patients 2–4 years after HSV/PCV in Leeds and Copenhagen, not a single proven case of recurrent duodenal ulceration was found, although 2 patients (2 per cent) in Copenhagen had developed gastric ulceration. Pain of ulcer type was experienced at some time during follow-up by 6 per cent of patients in Leeds, but in some of these it was mild or transient. These patients were investigated in the usual way by barium meal examination, gastroduodenoscopy and insulin/pentagastrin tests. No definite sign of ulceration was found in any of them and their acid outputs were found to be little different from those of patients who did not complain of pain. Two patients early in the series in Leeds underwent laparotomy because of suspicion of recurrent ulceration. The interior of the duodenum was inspected at operation and no mucosal defect was found : an antrectomy was performed in one patient and a pyloroplasty in the other. None of the patients in Leeds has perforated or bled significantly.

In other centres, the incidence of recurrent ulceration after HSV has varied from 0 to 22 per cent. Thus, Liavag and Roland (1973) reported 250 HSV operations in the previous 3 years with no recurrent ulceration. Grassi et al. (1973) reported 79 patients after HSV with only 1 recurrence. Moberg and Hedenstedt (1973) followed up 48 patients for a minimum period of 3 years after HSV and found 3 definite recurrences (6 per cent) which all occurred within the first year after operation. Wastell et al. (1972) report 2 recurrences (13 per cent) after a short period of follow-up of 16 patients, but the incidence of incomplete vagotomy as shown by the insulin test 1 week after HSV was no less than 28 per cent. Wastell et al. now have a much larger series of HSVs and the incidence of recurrence is lower. In Copenhagen, Kronborg and Madsen (1975) found that no fewer than 58 per cent of their patients had positive Hollander tests 10 days after both HSV and SV. The incidence of recurrent ulceration after HSV in their series was 22 per cent (Madsen and Kronborg, 1973; Kronborg and Madsen, 1975). An incidence of recurrence of 20 per cent within 18 months of HSV in 20 patients was reported by Liedberg and Oscarson (1973). In this pilot series, however, basal acid output (BAO) was reduced by only 40 per cent, maximal acid output (MAO) by only 33 per cent, while the insulin test was positive in 83 per cent of patients 2 months after operation and in 100 per cent of patients after 1 year. These findings led to a modification in surgical technique, with the result that good results were obtained in 60 subsequent patients, BAO being reduced by 80 per cent and MAO by 58 per cent, while no further recurrent ulcers were found.

Thus, although the clinical reports are conflicting, a pattern seems to be emerging which is familiar from previous experience with truncal and selective vagotomy. When vagotomy is complete, as shown by an intra-operative test such as that of Burge (Burge and Frohn, 1969) or Grassi (1971), or by the insulin test performed 1 week after operation, recurrent ulceration is rare. When vagotomy is shown to be incomplete by the Hollander test 1 week after operation, the incidence of recurrent ulceration is relatively high (Johnston et al., 1967; F. Kennedy et al., 1973). These findings underline the need for meticulous dissection around the oesophagus during HSV, and for monitoring the completeness of vagotomy. The insulin test 1 week after operation provides such a 'quality control'. If this test is found to be positive in no more than 10–15 per cent of patients, probably nothing more need be done because the incidence of recurrent ulceration should be low. If the incidence of incomplete vagotomy is higher, however, the operative technique should be reassessed and consideration given to the use of some intraoperative test. Such tests have not secured wide acceptance, but they are unquestionably a more rational form of quality control than the insulin test, because if the vagotomy is found to be incomplete a determined effort can be made to complete it, and the outcome of the surgeon's endeavours can be assessed once more. It seems preferable to use these tests than to despair of vagotomy and subject a high proportion of patients to an unnecessary and potentially harmful antrectomy.

The incidence of recurrent ulceration after truncal vagotomy is similar to that reported after HSV, ranging from 3 to 23 per cent. There is little evidence so far that the incidence of recurrence after HSV is any higher than that which is found after truncal or selective vagotomy with a drainage procedure.

Should antrectomy be added in hypersecretors?

Debate continues about the need for 'selective' surgery for duodenal ulcer, in which the magnitude of the operation is related to the size of the pre-operative MAO. Kronborg (1974) and Robbs et al. (1974) found a high incidence (20–30 per cent) of recurrent ulceration after V+D for duodenal ulcer in patients who had high levels of MAO before operation. They suggested that vagotomy without gastric resection was inadequate surgical therapy for such hypersecretors and that an antrectomy was needed in addition. We have found, however, that after HSV the over-all clinical results were as good and abdominal pain no more frequent in patients who secreted more than 50 mEq of HCl/hour before operation than in patients whose MAO before operation was less than 50 mEq/hour (Johnston et al., 1975). Thus so far no evidence has been found that the addition of antrectomy is necessary in hypersecretors. HSV alone seems to be sufficient provided that the incidence of incomplete vagotomy can be kept low.

Over-all clinical results

Two years after HSV/PCV, 88 per cent of patients in Leeds and Copenhagen were judged to have achieved either an excellent or a very good clinical result (Visick grades 1 and 2; Amdrup et al., 1974). When patients were assessed in an identical manner after truncal or selective vagotomy with a drainage procedure in Leeds, only 68–70 per cent were found to be in Visick grades 1 and 2 (Goligher et al., 1968a, b, 1972). We wondered whether this 20 per cent superiority of HSV over V+D was due to the operation itself, to the surgeon performing the operation, or to the insulin-test status of the patient 1 week after operation. The answer was that to a large extent it was the HSV which was responsible for the difference, although elimination of positive insulin tests improved the results after V+D from 69 per cent good-to-excellent to about 75 per cent good-to-excellent. The superiority of HSV over V+D was attributable in large measure to the reduction in side-effects such as dumping, diarrhoea and bilious vomiting, with the result that relatively few patients were in Visick grade 3, the 'fair' or 'moderate' category, after HSV. Six per cent of patients were graded Visick 3, and 6 per cent Visick 4 (which indicates failure). The reasons for failure were gastric ulceration, which occurred in 2 patients in Copenhagen, suspected recurrent ulceration, and finally complaints of a wide variety of symptoms by 2 patients who seemed to be of a rather neurotic temperament and in whom thorough investigation revealed no abnormality. Similar encouraging results after HSV have been reported by De Miguel (1972), Hedenstedt et al. (1972), Imperati et al. (1972), Grassi et al. (1973), Liavag and Roland (1973) and Liedberg and Oscarson (1973). Discouraging reports have come from Wastell et al. (1972) and from Kronborg and Madsen (1975), who report both a high incidence of incomplete vagotomy and a high incidence of recurrent ulceration.

The preliminary results of prospective random trials are in agreement with these findings. In the trial by Kennedy et al. (personal communication, 1975), HSV gave better results than SV + GJ. In Kronborg and Madsen's trial (1975), HSV did not yield better over-all results than SV + P; however, *all* their HSV patients who had *negative insulin tests* 1 week after HSV achieved good-to-excellent results, and if the results of patients who had positive insulin tests 1 week after operation were excluded, the results after HSV were considerably better than the results after SV + P. In both these trials, the superiority of HSV over V + D was attributable to the significantly lower incidence of side-effects.

4. Long-term sequelae

When patients are followed up for 15–20 years after TV + GJ, weight loss, iron-deficiency anaemia, and in some centres even tuberculosis, are found to be common (Wheldon et al., 1970). Weight loss and iron-deficiency anaemia have been found to be less after V + P than after V + GJ (Wastell, 1974). Anaemia and loss of weight are of course well known sequelae of partial gastrectomy (PG), which in addition may give rise to bone disease (either osteoporosis or osteomalacia) and to carcinoma of the gastric stump. The latter is about six times as common in patients 25 years after PG as in controls who have not undergone gastrectomy (Stalsberg and Taksdal, 1971).

Since HSV has been in use for only 6 years, not enough time has elapsed for long-term problems to appear. Because it is more conservative than the standard operations, however, weight loss and anaemia should be no worse in the long term after HSV than after V + D, and might well be less common. Our finding that faecal fat excretion is significantly greater after V + D than after HSV (Edwards et al., 1974) suggests that absorption not only of fat, but of minerals and vitamins also, will be more efficient after HSV than after V + D. Since capacity for meals after HSV is at least as great as after V + D, we predict that weight loss and iron-deficiency anaemia will be less common in the long term after HSV than after V + D. Preliminary studies of body weight after the three types of vagotomy in Leeds (Bradley et al., 1975 unpublished) provide some support for this view, because after both TV and SV with a drainage procedure body weight did not change significantly compared with pre-operative body weight, whereas after HSV body weight increased significantly.

The choice of operation for duodenal ulcer

Let me try to sum up. We have seen that 'milling' of food and gastric emptying of solids are controlled by the terminal antrum, and that the pylorus is a true sphincter which helps to control gastric emptying and probably also to prevent reflux of bile salts into the stomach. All the standard operations destroy or bypass this sphincteric mechanism at the exit of the stomach and so produce side-effects. The crucial new finding has been that vagal release of gastrin is relatively unimportant in man, because gastrin levels have been found to be no higher after

HSV than after truncal vagotomy. Hence there seems to be no reason to dener-
vate the gastric antrum. A pyloroplasty or gastroenterostomy is performed merely
to permit the vagotomized stomach to empty, but since the stomach empties perfectly well after HSV without the assistance of a drainage procedure, why should
one be used? Thus the experimental evidence at the moment suggests that for
the first time in the long history of gastric surgery, the principal functions of the
stomach—those of a 'hopper' to receive the meal and of a 'mill' to grind it into
chyme—can, in the main, be preserved; that drainage procedures can be discarded and that side-effects of gastric surgery such as early dumping, diarrhoea
and bilious vomiting are now largely preventable.

So much for theory. In clinical practice, too, I think that HSV is at present
the operation of choice for duodenal ulcer. It is safer than any of the 'standard'
operations, produces significantly fewer side-effects and in the long term will
certainly cause less metabolic upset than V+A or PG, and will probably lead
to less disturbance than V+D also. The main imponderable is still the incidence
of recurrent ulceration after HSV, but that too is rapidly being defined. Apart
from the four determinants of success or failure already mentioned, a fifth factor
should be taken into consideration, and that is the number of options which are
left open if the first operation should fail. Here again HSV possesses advantages,
because after HSV any one of the standard operations can still be used on the
second occasion, whereas after V+A, for example, the options left are fewer.
In conclusion, I would suggest that, because HSV is more conservative than the
other operations and because it has yielded excellent clinical results for up to
$6\frac{1}{2}$ years, it should be the operation of choice for duodenal ulcer. I think that
HSV should be used until some other procedure is shown to be significantly
better, after due consideration has been given to the five factors of operative mortality, side-effects, recurrent ulceration, long-term sequelae and the strategy of
the second operation.

Question and answer session

Q. Don't you think it is rather dangerous to advocate the widespread use
of HSV at this stage? The results may be good in specialized centres, but
elsewhere they might prove disastrous!

A. Although initially Professor Goligher and I performed nearly all the HSVs
in Leeds, the registrars and lecturers now do many of them, without much
difficulty, and their insulin test results are satisfactory. HSV is not a particularly difficult operation and is well within the competence of any
general surgeon who does a good deal of gastric surgery. Obviously, he
should begin with thin patients and he should preferably learn at first-
hand from someone who is familiar with the technique. I cannot over-
emphasize the importance of making sure that the vagotomy of the
parietal cell mass is complete, which in essence is a matter of taking
enough time to clear all fibres from at least 5 cm of the distal oesophagus.

Q. How long does the operation take? Surely the game is hardly worth the
candle in obese patients?

A. Sixty to 90 minutes. Obese patients presumably need their gastric reservoir and antral 'mill' just as much as thin patients. I have never excluded

patients on the grounds of obesity. You need a long incision, good retraction (especially of the rib cage) and a modicum of perseverance. Many such cases are technically easy, particularly if the costal angle is wide.

Q. Which elective cases are unsuitable for HSV?

A. The aged and/or the decrepit. In general, patients over 70 years of age and those in cardiac or respiratory failure are excluded. About 2 per cent of my elective cases are excluded on these grounds. I then use the quicker method of truncal vagotomy with a drainage procedure.

Q. How did you treat your 2 cases of recurrent ulceration after HSV?

A. Conservatively, because both were elderly, not very fit and neither had severe pain. Such patients should have serum gastrin determinations to exclude the possibility of Zollinger–Ellison syndrome (ZES) and an insulin/pentagastrin test to find out if the vagotomy is grossly incomplete. At re-operation, I would do an antrectomy, preferably with a Billroth I link-up, plus a (truncal) re-vagotomy provided that access to the oesophagus was not too difficult. If the insulin test was strongly positive and re-vagotomy proved impossible, I would do a Polya partial gastrectomy.

Gastric ulcer

The aetiology of gastric ulcer remains obscure. Admittedly, anything which produces gastric stasis—such as vagotomy or pyloric stenosis—tends to lead to gastric ulceration, but to admit that stasis produces ulcers is not to admit that ulcers are due to stasis! Indeed, very few of our patients with gastric ulceration have demonstrable gastric stasis. The classic Dragstedt theory (1956), which incriminates antral stasis, excessive release of gastrin and hypersecretion of acid, is not convincing; because stasis is often absent, secretion of acid is usually normal or low and high gastrin levels may merely be secondary to high intragastric pH. Even after allowance is made for back-diffusion of hydrogen ions (Davenport, 1968), hypersecretion of acid and pepsin is hardly likely to be the sole aetiological factor. The contending theory (du Plessis, 1965; Capper, 1967), that bile reflux breaks the mucus barrier and facilitates acid–pepsin attack, seems more convincing, but cannot be the full explanation either, because gastric ulcers are rare in the vicinity of a gastroenterostomy stoma, where there is no lack of bile. Probably there is no single cause. Acid and pepsin are certainly important contributory factors, first because where there is no acid there is no peptic ulcer, and secondly because acid has been shown to potentiate the harmful effects of alcohol, aspirin and bile on the gastric mucosa (Davenport, 1969; Menguy and Max, 1970).

Although V+P has been shown to bring about the healing of the majority of benign gastric ulcers (Forrest, 1969), Billroth I gastrectomy remains the treatment of choice for most patients. Patients with gastric ulcer have acid outputs which are within the normal range, but vagotomy presumably leads to healing of the ulcer by reducing the outputs of acid and pepsin. The incidence of recurrent ulceration is higher after vagotomy (2–20 per cent) than after gastrectomy (2–5 per cent; Forrest, 1969). In a prospective controlled trial of vagotomy with pyloroplasty versus Billroth I gastrectomy for gastric ulcer, Duthie and Kwong (1973) found that gastrectomy gave better over-all results than did vagotomy.

Recurrent ulceration was found in 4 per cent of patients after gastrectomy, compared with 10 per cent after vagotomy. Seventy-eight per cent of patients obtained a good clinical result (Visick grades 1 and 2) after gastrectomy, compared with 68 per cent after vagotomy. Thus, at present, Billroth I gastrectomy remains the treatment of choice. The fact that between 2 and 20 per cent of gastric ulcers which were thought to be benign before operation eventually are shown histologically to be malignant (Forrest, 1969) lends further weight to the argument in favour of gastrectomy and against vagotomy. The prognosis after gastrectomy of patients with such occult ulcer-cancers is much better than that of patients with other types of gastric cancer (Brown et al., 1961), and to deny them a chance of cure by using vagotomy is indeed a tragic error. If vagotomy is used in the treatment of gastric ulcer, it is essential that four-quadrant biopsies be taken from the epithelial margin of the ulcer, and if possible the entire epithelial margin of the ulcer should be excised and submitted immediately to frozen-section examination by an experienced pathologist.

The gastric ulcer that is situated high on the lesser curve presents a difficult problem because gastrectomy may carry a significant mortality and morbidity. Clarke et al. (1972a) treated 21 such ulcers by vagotomy and pyloroplasty, with no deaths, and only 1 patient subsequently developed a recurrent ulcer. These authors concluded that for the high and difficult gastric ulcer and for the bleeding gastric ulcer, vagotomy and pyloroplasty was an acceptable alternative to partial gastrectomy. Another alternative is to use the Kelling–Madlener procedure, a distal gastric resection in which the ulcer is left in situ. This, too, nearly always leads to healing of the ulcer provided that it is benign. In another study (Kennedy et al., 1972), a recurrence rate of 13 per cent was found in 33 patients whose lesser curve gastric ulcer had been treated by vagotomy with a drainage procedure.

We have used HSV in the treatment of benign gastric ulceration for the past 7 years. Of 55 patients who have been treated by HSV, 35 had gastric ulcer alone and 20 combined gastric and duodenal ulceration. The series is not quite consecutive because a few patients were excluded on account of anticipated technical difficulties, suspicion that the ulcer was malignant, or because of the patient's poor general condition (Johnston et al., 1972b). Great care was taken to ensure that only patients with benign ulcers were treated in this way. For final confirmation that the ulcer was benign at the time of operation, a gastrotomy was performed along the greater curvature and the ulcer was excised, usually in toto, and submitted to immediate frozen-section examination by an experienced pathologist. In the few cases where the ulcer was close to the pylorus, or very large or inaccessible, large biopsies were taken but the whole ulcer was not excised. In none of these 55 cases was carcinoma diagnosed by the pathologist, either on frozen-section examination or after study of the paraffin sections.

There was 1 operative death after HSV. Gastric secretory testing more than 1 year after operation showed that most of the patients had basal achlorhydria, that the maximal response to pentagastrin had been reduced by 80 per cent and that there was virtually no response either to insulin or to a test meal of meat extract (M. J. Greenall, 1975, unpublished). Follow-up barium meal examinations in 35 patients revealed no evidence of gastric stasis or of recurrent ulceration. Thus HSV may provide effective treatment for gastric ulceration, both by greatly reducing acid and pepsin secretion and perhaps by speeding up gastric emptying of liquids, and thus counteracting any pre-existing tendency to gastric stasis. The over-all results to date have been moderately encouraging. The clinical results in patients with combined gastric and duodenal ulcer are similar to those of patients who have undergone HSV for duodenal ulcer (90 per cent Visick grades 1 and 2). Of the patients who underwent HSV for gastric ulcer alone, 76 per cent are in Visick grades 1 or 2 (excellent-to-good), a result which is far from brilliant, but which is almost identical to that which is found after Billroth I gastrectomy for gastric ulcer in Leeds. Good clinical results after HSV for gastric ulcer have also been reported by Hedenstedt (1973) and Hedenstedt and Moberg (1974) and by Burge (1975, personal communication). For these reasons, we have begun a controlled prospective random trial of HSV versus PG for gastric ulcer.

Perforation

Perforated duodenal ulcer

Treatment may be operative or non-operative. Operative treatment can either be definitive, to cure the ulcer, or may merely take the form of simple suture of the perforation.

Conservative or non-operative treatment by means of 'suck, drip and anti-biotics' (Taylor, 1957; Elliott and Lane, 1959) is reserved for the small minority of patients who are unfit for operation because of advanced age, chronic cardio-respiratory insufficiency or shock due to long delay between perforation and the inception of treatment. The diagnosis must not be in doubt, because the results of conservative treatment for perforation of other viscera such as the colon are not good. Conservative treatment may also be indicated when surgical or anaes-thetic services are not available; on board ship, for example, or in remote parts of the world.

Operative treatment is indicated for about 95 per cent of patients. Most patients in Britain arrive in hospital within a few hours of perforating and need little pre-operative treatment apart from the administration of morphine and aspiration of the gastric contents. Others are shocked and require the intravenous infusion of several litres of water, electrolytes and either plasma or dextran.

Simple suture of the perforation, without vagotomy, should be used in patients who have no previous history of epigastric pain, or else only a brief history of pain. Simple suture may also be used in very ill, elderly patients, but such patients probably do better with non-operative treatment. Simple suture should also be used if the surgeon is inexperienced. *Definitive* treatment in the form of HSV, TV+P or TV+GJ should be used if the patient has a long (more than 1 year) history of ulcer or if he has previously perforated or bled from his ulcer, because if the perforation is merely sutured he is very likely to develop recurrent trouble. Such definitive treatment of active, chronic ulcer is little—if any—more risky than simple suture. Jordan et al. (1974), for example, performed 535 emer-gency partial gastrectomies (with or without vagotomy) for perforated peptic ulcer with an operative mortality of only 2·2 per cent, while many years earlier Lowdon (1952) reported that 51 selected patients out of a total of only 65 with perforation had been treated by partial gastrectomy without mortality. With proper selection of cases, the operative mortality of V + P or V + GJ for perforation should be less than 1 per cent (Hamilton and Harbrecht, 1967; Khan and Ralston, 1970). I use HSV plus suture of the perforation in favourable cases (Johnston et al., 1973c): that is, in patients who have perforated less than 12 hours previously, who are not shocked, are less than 60 years of age, and have no history of cardiac or respiratory illness. Twelve patients treated in this way in the past 5 years have achieved clinical results which are similar to those of patients treated electively by HSV for duodenal ulcer.

In summary, there is no single correct method for the treatment of a patient with perforated duodenal ulcer. The method which is chosen will depend upon the patient (how old? how fit? how fat? how long perforated?), the ulcer (how chronic?) and, not least, the surgeon (how experienced?).

Perforated gastric ulcer

The over-all mortality of perforated gastric ulcer ranges from 20 to 40 per cent (Taylor, 1957; Gall and Talbot, 1964; Rees and Thorbjarnarson, 1973), compared with 3–10 per cent for perforated duodenal ulcer. The high mortality is due to a variety of factors, such as the advanced age and poor general condition of many of the patients, the large size of the perforation, gross contamination of the peritoneal cavity with food and bacteria, haemorrhage from the ulcer, carcinoma in a few of the ulcers, and so on.

The results of conservative management are poor (Gall and Talbot, 1964) and operative treatment is advisable. It is difficult to be dogmatic about the type of operation which should be performed, because this once again depends upon the patient, the ulcer and the surgeon. For example, it would be unwise for an inexperienced registrar to attempt to perform a high gastrectomy in an aged and decrepit patient. Simple suture of the perforation is indicated if the ulcer is 'acute' rather than chronic or if the patient is desperately ill. Definitive treatment, usually in the form of a partial gastrectomy, is indicated for perforation accompanied by haemorrhage, for large perforated ulcers and for perforated ulcer–cancer. Suture of the perforation, plus biopsy of the ulcer and truncal vagotomy and gastroenterostomy should be used in selected cases: for example, in elderly, unfit patients with perforation of a chronic ulcer high up in the stomach, resection of which would be hazardous.

Haemorrhage

I will confine my remarks to the subjects of bleeding from chronic peptic ulcer and from acute gastric erosions. In Britain, about 30,000–40,000 patients per annum are admitted to hospital with acute upper gastrointestinal haemorrhage and 3,000–6,000 of them die (Forrest and Finlayson, 1974). Chronic peptic ulcer is the source of bleeding in about 50 per cent of these patients, and acute erosions in from 10 to 35 per cent.

The first essential is to replace as quickly as possible the blood which has been lost. At least 4 units of blood should then be held in the blood bank in case bleeding recurs. The patient should be watched carefully both by a physician and by a surgeon, who should visit him several times a day. His pulse, blood pressure, urine output, haematocrit and, ideally, central venous pressure should be measured at frequent intervals.

The source of the bleeding should be pinpointed within a few hours of the patient's admission to hospital, by means of oesophago-gastro-duodenoscopy (OGD), supplemented if necessary by barium meal examination. The history alone may be misleading. For example, many patients with cirrhosis of the liver bleed not from varices but from chronic peptic ulcer or gastric erosions, while patients who are known to have a peptic ulcer may not be bleeding from that ulcer. Occasionally, if the patient is bleeding actively and neither OGD nor the barium meal demonstrates a lesion, angiography may be used, not only to reveal the source of haemorrhage but also on occasion to permit the local infusion of vasopressin, which may lead to cessation of the bleeding, temporarily at least.

The timing of surgical intervention is vital. Transfusion of more than 10 units of blood within 24 hours is associated with a high mortality. Thus, if bleeding from a chronic peptic ulcer or from acute erosions does not stop, an operation should be performed long before 10 units of blood have been transfused. Again, patients over the age of 55 whose bleeding stops and then begins again should usually undergo operation. Indeed, in an elderly patient who is bleeding from a chronic ulcer, there is much to be said for early operative intervention after the initial resuscitation by blood transfusion, without waiting for the onset of a further episode of bleeding. Haemorrhage from a gastric ulcer carries a greater risk to life than haemorrhage from a duodenal ulcer and is usually an indication for early surgical intervention, whatever the patient's age. Finally, haemorrhage from acute gastric erosions is associated with a high mortality (Schiller et al., 1970), which may be due in part to delay in seeking surgical aid and to the consequent transfusion of excessive amounts of 'old' bank blood. While these are exceptionally difficult cases to treat, and a conservative regimen with blood transfusion, gastric lavage with iced saline, and perhaps infusion of vasopressin should certainly be pursued initially, it seems possible that earlier surgical intervention and the avoidance of massive blood transfusion might lower the mortality.

What type of operation should be performed? For bleeding duodenal ulcer, there is now little doubt that vagotomy, pyloroplasty and under-running of the bleeding point carries a lower mortality (3–10 per cent) than does partial gastrectomy (5–20 per cent) (Smith and Farris, 1958; Carruthers et al., 1967; Schiller et al., 1970; Boulos et al., 1971). For bleeding gastric ulcer, partial gastrectomy is probably still the most commonly used procedure, but the mortality is high, ranging from 10 to 20 per cent. Other reports (Schiller et al., 1970; Hegarty et al., 1973) suggest that it is considerably safer to suture the bleeding point and to perform vagotomy with a drainage procedure. Certainly in an elderly, unfit patient with an ulcer high on the lesser curve, the latter policy has much to commend it. For acute erosions, under-running of the erosions plus vagotomy with a drainage procedure is advisable when the erosions are few in number, but for diffuse erosive gastritis, partial gastrectomy with vagotomy may be necessary. Very rarely, nothing short of total gastrectomy will arrest the haemorrhage.

That is the general strategy. Let me now describe some of the surgical manœuvres in more detail. To recapitulate, first of all blood is transfused until, ideally, the patient's skin is warm and pink, his blood pressure stable and his urinary output good. Of course, this ideal state cannot always be achieved. The source of bleeding is defined by means of endoscopy. Next, the right time is chosen at which to operate. That is often within 24 hours of the patient's admission to hospital, before the vital organs have suffered repeated episodes of anoxia and before dangerous amounts of old bank blood have been transfused. When you do operate, get in quickly through a midline epigastric incision. Do not waste time making a paramedian incision in a patient who is bleeding. Although we have talked about the treatment being V + P plus under-running of the vessel, in practice the ulcer should be exposed as the first step in the operation and the vessel in its base under-run, after which the operation is completed by V + P. In these emergency conditions, and especially if the patient is shocked, elderly or still actively bleeding, there is no doubt that the vagotomy should be truncal in type. I use truncal vagotomy in about two-thirds of my patients with bleeding peptic ulcer. However, quite often at operation the bleeding is found to have stopped. If, in addition, the patient is relatively young, slim and fit, the operative risk should be little greater than that of an elective procedure and then I think it is justifiable, and indeed desirable, to take an extra 30 minutes and perform an HSV rather than a truncal vagotomy.

Since the bleeding vessel is embedded in the fibrous base of the ulcer, a strong needle is required so that it may be under-run effectively. An O Mersilene suture mounted on an atraumatic round-bodied needle serves this purpose well.

It must be confessed that even in the best-organized departments, it can still happen that at the time of operation you do not know where the bleeding is coming from. You open the abdomen and find—nothing! What next? Do *not* perform a wide gastroduedenotomy, because this commits you to subsequent pyloroplasty and thus to the destruction of the stomach's sphincteric mechanism. Instead, using the diathermy blade, make a longitudinal gastrotomy along the greater curvature in the middle third of the stomach, taking care to coagulate the large vessels which are encountered in the submucosa. The incision should not be made in the middle of the anterior wall, because if an HSV is subsequently performed the portion of the anterior wall of the stomach between lesser curve and the gastrotomy incision might undergo necrosis. The gastrotomy should begin well below the lowermost short gastric artery and end 7 or 8 cm from the pylorus, so that the 'antral mill' is not damaged. Blood clot is evacuated from the stomach and the entire mucosal lining inspected, from oesophagus to pylorus. If an ulcer is found, its base is under-run. Then, the ulcer is excised, if it is small, and biopsied in several places if it is large. The base of such a large ulcer is then excluded from the lumen of the stomach by means of interrupted catgut sutures. If the ulcer seems likely to be malignant, it should be excised in toto by means of a partial gastrectomy, but it is somewhat unusual for a malignant ulcer to precipitate emergency surgery of this nature. If no source of bleeding is found in the stomach, I next perform a longitudinal duodenotomy, *distal* to the pylorus, and if a duodenal ulcer is found, under-run it. The duodenotomy is then sutured, as it is made, longitudinally. Edge-to-edge apposition is the aim, without inversion. Thus, the antro-pyloro-duodenal segment is left undamaged. Such tactics are of course only needed if the intention is to perform HSV. If truncal vagotomy with a drainage procedure is planned, the use of a wide gastroduodenotomy incision is perfectly in order.

Pyloric stenosis

The term 'pyloric' stenosis is a misnomer. The peptic stricture is nearly always distal to the pylorus, an important point because it means that the sphincteric mechanism in the terminal antrum and pyloric musculature is undamaged, although its function may be impaired by spasm and oedema associated with active ulceration. By no means all patients who present with copious vomiting and a succussion splash have 'permanent' fibrous stenosis of the duodenum. In many of them, effective gastric emptying returns after a period of rest in bed and gastric lavage, signifying that obstruction had been due in large measure to oedema and spasm. The stomach compensates for obstruction at its outlet by hypertrophy of its muscular wall and by hyperperistalsis, especially in the antrum. Such compensatory mechanisms are wasted by conventional surgical procedures such as truncal or selective vagotomy with drainage, which cut the parasympathetic supply to the antrum. In contrast, they are conserved and utilized by the operation of highly selective vagotomy (Johnston et al., 1973c).

When a patient is admitted to hospital with pyloric stenosis, food residues in the stomach should be removed by repeated gastric lavage, and intravenous infusions of water, salt, potassium and blood should be administered as required. Stenosis secondary to peptic ulceration should be distinguished from that due to carcinoma by means of barium meal examination, gastroscopy plus biopsy of any suspicious lesion in the antrum and by the measurement of basal and maximal (pentagastrin-stimulated) acid output. Although patients with pyloric stenosis due to peptic ulcer are often said to have low acid outputs because of gastritis, I find that they usually have the high BAO and MAO of duodenal ulceration, whereas patients with antral carcinoma usually, though not always, have low acid outputs.

Truncal vagotomy with gastroenterostomy or pyloroplasty is the standard form of surgical treatment, and it gives good results (Feggetter and Pringle, 1965; Ellis et al., 1966; De Matteis and Hermann, 1974). The Finney type of pyloroplasty has been found to 'drain' the dilated stomach effectively (De Matteis and Hermann, 1974). Vagotomy should be preferred to gastrectomy because it is safer, particularly in such an ill-nourished group of patients. Although they are good, however, the clinical results are still marred by the side-effects of complete gastric vagotomy plus a drainage procedure, with the result that only about 45 per cent of patients achieve a perfect, symptom-free, Visick grade 1, result.

Finding that gastric emptying was not delayed after HSV—and indeed that emptying of fluids was faster than normal—I began 5 years ago to use HSV in the treatment of *all* patients who had pyloric stenosis secondary to duodenal ulcer (Johnston et al., 1973c). Twenty-two patients have now been treated in this way. Two important technical points should be mentioned. The first is that gastric emptying will depend upon the propulsive power of the gastric antrum. Since the stomach is usually dilated, more than the normal 6 or 7 cm of distal stomach should be left innervated, the exact length depending upon the degree of gastric dilatation and upon the configuration of the terminations of the nerves of Latarjet. As a rough guide, however, between 7 and 10 cm of distal stomach should be left innervated. The second point is that the stenotic segment must be dilated. For this purpose, a small gastrotomy is made in the *denervated* portion of the stomach, the right index finger is introduced and its tip used slowly and gently to dilate the stenosis until the whole finger can be passed round into the second part of the duodenum. Passage of the proximal interphalangeal joint through the stenosis implies that the lumen will take a 14 or 16 Hegar's dilator. During the dilatation, unyielding fibrous tissue is felt to rupture and occasionally a perforation of the duodenum results, just distal to the pyloric ring. This is no cause for alarm, and all that is needed is to close the perforation carefully with two or three interrupted 2–0 catgut sutures, and perhaps to reinforce the closure with a tag of omentum. The terminal antrum and pylorus have never, in my experience, been ruptured. Hence, after operation, the patient with pyloric stenosis reaps the same benefit as do the patients with uncomplicated duodenal ulceration. Of the patients we have treated in this way, 75 per cent have no side-effects whatsoever; that is, they are in Visick grade 1. Only 2 of them developed re-stenosis as the ulcer healed and both of these patients have now obtained excellent clinical results after the addition of a drainage procedure. Many of these patients had a severe degree of pyloric stenosis. These results bear witness to the remarkable propulsive power of the gastric antrum, which by expelling food through the duodenum presumably gently dilates it so that re-stenosis seldom takes place. This method may therefore be worthy of further cautious trial, by surgeons who have extensive experience of HSV for uncomplicated duodenal ulcer, and in patients who, being relatively young and fit, could readily withstand a second operation to establish gastric drainage if the first operation should fail.

References

ALEXANDER-WILLIAMS J., DONOVAN I. A., GUNN I. F., BROWN A. and HARDING L. K. (1973) The effect of vagotomy on gastric emptying. *Proc. R. Soc. Med.* **66,** 1102–1103.

AMDRUP B. M. and GRIFFITH C. A. (1969a) Selective vagotomy of the parietal cell mass: Part I: with preservation of the innervated antrum and pylorus. *Ann. Surg.* **170,** 207–214.

AMDRUP B. M. and GRIFFITH C. A. (1969b) Selective vagotomy of the parietal cell mass: Part II: with suprapyloric mucosal antrectomy and suprapyloric antral resection. *Ann. Surg.* **170,** 215–220.

AMDRUP E. and JENSEN H.-E. (1970) Selective vagotomy of the parietal cell mass preserving innervation of the undrained antrum. *Gastroenterology* **59,** 522–527.

AMDRUP E. and JOHNSTON D. (1975) Name of the new vagotomy. *Gastroenterology* **68,** 206–207.

AMDRUP B. M., STEINØE K. and BILLE-BRAHE N. E. (1971) An experimental study of the incidence of gastric ulcers in rabbits following truncal vagotomy, selective gastric vagotomy, and highly selective gastric vagotomy. *Acta Chir. Scand.* **137,** 794–796.

AMDRUP E., JENSEN H.-E., JOHNSTON D., WALKER B. E. and GOLIGHER J. C. (1974) Clinical results of parietal cell vagotomy (highly selective vagotomy) two to four years after operation. *Ann. Surg.* **180,** 279–284.

BALDWIN J. N., HEER F. W., ALBO R., PELOSO O., RUBY L. and SILEN W. (1966) Effect of vagus nerve stimulation on hepatic secretion of bile in human subjects. *Am. J. Surg.* **111,** 66–69.

BARLOW T. E., BENTLEY F. H. and WALDER D. N. (1951) Arteries, veins and arteriovenous anastomoses in the human stomach. *Surg. Gynecol. Obstet.* **93,** 657–671.

BOULOS P. B., HARRIS J., WYLLIE J. H. and CLARK C. G. (1971) Conservative surgery in 100 patients with bleeding peptic ulcer. *Br. J. Surg.* **58,** 817–819.

BROWN P. M., CAINE J. C. and DOCKERTY M. B. (1961) Clinically 'benign' gastric ulcer found to be malignant at operation. *Surg. Gynecol. Obstet.* **112,** 82–88.

BURGE H. (1964) *Vagotomy.* London, Edward Arnold.

BURGE H. and FROHN M. J. N. (1969) The technique of bilateral selective vagotomy with the electrical stimulation test. *Br. J. Surg.* **56,** 452–460.

BURGE H., MACLEAN C., STEDEFORD R., PINN G. and HOLLANDERS D. (1969) Selective vagotomy without drainage. An interim report. *Br. Med. J.* **3,** 690–693.

BURSTALL P. A. and SCHOFIELD B. (1953) Secretory effects of psychic stimulation and insulin hypoglycaemia on Heidenhain gastric pouches in dogs. *J. Physiol. (Lond.)* **120,** 383–408.

BURSTALL P. A. and SCHOFIELD B. (1954) The effects of pyloric antrectomy on the secretory response of Heidenhain pouches in dogs to central vagal stimulation. *J. Physiol. (Lond.)* **123,** 168–186.

BUSHKIN F. L., WICKBORN G., DEFORD J. W. and WOODWARD E. R. (1974) Post-operative alkaline reflux gastritis. *Surg. Gynecol. Obstet.* **138,** 933–939.

CANNON W. B. (1898) The movements of the stomach studied by means of the Röntgen rays. *Am. J. Physiol.* **1,** 359–382.

CAPPER W. M. (1967) Factors in the pathogenesis of gastric ulcer. *Ann. R. Coll. Surg. Engl.* **40,** 21–35.

CARLSON H. C., CODE C. F. and NELSON R. A. (1966) Motor action of the canine gastro-duodenal junction: a cineradiographic, pressure and electric study. *Am. J. Dig. Dis.* **11,** 155–172.

CARRUTHERS R. K., GILES G. R., CLARK C. G. and GOLIGHER J. C. (1967) Conservative surgery for bleeding peptic ulcer. *Br. Med. J.* **1,** 80–82.

CLARKE R. J. and ALEXANDER-WILLIAMS J. (1973) The effect of preserving antral innervation and of a pyloroplasty on gastric emptying after vagotomy in man. *Gut* **14,** 300–307.

CLARKE R. J., LEWIS D. L. and WILLIAMS J. A. (1972a) Vagotomy and pyloroplasty for gastric ulcer. *Br. Med. J.* **2,** 369–371.

CLARKE R. J., MCFARLAND J. B. and WILLIAMS J. A. (1972b) Gastric stasis and gastric ulcer after selective vagotomy without a drainage procedure. *Br. Med. J.* **1,** 538–539.

CLAVE R. A. and GASPAR M. R. (1969) Incidence of gallbladder disease after vagotomy. *Am. J. Surg.* **118,** 169–176.

COBB J. S., BANK S. and MARKS I. N. (1971) Gastric emptying after vagotomy and pyloroplasty. Relation to some post-operative sequelae. *Am. J. Dig. Dis.* **16,** 207–215.

COLMER M. R., OWEN G. M. and SHIELDS R. (1973) Pattern of gastric emptying after vagotomy and pyloroplasty. *Br. Med. J.* **2,** 448–450.

COWIE A. G. A. and CLARK C. G. (1972) The lithogenic effect of vagotomy. *Br. J. Surg.* **59,** 365–367.

COX A. G. (1968) Comparison of symptoms after vagotomy with gastrojejunostomy and partial gastrectomy. *Br. Med. J.* **1,** 288–290.

COX A. G., BOND M. R., PODMORE D. A. and ROSE D. P. (1964) Aspects of nutrition after vagotomy and gastrojejunostomy. *Br. Med. J.* **1,** 465–469.

COX A. G., SPENCER J. and TINKER J. (1969) Clinical results reviewed. In: WILLIAMS J. A. and COX A. G. (ed.), *After Vagotomy.* London, Butterworths.

DAVENPORT H. W. (1968) Destruction of the gastric mucosal barrier by detergents and urea. *Gastroenterology* **54,** 175–181.

DAVENPORT H. W. (1969) Gastric mucosal haemorrhage in dogs. Effects of acid, aspirin and alcohol. *Gastroenterology* **56,** 439–449.

DAVIS M., GUPTA S. and ELDER J. B. (1973) The effect of vagotomy on the exocrine pancreatic secretory response to pentagastrin and to a meat meal in dogs. *Br. J. Surg.* **60,** 318.

DE MATTEIS R. A. and HERMANN R. E. (1947) Vagotomy and drainage for obstructing duodenal ulcers. Importance of adequate drainage. *Am. J. Surg.* **127,** 237–240.

DE MIGUEL J. (1972) Vagatomia gastrica proximal sin drenaje por ulcera peptica: ulteriores observaciones. *Gac. Méd. N.* **24,** 238–244.

DEVINE H. B. (1925) Basic principles and supreme difficulties in gastric surgery. *Surg. Gynecol. Obstet.* **40,** 1–16.

DRAGSTEDT L. R. (1956) A concept of the etiology of gastric and duodenal ulcers. *Gastroenterology* **30,** 208–214.

DRAGSTEDT L. R. and OWENS F. M. JR (1943) Supradiaphragmatic section of the vagus nerves to the stomach in the treatment of duodenal ulcer. *Proc. Soc. Exp. Biol. Med.* **53,** 152–154.

DREILING D. A., DRUCKERMAN L. J. and HOLLANDER F. (1952) The effect of complete vagisection and vagal stimulation on pancreatic secretion in man. *Gastroenterology* **20,** 578–586.

DU PLESSIS D. J. (1965) Pathogenesis of gastric ulceration. *Lancet* **1,** 974–978.

DUTHIE H. L. and KWONG N. K. (1973) Vagotomy or gastrectomy for gastric ulcer. *Br. Med. J.* **4,** 79–81.

EDWARDS J. P., LYNDON P. J., SMITH R. B. and JOHNSTON D. (1974) Faecal fat excretion after truncal, selective and highly selective vagotomy for duodenal ulcer. *Gut* **15,** 521–525.

EISELSBERG A. (1920) Zur behandlung des Ulcus ventriculi et duodeni. *(Langenbeck's) Arch. Klin. Chir.* **114,** 539–544.

ELLIOTT J. L. and LANE J. D. (1959) Perforated peptic ulcer treated by the non-operative method. *Am. J. Dig. Dis.* **4,** 950–958.

ELLIS H., STARER F., VENABLES C. and WARE C. (1966) Clinical and radiological study of vagotomy and gastric drainage in the treatment of pyloric stenosis due to duodenal ulceration. *Gut* **7,** 671–676.

FAWCETT A. N., JOHNSTON D. and DUTHIE H. L. (1969) Revagotomy for recurrent ulcer after vagotomy and drainage for duodenal ulcer. *Br. J. Surg.* **56,** 111–116.

FEGGETTER G. Y. and PRINGLE R. (1965) The relationship between the severity of duodenal ulceration and the results of bilateral vagotomy and gastrojejunostomy. *Br. J. Surg.* **52,** 691–693.

FERGUSON D. J., BILLINGS H., SWENSON D. and HOOVER G. (1960) Segmental gastrectomy with innervated antrum for duodenal ulcer. Results at one to five years. *Surgery* **47,** 548–556.

FISHER R. and COHEN S. (1973) Physiological characteristics of the human pyloric sphincter. *Gastroenterology* **64,** 67–75.

FLETCHER D. M. and CLARK C. G. (1969) Changes in canine bile-flow and composition after vagotomy. *Br. J. Surg.* **56,** 103–106.

FLYNN P. J. and LONGMIRE W. P. JR (1960) Subtotal gastrectomy with pyloric sphincter preservation. *Surg. Forum* **10,** 185–188.

FORREST A. P. M. (1956) The importance of the innervation of the pyloric antrum in the control of gastric secretion in dogs. *20th Int. Congr. Physiol. Abstract of Communications,* pp. 299–300. Brussels, Office Internationale de Librairie.

FORREST A. P. M. (1969) Gastric ulcer. In: WILLIAMS J. A. and COX A. G. (ed.), *After Vagotomy.* London, Butterworths, pp. 344–370.

FORREST J. A. H. and FINLAYSON N. D. C. (1974) The investigation of acute upper gastrointestinal haemorrhage. *Br. J. Hosp. Med.* **12,** 160–165.

FRIESEN S. R. and RIEGER E. (1960) A study of the role of the pylorus in the prevention of the 'dumping syndrome'. *Ann. Surg.* **151,** 517–529.

FRITZ M. E. and BROOKS F. P. (1963) Control of bile flow in the cholecystectomized dog. *Am. J. Physiol.* **204,** 825–828.

GALL W. J. and TALBOT C. H. (1964) Perforated gastric ulcer. *Br. J. Surg.* **51,** 500–503.

GAMBLE W. S. (1970) Impaired pancreozymin secretion after vagotomy and pyloroplasty. *J. Lab. Clin. Med.* **76,** 871.

GILLESPIE I. E. (1959) Influence of antral pH on gastric acid secretion in man. *Gastroenterology* **37,** 164–168.

GLANVILLE J. N. and DUTHIE H. L. (1964) Contraction of the gall bladder before and after total abdominal vagotomy. *Clin. Radiol.* **15,** 350–354.

GOLIGHER J. C., PULVERTAFT C. N., DE DOMBALS F. T., CONYERS J. H., DUTHIE H. L., FEATHER D. B., LATCHMORE A. J. C., SHOESMITH J. H., SMIDDY F. G.and WILLSON-PEPPER J. (1968a) Five- to eight-year results of Leeds/York controlled trial of elective surgery for duodenal ulcer. *Br. Med. J.* **2,** 781–787.

GOLIGHER J. C., PULVERTAFT C. N., DE DOMBALS F. T., CLARK C. G., CONYERS J. H., DUTHIE H. L., FEATHER D. B., LATCHMORE A. J. C., MATHESON T. S., SHOESMITH J. H., SMIDDY F. G. and WILLSON-PEPPER J. (1968b) Clinical comparison of vagotomy and pyloroplasty with other forms of elective surgery for duodenal ulcer. *Br. Med. J.* **2,** 787–789.

GOLIGHER, J. C., PULVERTAFT C. N., IRVIN T. T., JOHNSTON D., WALKER B., HALL R. A., WILLSON-PEPPER J.and MATHESON T. S. (1972) Five- to eight-year results of truncal vagotomy and pyloroplasty for duodenal ulcer. *Br. Med. J.* **1,** 7–13.

GRASSI G. (1971) A new test for complete nerve section during vagotomy. *Br. J. Surg.* **58,** 187–189.

GRASSI G., ORECCHIA C., SPUELZ B. and GRASSI G. B. (1973) Early results of the treatment of duodenal ulcer by ultra selective vagotomy without drainage. *Surg. Gynecol. Obstet.* **136,** 726–728.

GREENALL M. J., LYNDON P. J., GOLIGHER J. C. and JOHNSTON D. (1975) Long term effects of highly selective vagotomy on basal and maximal acid output in man. *Gastroenterology* **68,** 1421–1425.

GRIFFITH C. A. (1969) Significant functions of the hepatic and coeliac vagi. *Amer. J. Surg.* **118,** 251–259.

GRIFFITH C. A. and HARKINS H. N. (1957) Partial gastric vagotomy: an experimental study. *Gastroenterology* **32,** 96–102.

HAMILTON J. E. and HARBRECHT P. J. (1967) Growing indications for vagotomy in perforated peptic ulcer. *Surg. Gynecol. Obstet.* **124,** 61–64.

HANSKY J., KORMAN M. G., COWLEY D. J. and BARON J. H. (1971) Serum gastrin in duodenal ulcer: II. Effect of insulin hypoglycaemia. *Gut* **12,** 959–962.

HANSKY J. and KORMAN M. G. (1973) Immunoassay studies in peptic ulcer. In: SIRCUS W. (ed.) *Clinics in Gastroenterology: Vol. 2, Peptic Ulceration.* New York and London, Saunders, pp. 275–291.

HANSKY J., SOVENY C. and KORMAN M. G. (1972) Role of the vagus in insulin-mediated gastrin release. *Gastroenterology* **63,** 387–391.

HART W. (1966) Neue physiologische und anatomische Gesichtspunkte zur Frage der vagalen Innervation des Magen-Antrums und ihre Bedeutung für die Magenchirurgie. *Z. Gastroenterol..* **4,** 324–337.

HART W. (1968) Neue Erkenntnisse zur physiologischen und chirurgischen Bedeutung des Magenantrums. *(Langenbeck's) Arch. Klin. Chir.* **322,** 703–708.

HEDENSTEDT S. (1973) Treatment of benign gastric ulcer by selective proximal vagotomy (SPV) without drainage. *Scand. J. Gastroenterol.* **8,** Suppl. 20, 10.

HEDENSTEDT S., LUNDQUIST G. and MOBERG S. (1972) Selective proximal vagotomy (SPV) in the treatment of duodenal ulcer. *Acta Chir. Scand.* **138,** 591–596.

HEDENSTEDT S. and MOBERG S. (1974) Gastric ulcer treated with selective proximal vagotomy (SPV): a preliminary report. *Acta Chir. Scand.* **140,** 309–312.

HEGARTY M. M., GRIME R. T. and SCHOFIELD P. F. (1973) The management of upper gastrointestinal tract haemorrhage. *Br. J. Surg.* **60,** 275–279.

HERRINGTON J. L. JR (1969) Current operations for duodenal ulcer. In: HARKINS H. N. and

NYHUS L. M. (ed.), *Surgery of the Stomach and Duodenum*, 2nd edn. Boston, Little, Brown & Co., pp. 575–603.

HERRINGTON J. L. JR (1972) Current operations for duodenal ulcer. In : RAVITCH M. M. (ed.) *Current Problems in Surgery*. Chicago, Year Book Med. Publ., pp. 1–61.

HOLLE F. and HART W. (1967) Neue Wege der Chirurgie des Gastroduodenalulcus. *Med. Klin.* **62,** 441–450.

HUMPHREY C. S., DYKES J. R. W. and JOHNSTON D. (1975) The effect of truncal, selective and highly selective vagotomy on glucose tolerance and insulin secretion in patients with chronic duodenal ulcer. I. Effect of vagotomy on response to oral glucose. II. Comparison of responses to oral and intravenous glucose. *Br. Med. J.* **2,** 112–116.

HUMPHREY C. S., JOHNSTON D., WALKER B. E., PULVERTAFT C. N. and GOLIGHER J. C. (1972) Incidence of dumping after truncal and selective vagotomy with pyloroplasty and highly selective vagotomy without drainage procedure. *Br. Med. J.* **3,** 785–788.

HUMPHREY C. S. and WILKINSON A. R. (1972) The value of preserving the pylorus in the surgery of duodenal ulcer. *Br. J. Surg.* **59,** 779–783.

IMPERATI L., NATALE C. and MARLNACCHIO F. (1972) Acid-fundic selective vagotomy of the stomach without drainage in the treatment of duodenal ulcer: technique and results. *Br. J. Surg.* **59,** 602–605.

INTERONE C. V., DEL FINADO J. E., MILLER B., BOMBECK C. T. and NYHUS L. M. (1971) Parietal cell vagotomy: studies of gastric emptying and observations of protection from histamine-induced ulcer. *Arch. Surg.* **102,** 43–44.

ISENBERG J. I. and CSENDES A. (1972) Effect of octapeptide of cholecystokinin on canine pylorus pressure. *Am. J. Physiol.* **222,** 428–431.

JAFFE B. M., CLENDINNEN B. G., CLARKE R. J. and WILLIAMS J. A. (1974) The effect of selective and proximal vagotomy on serum gastrin. *Gastroenterology* **66,** 944–953.

JANSSON G. (1969) Vaso-vagal reflex relaxation of the stomach in the cat. *Acta Physiol. Scand.* **75,** 245–252.

JEPSON K., LARI J., HUMPHREY C. S., SMITH R. B., WILKINSON A. R. and JOHNSTON D. (1973) A comparison of the effects of truncal, selective and highly selective vagotomy on maximal acid output in response to pentagastrin. *Ann. Surg.* **178,** 769–772.

JOHNSON F. E. and BOYDEN E. A. (1952) The effect of double vagotomy on the motor activity of the human gall bladder. *Surgery* **32,** 591–601.

JOHNSTON D. (1972) *Highly Selective Vagotomy*. MD Thesis, Glasgow University.

JOHNSTON D. (1975) Operative mortality and post-operative morbidity of highly selective vagotomy. *Br. J. Surg.* **62,** 160.

JOHNSTON D. and GOLIGHER J. C. (1971) The influence of the individual surgeon and of the type of vagotomy upon the insulin test after vagotomy. *Gut* **12,** 963–967.

JOHNSTON D., HUMPHREY C. S., WALKER B. E., PULVERTAFT C. N. and GOLIGHER J. C. (1972a) Vagotomy without diarrhoea. *Br. Med. J.* **3,** 788–790.

JOHNSTON D., HUMPHREY C. S., SMITH R. B. and WILKINSON A. R. (1972b) Treatment of gastric ulcer by highly selective vagotomy without a drainage procedure: an interim report. *Br. J. Surg.* **59,** 787–792.

JOHNSTON D., LYNDON P. J., SMITH R. B. and HUMPHREY C. S. (1973c) Highly selective vagotomy without a drainage procedure in the treatment of haemorrhage, perforation and pyloric stenosis due to peptic ulcer. *Br. J. Surg.* **60,** 790–797.

JOHNSTON D., PICKFORD I. R., WALKER B. E. and GOLIGHER J. C. (1975) Highly selective vagotomy for duodenal ulcer: do hypersecretors need antrectomy? *Br. Med. J.* **1,** 716–718.

JOHNSTON D., THOMAS D. G., CHECKETTS R. G. and DUTHIE H. L. (1967) An assessment of post-operative testing for completeness of vagotomy. *Br. J. Surg.* **54,** 831–833.

JOHNSTON D. and WILKINSON A. R. (1969) Selective vagotomy with innervated antrum without drainage procedure for duodenal ulcer. *Br. J. Surg.* **56,** 626.

JOHNSTON D. and WILKINSON A. R. (1970) Highly selective vagotomy without a drainage procedure in the treatment of duodenal ulcer. *Br. J. Surg.* **57,** 289–296.

JOHNSTON D., WILKINSON A. R., HUMPHREY C. S., SMITH R. B., GOLIGHER J. C., KRAGELUND E. and AMDRUP E. (1973a) Serial studies of gastric secretion in patients after highly selective (parietal cell) vagotomy without a drainage procedure for duodenal ulcer. I. Effect of highly selective vagotomy on basal and pentagastrin-stimulated maximal acid output. *Gastroenterology* **64,** 1–11.

JOHNSTON D., WILKINSON A. R., HUMPHREY C. S., SMITH R. B., GOLIGHER J. C., KRAGELUND E. and AMDRUP E. (1973b) Serial studies of gastric secretion in patients after highly selective (parietal cell) vagotomy without a drainage procedure for duodenal ulcer. II. The insulin test after highly selective vagotomy. *Gastroenterology* **64,** 12–21.

JORDAN G. L. JR, DeBAKEY M. E. and DUNCAN J. M. JR. (1974) Surgical management of perforated peptic ulcer. *Ann. Surg.* **179,** 628–633.

JORDAN P. H. (1974) A follow-up report of a prospective evaluation of vagotomy-pyloroplasty and vagotomy-antrectomy for treatment of duodenal ulcer. *Ann. Surg.* **180,** 259–264.

JORDAN P. H. and CONDON R. E. (1970) A prospective evaluation of vagotomy-pyloroplasty and vagotomy-antrectomy for treatment of duodenal ulcer. *Ann. Surg.* **172,** 547–563.

KAY A. W. (1959) The pyloric antrum and peptic ulceration. *Proc. World Congr. Gastroenterol., Washington*, 1958. Baltimore, Williams and Wilkins, p. 833–836.

KAYNAN A., BEN-ARI G., KARK A. E. and RUDICK J. (1973) Effects of parietal cell vagotomy on acid and pepsin secretion in gastric fistula dogs. *Ann. Surg.* **178,** 204–208.

KELLY K. A. and CODE C. F. (1969) Effect of transthoracic vagotomy on canine gastric electrical activity. *Gastroenterology* **57,** 51–58.

KELLY K. A., NYHUS L. M. and HARKINS H. N. (1964) The vagal nerve and the intestinal phase of gastric secretion. *Gastroenterology* **46,** 163–166.

KENNEDY T. (1973) Evaluation of selective vagotomy. In: COX A. G. and ALEXANDER-WILLIAMS J. (ed.), *Vagotomy on Trial*. London, Heinemann, p. 95.

KENNEDY T. (1974) Which vagotomy? Which drainage? *Proc. R. Soc. Med.* **67,** 3–4.

KENNEDY T. and CONNELL A. M. (1969) Selective or truncal vagotomy. *Lancet* **1,** 899–901.

KENNEDY T., CONNELL A. M., LOVE A. H. G., MACRAE K. D. and SPENCER E. F. A. (1973b) Selective or truncal vagotomy? Five-year results of a double-blind, randomized, controlled trial. *Br. J. Surg.* **60,** 944–948.

KENNEDY T., JOHNSTON G. W., LOVE A. H. G., CONNELL A. M. and SPENCER E. F. A. (1973a) Pyloroplasty versus gastrojejunostomy. Results of a double-blind, randomized, controlled trial. *Br. J. Surg.* **60,** 949–952.

KENNEDY T., KELLY J. M. and GEORGE J. D. (1972) Vagotomy for gastric ulcer. *Br. Med. J.* **2,** 371–373.

KENNEDY F., MACKAY C., BEDI B. S. and KAY A. W. (1973) Truncal vagotomy and drainage for chronic duodenal ulcer disease: a controlled trial. *Br. Med. J.* **2,** 71–75.

KHAN I. H. and RALSTON G. J. (1970) Perforated duodenal ulcer treated by vagotomy and drainage. *J. R. Coll. Surg. Edinb.* **15,** 41–44.

KILLEN D. A. and SYMBAS P. N. (1962) Effect of preservation of the pyloric sphincter during antrectomy on post-operative gastric emptying. *Am. J. Surg.* **104,** 836–842.

KIRK R. M. (1970) The size of the pyloroduodenal canal: its relation to the cause and treatment of peptic ulcer. *Proc. R. Soc. Med.* **63,** 46–48.

KLEMPA I., HOLLE F., BRÜCKNER W., WELSCH K. H., HÄNDLE H. and VON WOLFF A. (1971) The effect of selective proximal vagotomy and pyloroplasty on gastric secretion and motility in the dog. *Arch. Surg.* **103,** 713–719.

KORMAN M. G., HANSKY J., COUPLAND G. A. E. and CUMBERLAND V. H. (1973a) Gastrin studies after parietal cell vagotomy: is drainage necessary? *Digestion* **8,** 1–7.

KORMAN M. G., HANSKY J., COUPLAND G. A. E. and CUMBERLAND V. H. (1973b) Serum gastrin response to insulin hypoglycaemia : studies after parietal cell vagotomy and after selective gastric vagotomy. *Scand. J. Gastroenterol.* **8,** 235–239.

KØSTER J. and MADSEN P. (1970) The intragastric pressure before and immediately after truncal vagotomy. *Scand. J. Gastroenterol.* **5,** 381–383.

KRAFT R. O., FRY W. J., WILHELM K. G. and RANSOM M. K. (1967) Selective gastric vagotomy : a critical reappraisal. *Arch. Surg.* **95,** 625–630.

KRAFT R. O., KIRSH M. M., KITTLESON A. C., ERNST C. B., POLLARD H. M. and RANSOME H. K. (1965) Metabolic studies in patients subsequent to selective gastric vagotomy. *Surg. Gynecol. Obstet.* **120,** 472–476.

KRONBORG O. (1974) Gastric acid secretion and risk of recurrence of duodenal ulcer within 6–8 years after truncal vagotomy and drainage. *Gut* **15,** 714–719.

KRONBORG O. and MADSEN P. (1975) A controlled randomized trial of highly selective vagotomy versus selective vagotomy and pyloroplasty in the treatment of duodenal ulcer. *Gut* **16,** 268–271.

KRONBORG O., STADIL F., REHFELD J. and CHRISTIANSEN P. M. (1973) Relationship between serum gastrin concentration and gastric acid secretion in duodenal ulcer patients before and after selective and highly selective vagotomy. *Scand. J. Gastroenterol.* **8,** 491–496.

LANDOR J. H. (1964) The effect of extragastric vagotomy on Heidenhain pouch secretion in dogs. *Am. J. Dig. Dis.* **9,** 256–269.

LIAVAG I. and ROLAND M. (1973) Selective proximal vagotomy in the treatment of gastro-duodenal ulcers. *Scand. J. Gastroenterol.* **8,** Suppl. 20, 10–11.

LIEDBERG G. and OSCARSON J. (1973) Selective proximal vagotomy—short-term follow-up of 80 patients. *Scand. J. Gastroenterol.* **8,** Suppl. 20, 12.

LOWDON A. G. R. (1952) The treatment of acute perforated peptic ulcer by primary partial gastrectomy. *Lancet* **1,** 1270–1274.

LYNDON P. J., GREENALL M. J., SMITH R. B., GOLIGHER J. C. and JOHNSTON D. (1975) Serial insulin tests over a five year period after highly selective vagotomy for duodenal ulcer. *Gastroenterology* **69,** 1188–1195.

MCKELVEY S. T. D. (1970) Gastric incontinence and post-vagotomy diarrhoea. *Br. J. Surg.* **57,** 741–747.

MCKELVEY S. T. D., CONNELL A. M. and KENNEDY T. L. (1969) Gastric emptying and transit time as factors in post-vagotomy diarrhoea. *Gut* **10,** 1047.

MCKELVEY S. T. D., TONER D., CONNELL A. M. and KENNEDY T. L. (1973) Coeliac and hepatic nerve function following selective vagotomy. *Br. J. Surg.* **60,** 219–221.

MCKEOWN K. C. (1972) A prospective study of the immediate and long-term results of Polya gastrectomy for duodenal ulcer. *Br. J. Surg.* **59,** 849–868.

MADSEN P. and KRONBORG O. (1973) A double-blind trial of highly selective vagotomy without drainage and selective vagotomy with pyloroplasty in the treatment of duodenal ulcer. *Scand. J. Gastroent* **8,** Suppl. 20, 12–13.

MADSEN P., KRONBORG O. and FELDT-RASMUSSEN K. (1973) The gastric emptying and small intestinal transit after highly selective vagotomy without drainage and selective vagotomy with pyloroplasty. *Scand. J. Gastroenterol.* **8,** 541–543.

MAKI T., SHIRATORI T., HATAFUKU T. and SUGAWARA K. (1967) Pylorus-preserving gastrectomy as an improved operation for gastric ulcer. *Surgery* **61,** 838–845.

MALAGELADA J. R., GO V. L. W. and SUMMERSKILL W. H. J. (1974) Altered pancreatic and biliary function after vagotomy and pyloroplasty. *Gastroenterology* **66,** 22–27.

MASON M. C., GILES G. R., GRAHAM N. G., CLARK C. G. and GOLIGHER J. C. (1968) An early assessment of selective and total vagotomy. *Br. J. Surg.* **55,** 677–680.

MENGUY R. and MAX H. M. (1970) Influence of bile on the canine gastric mucosa. *Am. J. Surg.* **199,** 177–182.

MIDDLETON M. D., KELLY K. A., NYHUS L. M. and HARKINS H. N. (1965) Selective vagal effects on the intestinal phase of gastric secretion. *Gut.* **6,** 296–300.

MILLER M. C. (1968) Cholelithiasis developing after vagotomy: a preliminary report. *Can. Med. Assoc. J.* **98,** 350–354.

MOBERG S., CARLBERGER G., BÁRÁNY F. and LUNDH G. (1972) Gastric emptying in peptic ulcer patients before and after partial gastrectomy and selective proximal vagotomy. *Rendic. Gastroenterol.* **4,** 1–7.

MOBERG S. and HEDENSTEDT S. (1973) Selective proximal vagotomy—a three year follow up. *Scand. J. Gastroenterol.* **8,** Suppl. 20, 9.

MORELAND H. J. S. and JOHNSON L. R. (1971) Effect of vagotomy on pancreatic secretion stimulated by endogenous and exogenous secretin. *Gastroenterology* **60,** 425–431.

NELSEN T. S., EIGENBRODT E. H., KEOSHIAN L. A., BUNKER C. and JOHNSON L. (1967) Alterations in muscular and electrical activity of the stomach following vagotomy. *Arch. Surg.* **94,** 821–835.

NEWCOMBE J. F. (1973) Fatality after highly selective vagotomy. *Br. Med. J.* **1,** 610.

NIELSEN J. R. (1964) The development of cholelithiasis following vagotomy. *Am. J. Dig. Dis.* **9,** 506–508.

NOBLES E. R. (1966) Vagotomy and gastroenterostomy: 15-year follow-up of 175 patients. *Am. Surg.* **32,** 177–182.

NOVIS B. H., BANK S. and MARKS I. N. (1971) The cephalic phase of pancreatic secretion in man. *Scand. J. Gastroenterol.* **6,** 417–422.

NYHUS L. M., CHAPMAN N. D., DEVITO R. V. and HARKINS H. N. (1960) The control of gastrin release. An experimental study illustrating a new concept. *Gastroenterology* **39,** 582–589.

OBERHELMAN H. A., RIGLER S. P. and DRAGSTEDT L. R. (1957) Significance of innervation in the function of the gastric antrum. *Am. J. Physiol.* **190,** 391–395.

OBERHELMAN H. A., WOODWARD E. R., ZUBIRAN J. M. and DRAGSTEDT L. R. (1952) Physiology of the gastric antrum. *Am. J. Physiol.* **169,** 738–748.

OCHSNER A., ZEHNDER P. R. and TRAMMELL S. W. (1970) The surgical treatment of peptic ulcer: a critical analysis of results from subtotal gastrectomy and from vagotomy plus partial gastrectomy. *Surgery* **67,** 1017–1028.

PARKIN G. J. S., SMITH R. B. and JOHNSTON D. (1973) Gall bladder volume and contractility after truncal, selective and highly selective (parietal cell) vagotomy in man. *Ann. Surg.* **178,** 581–586.

PAYNE R. A. and KAY A. W. (1962) The effect of vagotomy on the maximal acid secretory response to histamine in man. *Clin. Sci.* **22,** 373–382.

PEDERSEN G. and AMDRUP E. (1970) The gastrointestinal passage of a physiological contrast medium in duodenal ulcer patients before and after vagotomy of the parietal cell mass with preserved antral innervation or a selective gastric vagotomy with Finney pyloroplasty. In: *Advance abstracts, 4th Wld Congr. Gastroenterology.* Copenhagen, Danish Gastroent. Ass., p. 433.

PE THEIN M. and SCHOFIELD B. (1959) Release of gastrin from the pyloric antrum following vagal stimulation by sham feeding. *J. Physiol. (Lond.)* **148,** 291–305.

PFEFFER R. B., STEPHENSON H. E. and HINTON J. W. (1952) The effect of thoracolumbar sympathectomy and vagus resection on pancreatic function in man. *Ann. Surg.* **136,** 585–594.

POSTLETHWAIT R. W. (1973) Five year follow-up results of operations for duodenal ulcer. *Surg. Gynecol. Obstet.* **137,** 387–392.

REES J. R. and THORBJARNARSON B. (1973) Perforated gastric ulcer. *Am. J. Surg.* **126,** 93–97.

RHODES J., BARNADO D. E., PHILLIPS S. F., ROVELSTAD A. and HOFMANN A. F. (1969) Increased reflux of bile into the stomach in patients with gastric ulcer. *Gastroenterology* **57,** 241–252.

ROBBS J. V., BANK S., MARKS I. N., LOUW J. H. (1973) Selection of operation for duodenal ulcer based on acid secretory studies: a reappraisal. *Br. J. Surg.* **60,** 601–605.

RUDICK J. and HUTCHISON J. S. F. (1964) Effects of vagal nerve section on the biliary system. *Lancet* **1**, 579–581.

SARLES H., DANI R., PREZELIN G., SOUVILLE C. and FIGARELLA C. (1968) Cephalic phase of pancreatic secretion in man. *Gut* **9**, 214–221.

SAWYERS J. L., SCOTT H. W., EDWARDS W. H., SHULL H. J. and LAW D. H. (1968) Comparative studies of the clinical effects of truncal and selective gastric vagotomy. *Am. J. Surg.* **115**, 165–172.

SCHEIN C. J., ROSEN R. G., WARREN A. and GUEDMAN M. L. (1969) A vagal factor in cholecystitis. *Surgery* **66**, 345–352.

SCHILLER K. F. R., TRUELOVE S. G. and WILLIAMS D. G. (1970) Haematemesis and melaena, with special reference to factors influencing the outcome. *Br. Med. J.* **2**, 7–14.

SHIINA E. and GRIFFITH C. A. (1969) Selective and total vagotomy without drainage: a comparative study of gastric secretion and motility in dogs. *Ann. Surg.* **169**, 326–333.

SMALL W. P. (1973) The long term results of peptic ulcer surgery. In: SIRCUS W. (ed.), *Clinics in Gastroenterology*: Vol. 2, *Peptic Ulceration*. New York and London, Saunders, p. 243.

SMITH G. K. and FARRIS J. M. (1958) Rationale of vagotomy and pyloroplasty in management of bleeding duodenal ulcer. *JAMA* **166**, 878–881.

SMITH R. B., EDWARDS J. P. and JOHNSTON D. (1973) Does the vagal nerve supply to the pancreas matter in man? *Br. J. Surg.* **60**, 318.

SMITHWICK R. H., HARROWER H. W. and FARMER D. A. (1961) Hemigastrectomy and vagotomy in the treatment of duodenal ulcer. *Am. J. Surg.* **101**, 325–335.

STADAAS J. and AUNE S. (1970) Intragastric pressure/volume relationship before and after vagotomy. *Acta Chir. Scand.* **136**, 611–612.

STADIL F. (1972) Effect of vagotomy on gastrin release during insulin hypoglycaemia in ulcer patients. *Scand. J. Gastroenterol.* **7**, 225–231.

STADIL F. and REHFELD J. H. (1974) Gastrin response to insulin after selective, highly selective and truncal vagotomy. *Gastroenterology* **66**, 7–15.

STALSBERG H. and TAKSDAL S. (1971) Stomach cancer following gastric surgery for benign conditions. *Lancet* **2**, 1175–1177.

STAVNEY L. S., KATO T., GRIFFITHS C. A., NYHUS L. M. and HARKINS H. N. (1963) A physiologic study of motility changes following selective gastric vagotomy. *J. Surg. Res.* **3**, 390–394.

STENING G. F. and GROSSMAN M. I. (1970) Gastric acid response to pentagastrin and histamine after extra-gastric vagotomy in dogs. *Gastroenterology* **59**, 364–371.

STERN D. H. and WALSH J. H. (1973) Gastrin release in post-operative ulcer subjects: evidence for release of duodenal gastrin. *Gastroenterology* **64**, 363–369.

STODDARD C. J., BROWN B. H., WHITTAKER G. E., WATERFALL W. E. and DUTHIE H. L. (1973) Effects of varying the extent of vagotomy on the myoelectrical and motor activity of the stomach in man. *Br. J. Surg.* **60**, 307.

TANTURI C. A. and IVY A. C. (1938) On the existence of secretory nerves in the vagi for reflex excitation and inhibition of bile secretion. *Am. J. Physiol.* **121**, 270–283.

TAYLOR H. (1957) The non-surgical treatment of perforated peptic ulcer. *Gastroenterology* **33**, 353–368.

TOMPKINS R. K., KRAFT A. R., ZIMMERMAN E., LICHTENSTEIN J. E. and ZOLLINGER R. M. (1972) Clinical and biochemical evidence of increased gallstone formation after complete vagotomy. *Surgery* **71**, 196–202.

TOVEY F. I. (1969) A comparison of Polya gastrectomy, total and selective vagotomy, and of pyloroplasty and gastrojejunostomy. *Br. J. Surg.* **56**, 281–286.

UVNÄS B. (1942) The part played by the pyloric region in the cephalic phase of gastric secretion. *Acta Physiol. Scand.* **4**, Suppl. 13.

WASTELL, C. (1966) Excretion of fat after vagotomy alone and in combination with pyloroplasty: an experimental study. *Br. Med. J.* **1**, 1198–1199.

WASTELL C. (1974) Gastric drainage: pyloroplasty or gastrojejunostomy? In: WASTELL C. (ed.), *Westminster Hospital Symposium on Chronic Duodenal Ulcer*. London, Butterworths, pp. 259–269.

WASTELL C., COLIN J. F., MACNAUGHTON J. I. and GLEESON J. (1972) Selective proximal vagotomy with and without pyloroplasty. *Br. Med. J.* **1,** 28–30.

WASTELL C. and ELLIS H. (1966) Faecal fat excretion and stool colour after vagotomy and pyloroplasty. *Br. Med. J.* **1,** 1194–1197.

WHELDON E. J., VENABLES C. W. and JOHNSTON I. D. A. (1970) Late metabolic sequelae of vagotomy and gastroenterostomy. *Lancet* **1,** 437–440.

WILBUR B. G. and KELLY K. A. (1973) Effect of proximal gastric, complete gastric, and truncal vagotomy on canine gastric electric activity, motility and emptying. *Ann. Surg.* **178,** 295–303.

WILKINSON A. R. and JOHNSTON D. (1973) Effect of truncal, selective and highly selective vagotomy on gastric emptying and intestinal transit of a food-barium meal in man. *Ann. Surg.* **178,** 190–193.

WILLIAMS E. J. and IRVINE W. T. (1966) Functional and metabolic effects of total and selective vagotomy. *Lancet* **1,** 1053–1057.

WOHLRABE D. E. and KELLY W. D. (1959a) Motility studies of isolated antral pouches before and after vagus denervation. *J. Appl. Physiol.* **14,** 22–26.

WOHLRABE D. E. and KELLY W. D. (1959b) Studies on the role of nervous mechanisms in antral function. *Surg. Forum* **9,** 430–433.

WOMACK N. A. (1969) Blood flow through the stomach: clinical aspects. *Am. J. Surg.* **117,** 771–780.

WOODWARD E. R., LYON E. S., LANDOR J. and DRAGSTEDT L. R. (1954) The physiology of the gastric antrum: experimental studies on isolated antrum pouches in dogs. *Gastroenterology* **27,** 766–785.

9

Presentation and Management of Stones in the Common Bile Duct

B. H. Hand, MS, FRCS

It has been reported that something of the order of 10 per cent of people over 50 years of age in Europe and North America are likely to have gallstones, and there is evidence that the incidence is increasing and that more male patients and younger people develop them than hitherto. Cholecystectomy is, therefore, a common operation. An average of the larger published series indicates that stones are present in the bile ducts of some 10–12 per cent of patients who come to cholecystectomy. Exploration of the common bile duct is, therefore, frequently performed.

The common bile duct is a delicate structure and operations upon it should never be performed without adequate training, a sound knowledge of anatomy, adequate facilities and good lighting, proper assistance and, in my view, radiological services in the operating theatre. We must remember that the patients concerned are often young and suffering from a benign and essentially curable condition (Hand, 1973).

The literature on biliary surgery shows that duct exploration may be associated with a slightly higher mortality than cholecystectomy alone. There is definitely a higher morbidity rate in respect of chest and biliary complications and therefore a longer length of stay in hospital (Bartlett and Waddell, 1958; Colcock, 1958; Hight et al., 1959; Havard, 1960; Nienhuis, 1961). It is higher still if re-exploration for residual stone is required. We must accept that published figures are somewhat loaded by the fact that exploration of the common bile duct in a jaundiced patient is a more serious operation and it does not prove that unnecessary exploration in a non-jaundiced patient is accompanied by such an appreciable increase in mortality or morbidity.

However, these figures tend to emanate from so-called centres of excellence and I venture to suggest they could well be worse up and down the country.

It behoves us, therefore, never to leave unexplored a duct which contains calculi, to ensure that the ducts are completely cleared of stones, and at the same time we must try to avoid unnecessary duct exploration.

Stones usually reach the common bile duct via the cystic duct and at this time are usually small. However, once in the duct they increase in size by deposition of pigment around the typical faceted basic make-up. Occasionally they reach the common bile duct by ulceration of Hartmann's pouch into the common hepatic duct.

Stones may form in the bile ducts due to the presence of parasites and foreign bodies, in the presence of obstruction by other stones or fibrosis of the terminal portions of the duct, and also in some cases of haemolytic anaemia. But we must not be deluded by the self-indulgent postulation, without these circumstances, that stones form subsequent to cholecystectomy. Most, if not all, let us be honest, are the result of errors in technique.

Stones in the bile duct present clinically in the following circumstances:

1. At primary operation in:
   (a) a jaundiced patient;
   (b) a non-jaundiced patient.
2. On subsequent occasions, usually referred to as residual stones.
3. Post-operatively at T tube cholangiography after 1 or 2, above.

Primary operation

Jaundiced patient

Let us consider first the jaundiced patient. It must be appreciated that while in most cases there is characteristic painful and fluctuating jaundice associated with pruritus and a past history of flatulent dyspepsia, there is a hard core of patients in whom it is very difficult to distinguish between organic obstruction and medical causes of jaundice, in particular intrahepatic cholestasis. It is clearly important to avoid anaesthesia and operation in the medical cases and further-more it is also very useful to differentiate pre-operatively between calculus, fibrotic or malignant obstruction in the surgical cases if we can.

Briefly then, as space does not permit a full discussion on the differential diag-nosis of jaundice, what investigations can help in indicating that organic obstruc-tion is present?

1. Biochemical

Blood   The serum bilirubin, mainly conjugated, is raised, but if later hepato-cellular damage occurs, the ratio of conjugated to free is reduced. The alkaline phosphatase is always raised, but this does not distinguish between intrahepatic cholestasis and extrahepatic organic obstruction, though high values of over 30 units are uncommon in the early stages of viral hepatitis. The serum cholesterol rises leading to increase in β and α_2 globulins. Albumin tends to fall in hepato-cellular damage from any cause after 2–3 weeks. The flocculation tests are entirely non-specific but are usually little affected in obstructive jaundice because the γ globulins tend to be normal. The serum transaminases are either normal or only slightly raised unless ascending cholangitis is present to any extent.

Urine   Both bile pigments and salts are present in amounts related to the degree of jaundice. Urbilinogen is absent only if obstruction is complete; this test may be helpful when the jaundice is fluctuating.

2. Haematological

A full blood count is desirable to exclude haemolytic anaemia, especially in patients of Mediterranean countries. We must remember that these patients do form pigment stones which may be in the common bile duct, and a mixed investigatory picture can be obtained. A leucocytosis occurs in cholangitis. The prothrombin time in obstructive jaundice is lowered but, although not reduced enough to produce spontaneous bleeding, it may be sufficient to cause increased bleeding at operation.

3. Histological

Material may be obtained by aspiration liver biopsy and, in most instances, if required, will have been done by our medical colleagues before referring the case.

4. Radiological

Cholecystography and intravenous cholangiography are frequently unhelpful if the serum bilirubin is above 50 umol/l (3 mg%), and in the more deeply jaundiced it may be dangerous (Craft and Swales, 1967). Direct cholangiography has been performed by direct puncture of the gall bladder visualized on peritoneoscopy; but this is potentially dangerous by producing biliary peritonitis and has been superseded by the percutaneous method. Greater safety may be achieved by utilizing the drip method of injecting iodipamide (Nolan and Gibson, 1970).

Percutaneous transhepatic cholangiography

This test is not one to be performed routinely but only in those cases where there is real doubt as to the diagnosis, since haemorrhage, biliary peritonitis and gram-negative septicaemia may occur in the obstructed patient. The patient should receive vitamin K for several days before the test. It should be performed in the x-ray department under local anaesthetic plus sedation, and the operating theatre must be available within a few hours if required. A flexible needle or preferably a Shaldon's needle (plastic covered) is inserted, with respiration inhibited, 2 cm below and to the right of the xiphisternum in an upwards and backwards direction for 10 cm. The needle is then removed and, with the patient breathing shallowly, the Polythene cover is slowly withdrawn while aspirating until bile is obtained. As much bile is aspirated as possible, a specimen sent for culture, then 20 ml of some suitable dye (such as sodiumdiatrizoate Hypaque 25%) is injected while observing the screen of the image intensifier, and suitable exposures made. When the test is complete the dye and remaining bile are allowed to drain freely. In the event of a negative tap, the procedure may be repeated three times. Failure to enter a bile duct indicates a non-obstructive lesion and removal of the tube is considered safe: operation is thus avoided (Shaldon et al., 1962; Dodd, 1967).

If the bile looks infected on aspiration, an antibiotic is given pending sensitivity results of the culture (Keighley et al., 1973).

Ascending cholangiography

A more recent approach to the jaundiced case has been made possible by the fibre-optic flexible duodenoscope with an angled mechanism permitting direct cannulation of the papilla of Vater. This instrument is expensive and as yet only a few hospitals have specialized endoscopy departments. In any case, it should be employed only in the difficult diagnostic problem. It is performed under local anaesthetic with sedation. Silicone is introduced into the duodenum to prevent frothing and hyoscine given intramuscularly to reduce peristalsis (Cotton et al., 1972).

After some, or all, of these tests, we hope we are left with a jaundice patient who is a surgical problem and with luck we will in some cases have distinguished between calculus, fibrotic or malignant disease as the cause.

If we are satisfied that the jaundice is obstructive and likely to be due to calculus, there is no great urgency to operate for a week or two, during which time the stone may disimpact and the jaundice subside. This will permit a fuller investigation and render the operation safer at a later date.

If, however, the jaundice does not relent and operation is required, vitamin K i.m. 10 mg daily is prescribed for about 3 days pre-operatively. Remember, also, that after decompression the jaundice usually deepens and it is advisable to continue vitamin K post operatively for a week or so to avert the possible danger of a secondary haemorrhage.

In all but mild degrees of jaundice it has been shown that there is an increased incidence of anuria or oliguria post-operatively. This risk can be reduced by administration of 500 ml of 10% mannitol immediately pre-operatively and continued as a 5% solution during and after operation, as indicated by the urinary output; accurate measurement is best provided with an indwelling urethral catheter (Dawson, 1968).

If cholangitis is present, pre- and post-operative antibiotics are necessary. It has recently been suggested that, in a jaundiced patient, ampicillin, tetracycline and rifampicin may not be excreted by the liver as well as we had thought, and that gentamicin or cephaloridine is better.

Non-jaundiced patient

In a patient who is not jaundiced at the time of operation we still have to decide whether there are stones in the common bile duct. In other words, this question must be asked in all patients with gallstones.

Clinical observations

There may be no special indications, rarely even an absence of pain. There may be a past history of biliary colic, usually not an intermittent pain but continuous with exacerbations, often in the epigastrium and accompanied by vomiting. There is usually no pyrexia; but in retrospect, mild attacks of cholecystitis may be confused with colic. There is no difference in the type of pain if a stone is impacted in the cystic duct or lies in the common bile duct. Furthermore, during the attack of colic the stone may have passed into the duodenum and the ducts are clear by the time the patient comes to operation. A past history of jaundice may be confusing. The dirty grey colour of a nauseated patient in pain may be thought to be yellow; the patient may be a bit dehydrated so the urine is concentrated and darker than normal; some diarrhoea may occur and pale stools are passed after the attack. The patients may not have been seen by the general practitioner during the attack and, even if they have, liver function tests have often been omitted and confirmation of jaundice and its type is thereby missed.

Charcot's intermittent hepatic fever or the tetrad of intermittent pain, intermittent jaundice, intermittent pyrexia and loss of weight is characteristic of ascending cholangitis and indicates biliary obstruction.

Acute or recurrent pancreatitis may be induced by a stone in the common bile duct, but also occurs from spasm of the sphincter even when the stones are confined to the gall bladder.

Radiographic evidence

Only 10–15 per cent of all gallstones are radio-opaque on plain abdominal x-ray. It is rare to find a radio-opaque stone in the bile ducts because bile salts and not calcium seem to be deposited once they have left the gall bladder.

With modern techniques of oral cholecystography the common bile duct is visualized quite often when the gall bladder has concentrated the dye, but not usually when the ducts are dilated. This test, introduced by Graham and Cole in 1924, made the pre-operative diagnosis of gallstones reliable for the first time.

In 1953 intravenous cholangiography with iodipamide was introduced and it was hoped that this would solve the problem of the detection of duct stones. But later, even with the stronger preparation of iodipamide (Biligrafin forte) and with tomography, positive evidence of filling defects is all too infrequent and we usually have to be content with visualization and measurement of the diameter of the bile ducts. Some have given intravenous morphine to cause spasm of the sphincter and hold the dye in the bile duct in the hope of better visualization of filling defects.

Operative

Any of the following findings will provide evidence in support of the presence of duct stones.

1. A palpable stone in the duct.

2. A dilated duct, which is not always an easy factor to assess due to the variation in normal calibre. It is especially difficult if there is a long parallel entry of the cystic duct.

3. The presence of thickened and opaque bile ducts.

4. If there are no stones in the gall bladder and it is fibrosed.

5. The existence of turbid bile in the ducts.

6. If multiple stones are palpable in the gall bladder, especially if some are small and the cystic duct is patent or even dilated.

Operative cholangiography

If you accept the wide range of indications of the presence of duct stones outlined above—be they clinical, biochemical, radiological or operative in the non-jaundiced patient—you will conclude that some 60 per cent of ducts would seem to require exploration. In fact, we know that stones will be present in only 10–15 per cent of cases. It follows that, in the absence of jaundice at the time of operation, most of the factors mentioned above are no more than relative indications for duct exploration.

We therefore require something additional during the operation to help us to decide whether or not to explore the duct. This, in my view, is where operative cholangiography comes to our aid. Although this test has been used for over 25 years and has become increasingly popular in the last 10 years, it is still not accepted universally in spite of a wealth of literature strongly in favour of it when properly performed.

A new and rather novel technique has recently been described of a transjugular approach to the liver. A special needle–catheter combination is passed into the jugular vein and introduced via the heart into the hepatic veins, permitting a liver biopsy and a cholangiogram without transgressing the peritoneal cavity (Rösch et al., 1973).

Certain criteria are essential for success in operative cholangiography if standardized and reliable results are to be obtained. You need constant practice, so it must become a routine procedure; it is no good merely performing it occasionally in a difficult case. There must be close co-operation between the surgeon, anaesthetist, radiographer and scrub nurse, and finally the details of the technique must be followed scrupulously.

Pre-exploratory cholangiography is performed in order to decide whether duct exploration is necessary. After the duct has been explored, post-exploratory cholangiography is utilized to determine whether the bile ducts have been cleared of stones.

The literature abounds with articles and monographs on the subject of operative cholangiography and a full consideration of the technique and all its pitfalls would take a whole article. A great deal of information, together with numerous references, can be found in Schulenberg's monograph (1966).

I feel bound to mention some of the essential points of the method I have employed for nearly 25 years (Le Quesne, 1964).

The patient lies on an operating table with a radiolucent top or on a box tunnel into which the plates can be inserted, preferably from the head end. Towels are fixed with sutures and not clips. After identification of the cystic, common bile and common hepatic ducts and the cystic artery, the last-named is tied. The cystic duct is palpated to ensure there are no stones in it. A ligature is then tied round the proximal end of the cystic duct to prevent stones in the gall bladder being dislodged. The cystic duct is opened close to the common bile duct and a probe is passed to facilitate insertion of a ureteric catheter or one of the varieties of plastic tube now available (*British Medical Journal*, 1969), which has previously been filled with normal saline from a 20-ml syringe to exclude all air bubbles. All instruments and swabs are removed, and if a Ryle's tube is in the stomach, it is withdrawn so that its tip is clear of the duct system. It is desirable to bring the outer end of the catheter through the abdominal wall via a stab incision (which can be used later for the corrugated drain) in order to bring it well clear of the duct system on the x-ray film. The wound is covered with a pack and the table is then tilted 15 degrees downwards to the right to place the duodenum clear of the transverse processes of the lumbar vertebrae. The plate is positioned and the x-ray machine centred. The syringe with normal saline is replaced by a 2-ml syringe containing sodium diatrizoate 25%, again aspirating any air bubbles. Stronger solutions may over-opacify the bile ducts and obscure small stones. The injection must be slow to avoid sudden distension of the bile duct, which will induce sphincter spasm and prevent free flow. The initial volume must be small so that, if free flow occurs into the duodenum, too much dye in the latter will not overlie and obscure the lower reaches of the ducts. When the surgeon is ready the anaesthetist, who is responsible for inhibiting respiration at the moment of exposure, does the countdown so as to ensure that the injection, the apnoea and the exposure are simultaneous; this is vital.

If the common bile duct is wide, more than 2 ml will be required for the first

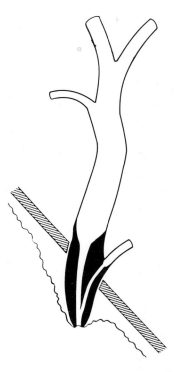

Fig. 9.1 A diagrammatic representation of the common bile duct, showing the notch which divides it into an upper wide-lumened thin-walled portion and a lower narrow-lumened thick-walled portion. The lower portion is seen to lie mainly in the submucous layer of the duodenum. (Reproduced from Hand, 1963, *Br. J. Surg.* **50,** 486–494, by courtesy of the Editor.)

exposure in order to fill the system. A second injection is performed and x-rays taken in the same way, using a further 7–8 ml. A third film is sometimes required if the whole duct system is not opacified; in particular the intrahepatic ducts must be filled because some 10 per cent of those patients with stones in the extrahepatic ducts will also have stones in the ducts within the liver.

The interpretation of the films requires, first, a knowledge of anatomy and, secondly, a knowledge of the factors which indicate the presence of stones.

The common bile duct described in anatomy books is divided into a supraduodenal, a retroduodenal, an intrapancreatic and an intraduodenal portion. For the biliary surgeon it is far more usefully divided into two portions—an upper, longer, thin-walled wide-lumened portion, and a shorter, lower, thick-walled narrow-lumened portion. The wall of the upper part is composed mainly of fibrous and elastic tissue with minimal longitudinal muscle; the lower portion, composed predominantly of muscle, corresponds to the sphincter mechanism. The junction of these two portions lies some 2 mm outside the duodenal wall and is characterized radiologically by a notch (Hand, 1963). Figure 9.1 shows a diagrammatic representation of this. Figure 9.2 is a post-mortem cholangiogram, showing the anatomy particularly well. Large and medium-sized stones are, of course, held up above the notch, whereas small stones may pass further on but tend to be held up in the narrowest portion of the duct which lies just above its junction

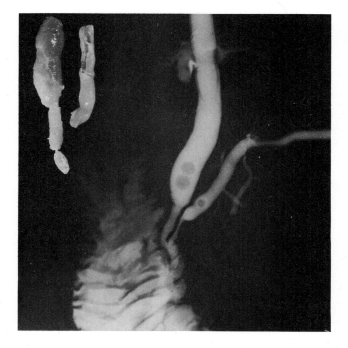

Fig. 9.2 A post-mortem cholangiogram and cast of the common bile and pancreatic ducts showing the features described in Fig. 9.1. (Reproduced from Hand, 1963, *Br. J. Surg.* **50,** 486–494, by courtesy of the Editor.)

with the pancreatic duct. It is uncommon to find them in the common channel or impacted at the orifice of the papilla.

A normal cholangiogram should reveal the following information:

1. Free flow into the duodenum, preferably in all films.
2. Visualization of the terminal narrow segment.

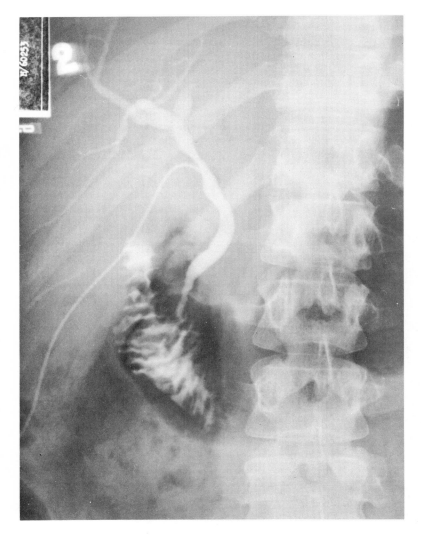

Fig. 9.3 The second film of a normal operative cholangiogram; 8 ml of contrast had been injected. Free flow has occurred, the duct is of normal calibre, there are no filling defects, the lower end is visualized clear of the contrast in the duodenum and the intrahepatic radicles have been filled. The notch is identifiable.

3. A normal calibre duct, the maximum diameter being 10 mm or, at the most, 12 mm.
4. No filling defects.
5. Filling of the intrahepatic ducts without over-distension.

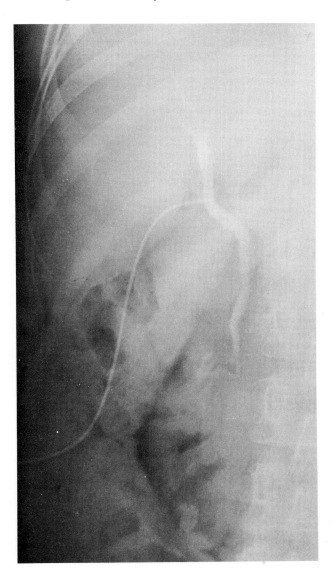

Fig. 9.4 The first film of a normal cholangiogram, using 2 ml of contrast. Note how well the lower end is visualized, and even with this small volume, flow into the duodenum has occurred.

6. Reflux up the pancreatic duct is of no significance and does not seem to induce pancreatitis post-operatively.

Figure 9.3 shows the second film of a normal pre-exploratory cholangiogram. Figures 9.4 and 9.5 are the first and second films of a normal pre-exploratory cholangiogram showing pancreatic duct reflux.

Air bubbles or sphincter spasm with failure to flow will produce false positive results. The test can be repeated after a gentle washout with normal saline, and sphincter spasm can be relaxed by inhalation of amyl nitrite during the repeat x-rays.

This test, like any other, is not 100 per cent reliable and must not take the place of overwhelming clinical evidence. The particular value of operative cholangiography is to confirm that the duct is free of stones when there are either no indications to explore or when these are only relative. In practised hands unnecessary duct exploration is avoided in at least 40 per cent of cases. It may reveal entirely unsuspected calculi in possibly 3 per cent of cases. Furthermore, it will reliably confirm the clinical impression that there are stones in the duct and that exploration is necessary. With skill and practice, false positive x-rays amount to only 5 per cent.

There is also a bonus from the test in that anatomical anomalies are revealed, such as so-called accessory hepatic ducts, low junction of hepatic ducts, low or spiral entry of the cystic duct, entry of cystic duct into right hepatic duct. Furthermore, it will confirm that so far in the operation the bile duct is undamaged!

Manometry or choledochometrography

In this test, which has been used in the detection of bile duct stones, known volumes of fluid are introduced into the bile duct at a known pressure over a fixed period of time. The pressure change pattern produced in the bile duct is recorded on a smoked drum. Those surgeons with experience of the procedure can interpret the curves produced in terms of organic obstruction, hypertonicity or hypotonicity of the sphincter (Mallet-Guy, 1952).

In a Hunterian lecture, Daniel (1972) concluded that the test is of value though it has so far received little support in Britain.

Ultrasonics

Although some success has been achieved in the detection of gall bladder calculi by ultrasonics when conventional methods have failed or are not applicable (Doust and Maklad, 1974), it is clearly considerably more difficult when applied to the detection of bile duct stones (Knight and Newell, 1963).

Operative technique of exploration of the common bile duct

After the exploratory cholangiogram has been performed the gall bladder is dissected off the liver and the bed reperitonealized while the operative cholangiogram films are being developed. If no exploration is required the cystic duct is tied flush, the gall bladder removed and the wound closed with drainage of the gall bladder bed.

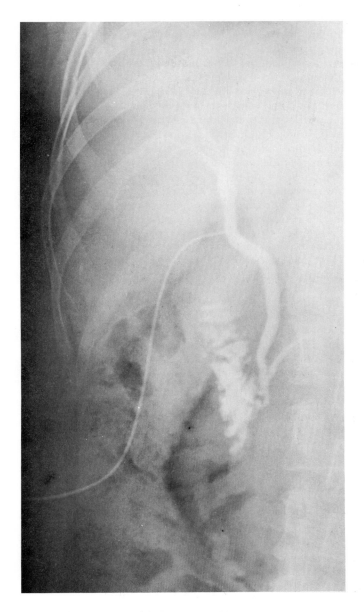

Fig. 9.5 The second film on the same subject as Fig. 9.4, using a total of 7 ml of contrast. Greater intrahepatic filling and flow into the duodenum has occurred. Pancreatic duct reflux has taken place.

If duct exploration is required the surgeon should now move to the left side of the patient, and the duodenum and head of pancreas are mobilized by Kocher's manoeuvre. Preliminary palpation of the ducts can now be performed with the thumb and forefinger of the left hand.

Stay sutures are then inserted into the common bile or common hepatic ducts at a convenient point dependent upon the level of entry of the cystic duct, sufficiently distant from both the porta hepatis and the duodenum. The duct is opened with a small scalpel on a long handle with traction of the stay sutures to avoid damage to the posterior wall of the duct, and avoiding the longitudinal veins which lie on the wall of the duct. The incision is enlarged with fine scissors, but without cutting too close to the duodenum in case there is a high supraduodenal artery. When there is a long parallel or spiral insertion, care must be taken not to open into the cystic duct, instead of the bile duct; otherwise you will find you can only explore downwards and not upwards into the liver!

Exploration should be gentle, and sharp instruments like scoops avoided. Desjardins' forceps, suction and saline irrigation with a catheter are less traumatic. Irrigation is of value, especially if the stone breaks up. Most surgeons advise exploration upwards in the first instance, making sure that both left and right hepatic ducts are entered. Exploration downwards is facilitated by the use of fine gum elastic bougies up to size No. 8 or 9. The larger size Bake's dilators are, I consider, too traumatic. It is possible to feel stones against the bougie in the duct more easily than against the head of the pancreas, and with practice I am convinced it is possible to feel the sphincter mechanism of the intraduodenal portion of the duct surrounding the bougie and to locate the point where the bougie enters the lumen, in spite of many statements to the contrary. Overstretching of the papilla is to be avoided and I think it is probably one cause of a condition described in recent years of stenosing papillitis. This condition was reviewed in the *British Medical Journal* (1957).

The pre-exploratory cholangiogram will tell you that there are at least a certain number of stones in the ducts, but it is unreliable in indicating the exact number. If, after conscientious exploration, it is felt the duct is clear, a post-exploratory cholangiogram should be performed via a T tube inserted into the exploratory incision, the duct being closed around it with 000 plain atraumatic catgut sutures. While operative cholangiography, properly performed, is reliable in indicating when to explore the common bile duct, it is unfortunately less accurate in showing that the duct has been cleared of calculi. This is due to the fact that it is difficult to exclude all the air bubbles, some leakage may occur through the choledochotomy incision, and not infrequently the dye fails to flow into the duodenum, even when there are no residual calculi. This latter sign is regarded as an important one in the pre-exploratory test to indicate the existence of stones within the duct. Presumably sphincter spasm is the cause. Nevertheless, in spite of its deficiencies, the post-exploratory x-ray is worth while performing. If residual stones are seen the T tube is removed and a further exploration carried out.

In 1953 a rigid choledochoscope was introduced; later, in 1965, the flexible fibre-optic instrument superseded it in the detection of duct stones. It has been suggested that perhaps its best use is after duct exploration to assist in ensuring that the ducts have been completely cleared (Longland, 1973). This instrument is, of course, expensive and requires careful handling and maintenance and is likely to be available only in large gastroenterological centres.

In some cases the presence of stones may be known to be within the intrahepatic ducts, but cannot be delivered by any of the means described above. A modified Fogarty catheter has been designed which may help in delivery of these stones in the same manner in which the instrument has been used to evacuate arterial emboli (Fogarty et al., 1968).

However, if one is satisfied that the ducts have been cleared the wound can now be closed with corrugated tube drainage. The opportunity to check that the duct was cleared is provided by post-operative T tube cholangiography some 10 days after the operation. This opportunity is denied to those who feel that T tube drainage after choledochotomy is not only unnecessary but may actually damage the bile ducts. I cannot agree with this view.

If, following the technique of duct exploration described above, it is considered that stones or debris still remain in the intrahepatic or extrahepatic ducts, or there is fibrosis of the papilla preventing the passage of bougies into the duodenal lumen, there are two further procedures which can be performed. First, sphincterotomy, which will permit a wider through-and-through instrumentation and irrigation and leave the patient with a larger entry of the bile duct into the duodenum. Secondly, a choledochoduodenostomy may be carried out.

Sphincterotomy

Some confusion has developed between the terms sphincterotomy and sphincteroplasty. In the former operation only part of the sphincter mechanism is divided, whereas the latter is really a transduodenal choledochoduodenostomy with total division of the sphincter. A clear distinction with anatomical and technical details is described by Jones (1973).

Peel et al. (1974), while strongly advocating sphincterotomy for residual stone, have gone further to suggest that it should be the primary method of duct exploration rather than choledochotomy and not merely when the latter has failed. However, they did not feel the need to perform a sphincteroplasty.

There are a number of techniques of performing a sphincterotomy. One method is to pass a plastic or gum elastic bougie through the choledochotomy incision into the duodenum and locate the site of the papilla by palpation. The duodenum, having been previously mobilized by Kocher's manœuvre, is opened longitudinally or obliquely centred over the papilla. The bougie is pulled down so that the expanded end impacts in the papilla and by gentle traction the papilla can be pulled forwards through the duodenal incision. The bougie protects the pancreatic duct lying posteriorly or posteromedially and an incision can safely be made through the anterior wall of the papilla on to the bougie (Le Quesne, 1964). I personally favour suturing the cut edges with 3×0 plain atraumatic catgut to produce epithelial apposition and prevent fibrosis; this does not constitute sphincteroplasty. As the diameter of the orifice is increased the bougie will slip through and larger ones are then passed which, in turn, will impact as before; small cuts are made, suturing as you proceed until the stone is recovered. Usually at least a 5-mm and at the most a 10-mm incision is required. It is important not to make too large an incision, otherwise the whole sphincter mechanism will be divided and, since it extends outside the duodenal wall, a duodenal fistula will be produced unless the technique of sphincteroplasty is carefully followed. Remember the average length of the thickened segment (i.e. the sphincter) is 1·5 cm, with a range of 1–3 cm. After further exploration, and when the duct is considered clear, the duodenal wall is closed in two layers in such a way that duodenal narrowing is not produced. The duodenal closure should be drained externally. Post-operative gastric suction and intravenous replacement therapy are advisable following sphincterotomy.

Choledochoduodenostomy

Although described in the early part of this century, choledochoduodenostomy fell into disrepute because of the ascending cholangitis. Hosford (1957) drew attention to its value in selected cases. More recent evidence indicates that, provided the stoma is of the order of 2 cm in diameter, cholangitis does not occur. If the bile duct is narrower than this a lateral anastomosis may be performed (Madden, 1958; Capper, 1961).

Although there is clearly a place for choledochoduodenostomy in the management of duct stones, whether external or transduodenal (i.e. a sphincteroplasty), it is clearly unwise to bypass nature's sphincters if it can be avoided.

Residual calculi

So far the diagnosis and treatment of choledocholithiasis at the primary operation have been considered. Clearly the diagnosis of subsequent residual calculi will be reached by the same clinical, radiological and pathological observations already outlined. There is, however, one radiological fact, which is not generally appreciated, to which I would like to draw attention. It has been clearly demonstrated that the common bile duct does not dilate after cholecystectomy. This is contrary to Oddi's teaching which has been handed down for many years. Furthermore, the dilated duct does not demonstrably reduce in diameter after removal of the obstruction (Le Quesne et al., 1959). It follows that, if continued obstruction is to be postulated, an increase in diameter since the initial operation must be shown. When making the measurements, allowance for a magnification factor has to be made. This comparison is only possible if previous iodipamide or operative cholangiography has been performed.

Operative cholangiography is still possible in these patients by fixing a fine short-bevelled needle into the end of a ureteric catheter, which is inserted into the bile duct and held in place by a fine stay suture. However, if the previous surgeon has left a little stump of cystic duct it may be possible to find a way into the common bile duct through this.

Second operations are clearly technically more difficult than the first, and there is a temptation to perform a choledochoduodenostomy as an easier way out and perhaps avoid a third operation. It is in these patients that Peel et al. (1974) would consider it safer to explore the duct by transduodenal sphincterotomy.

Residual calculi found at T tube cholangiography

The discovery of residual calculi is an unfortunate one for both patient and surgeon. Re-exploration so soon after the first operation is difficult and accompanied by a higher mortality, and must be avoided if at all possible.

If the stone is small, it is reasonable to leave the T tube in place and spiggoted off and the patient can be sent home or to convalescence. This is quite safe for several weeks and with luck the stone will pass. Irrigation after inhalation with amyl nitrite or with xylocaine may assist its passage by producing a short period of relaxation of the sphincter mechanism. If possible, this should be done using an image intensifier.

Dissolution of stones

If the hopeful attitude fails or the stone is obviously too large to pass spontaneously, surgeons in the past have tried to dissolve or fragment them. Ether, alcohol, chloroform, citric acid, chenodeoxycholic acid, sodium phosphate and heparin, to mention but a few substances, have been tried. Indeed, Best et al. (1953) reported a review of the use of no less than 113 solutions that had been tried. Bearing in mind that the composition of these stones varies, this is hardly surprising. Generally speaking, dissolution methods have not been popular or successful, but recent work suggests that a combination of heparin and chenodeoxycholic acid may prove useful. This subject was reviewed recently by Bell (1974).

Closed removal

It has been shown that if the T tube is left in situ for 3–4 weeks a firm fibrous tract develops. It is possible, after removal of the T tube and under sedation, to utilize this tract for instrumentation under radiographic control, using an image intensifier. Desjardins' forceps, a modified Fogarty catheter and a Dormia basket have been successfully used to remove or fragment stones on occasions (Margarey, 1971; Burhenne, 1973; Galloway et al., 1973).

A recent advance, namely endoscopic papillotomy, performed by means of high frequency diathermy using a lateral viewing duodenoscope could possibly become the method of choice in the future (Classen and Safrany, 1975).

If all else fails, then re-exploration is necessary. There is no hurry if the T tube has been left in situ. If it has been removed, then operation may be required forthwith because of the development of a biliary fistula or ascending cholangitis.

References

BARTLETT M. K. and WADDELL W. R. (1958) Indications for common-duct exploration. Evaluation in 1,000 cases. *N. Engl. J. Med.* **258,** 164–167.

BELL G. D. (1974) The present position concerning gallstone dissolution. *Gut* **15,** 913–929.

BEST R. R., RASMUSSEN J. A. and WILSON C. E. (1953) An evaluation of solutions for fragmentation and dissolution of gallstones and their effect on liver and ductal tissue. *Ann. Surg.* **138,** 570–581.

BRITISH MEDICAL JOURNAL (1957) Stenosis of the sphincter of Oddi. **2,** 1044.

BRITISH MEDICAL JOURNAL (1969) Disposable operative cholangiogram cannula. **1,** 706–707.

BURHENNE H. J. (1973) Non-operative retained biliary tract stone extraction: a new roentgenologic technique. *Am. J. Roentgenol.* **117,** 388–399.

CAPPER W. M. (1961) External choledochoduodenostomy; an evaluation of 125 cases. *Br. J. Surg.* **49,** 292–300.

CLASSEN M. and SAFRANY L. (1975). Endoscopic papillotomy and removal of gall stones. *Br. Med. J.* **4,** 371–374.

COLCOCK B. P. (1958) Common duct stones. *Surg. Clin. North Am.* **38,** 663–672.

COTTON P. B., BLUMGART L. H., DAVIES G. T., PIERCE J. W., SALMON P. R., BURWOOD R. J., LAWRIE B. W. and READ A. E. (1972) Cannulation of papilla of Vater via fiber-duodenoscope: assessment of retrograde cholangiopancreatography in 60 patients. *Lancet* **1,** 53–58.

CRAFT I. L. and SWALES J. D. (1967) Renal failure after cholangiography. *Br. Med. J.* **2,** 736–738.

DANIEL O. (1972) The value of radiomanometry in bile duct surgery. *Ann. R. Coll. Surg. Engl.* **51,** 357–372.

DAWSON J. L. (1968) Acute post-operative renal failure in obstructive jaundice. *Ann. R. Coll. Surg. Engl.* **42,** 163–180.

DODD G. (1967) Percutaneous transhepatic cholangiography. *Surg. Clin. North Am.* **47,** 1095–1106.

DOUST B. P. and MAKLAD N. F. (1974) Ultrasonic B-mode examination of the gallbladder. Technique and criteria for the diagnosis of gallstones. *Radiology* **110,** 643–647.

FOGARTY T. J., KRIPPAEHNE W. W., DENNIS D. L. and FLETCHER W. S. (1968) Evaluation of an improved operative technique in common duct surgery. *Am. J. Surg.* **116,** 177–183.

GALLOWAY S. J., CASARELLA W. J. and SEAMAN W. B. (1973) The non-operative treatment of retained stones in the common bile duct. *Surg. Gynecol. Obstet.* **137,** 55–58.

GRAHAM E. A. and COLE W. H. (1924) Roentgenologic examination of the gallbladder. *JAMA* **82,** 613–614.

HAND B. H. (1963) An anatomical study of the choledochoduodenal area. *Br. J. Surg.* **50,** 486–494.

HAND B. H. (1973) Anatomy and function of the extrahepatic biliary system. *Clin. Gastroenterol.* **2,** 3–29.

HAVARD C. (1960) Non-malignant bile duct obstruction. *Ann. R. Coll. Surg. Engl.* **26,** 88–114.

HIGHT D., LINGLEY J. R. and HURTUBISE F. (1959) An evaluation of operative cholangiograms as a guide to common duct exploration. *Ann. Surg.* **150,** 1086–1091.

HOSFORD J. (1957) Treatment of stone in the common bile duct. *Br. Med. J.* **1,** 1202–1205.

JONES S. A. (1973) Sphincteroplasty (not sphincterotomy) in the treatment of biliary tract disease. *Surg. Clin. North Am.* **53,** 1123–1137.

KEIGHLEY M. R. B., WILSON G. and KELLY J. P. (1973) Fatal endotoxic shock of biliary tract origin complicating transhepatic cholangiography. *Br. Med. J.* **3,** 147–148.

KNIGHT P. R. and NEWELL J. A. (1963) Operative use of ultrasonics in cholelithiasis. *Lancet* **1,** 1023–1025.

LE QUESNE L. P. (1964) Choledocholithiasis. In: SMITH R. and SHERLOCK S. (ed.), *Surgery of the Gallbladder and Bile Ducts.* London, Butterworths, pp. 118–163.

LE QUESNE L. P., WHITESIDE C. G. and HAND B. H. (1959) The common bile duct after cholecystectomy. *Br. Med. J.* **1,** 329–332.

LONGLAND C. J. (1973) Choledochoscopy in choledocholithiasis. *Br. J. Surg.* **60,** 626–628.

MADDEN J. L. (1958) *Atlas of Technic in Surgery*. New York and London, Appleton-Century-Croft.

MALLET-GUY P. (1952) Value of peroperative manometric and roentgenographic examination in the diagnosis of pathologic changes and functional disturbances of the biliary tract. *Surg. Gynecol. Obstet.* **94,** 385–393.

MARGAREY C. J. (1971) Non-surgical removal of retained biliary calculi. *Lancet* **1,** 1044–1046.

NIENHUIS L. I. (1961) Routine operative cholangiography. *Ann. Surg.* **154,** 192–202.

NOLAN D. J. and GIBSON M. J. (1970) Improvements in intravenous cholangiography. *Br. J. Radiol.* **43,** 652–657.

PEEL A. L. G., HERMON-TAYLOR J. and RITCHIE H. D. (1974) Technique of transduodenal exploration of the common bile duct. Duodenoscopic appearances after biliary sphincterotomy. *Ann. R. Coll. Surg. Engl.* **55,** 236–244.

RÖSCH J. R., LAKIN P., ANTONOVIC R. and DOTTER C. T. (1973) Transjugular approach to liver biospy and transhepatic cholangiography. *N. Engl. J. Med.* **289,** 227–231.

SCHULENBURG C. A. R. (1966) *Operative Cholangiography*. London, Butterworths.

SHALDON S., BARBER K. M. and YOUNG W. B. (1962) Percutaneous transhepatic cholangiography. A modified technique. *Gastroenterology* **42,** 371–379.

SHEIN C. J., STERN N. Z., HURWITT E. S. and JACOBSON H. G. (1963) Cholangiography and biliary endoscopy as complementary methods of evaluating the bile ducts. *Am. J. Roentgenol.* **89,** 864–875.

10

Pancreatitis: Acute and Chronic

J. E. Trapnell, MD, FRCS

In this chapter it will not be possible to cover all aspects of this large subject, but we shall touch on those areas where new data have become available or where there is controversy. In fact, neither the acute nor the chronic relapsing forms of pancreatitis is common at the present time, but both are important clinically. Acute pancreatitis still carries an appreciable mortality and its management presents a variety of problems, while in the chronic forms of the disease the surgical treatment is complex and must be varied from case to case.

Acute pancreatitis

Although the actual cause of acute pancreatitis is still not known, it is obvious that the patient can only be treated scientifically if the pathological changes which develop in the gland are clearly understood. Originally a macroscopic description of oedema progressing to haemorrhage and then to necrosis was all that was available, but now, with a better understanding of the pathophysiology of the disease, a more sophisticated view can be presented.

   With the development of an episode of acute pancreatitis there is within the gland an explosive release of enzymes. These may be contained locally or may spill over into the general circulation. In one respect amylase is the most important of these, for it is the linchpin in the biochemical confirmation of a clinical diagnosis. However, this particular enzyme system, even in high concentration, is quite harmless to the patient. Lipase is also released and is involved in some complicated mechanism, not fully understood, in the development of fat necrosis. It is, however, the proteases which cause the main tissue damage and which make acute pancreatitis so dangerous. Some of the individual enzymes have been named and have been synthesized and their actions are understood. Trypsin, chymotrypsin, carboxypeptidase, elastase and lysolecithin fall into this category. The kinins—kallikrein and bradykinin—are also important (Ryan et al., 1965; Nugent et al., 1966). The physiological role of this group has not yet been elucidated, but they play a critical role in the pathological changes which occur in acute pancreatitis, for they are highly vasoactive. In addition, a whole range of short chain peptides are released which have barely been identified. In the past there has been a tendency to concentrate attention on one or other of these particular systems, but if one takes a wider, more balanced view it is immediately apparent that within this 'broth' it is not so much the individual constituent which is important but the over-all effect of the 'witches' brew' which is produced. This is vasoactive and highly destructive of tissue.

These dangerous substances may wreak their havoc locally where they produce increased tissue permeability and tissue necrosis. There is, therefore, a leak of a large amount of fluid into the pancreas, the peri-pancreatic and retroperitoneal tissues. Clinically this is seen as oedema in and around the gland, increased lymphatic flow and a peritoneal exudate, all resulting in a loss of extracellular fluid volume. In severe cases of pancreatitis as much as 5–6 litres of fluid may be effectively lost from the circulation in this way (Anderson et al., 1967; Nugent et al., 1969). A further local action resulting from the release of this enzyme-rich fluid is irritation and disorganization of the coeliac plexus. This, together with the oedema-distension of the gland tissue, is responsible for the very severe pain which is a salient feature in the majority of cases of acute pancreatitis.

In the last 4 or 5 years it has come to be recognized that acute pancreatitis is very often a multi-organ disease, for when the proteolytic enzyme systems fail to be contained in the vicinity of the gland by the body's own defence mechanisms, much more serious and more widespread effects are produced. The kinins are implicated in an alteration of the coagulation mechanism which takes the form of a consumptive coagulopathy (Kwaan et al., 1971). A degree of liver damage is present in nearly all cases of acute pancreatitis. This is reflected in the disturbance of liver enzyme patterns and it is also important clinically because in the investigation of these patients a cholecystogram cannot be performed within a month of the acute attack for, during this period of time, owing to the altered liver function, non-function of the gall bladder may be observed when in fact there is no biliary tract disease present. Then there is also a direct enzymic effect on the heart, the so-called myocardial depressant factor (Lefer et al., 1971). This probably accounts for the ECG changes which may be seen in the more severe cases and which are very similar to the changes occurring in ischaemic heart disease. This is perhaps not surprising because the effect of this enzyme release is basically vasoactive. The lungs are also affected. The mechanism here is not absolutely clear. It may be a primary effect on the alveoli themselves, for there is an alteration in pulmonary compliance and resistance (Ranson et al,, 1974). It is also possible that these changes may result from microembolism within the alveoli (Gupta, 1971). Finally, there is a direct effect on the kidneys. Renal failure is a well recognized complication of acute pancreatitis (Gordon and Calne, 1972; Imrie, 1974). Originally it was thought that this resulted purely from hypovolaemia. It then began to be apparent that there was a renal as well as a prerenal element and it was therefore suggested (Kwaan et al., 1971) that the damage was produced by microembolism. Quite recently Werner et al. (1974), in a well designed clinical study, have demonstrated a local pressor mechanism which may produce alteration in renal blood flow and glomerular filtration rates.

Aetiology

In spite of the fact that an enormous amount of experimental work has been carried out, the exact mechanism which triggers these pathological changes has not yet been elucidated. It is, however, recognized that a variety of other conditions predispose to acute pancreatitis—some commonly, some only rarely—and that these aetiologically related conditions also govern the natural history of the illness.

The present spectrum of these factors in Great Britain is fairly well represented by our own review of cases seen in Bristol over a 20-year period up to 1969 (Trapnell, 1972). There were, during this time, 590 patients with acute pancreatitis and the aetiological background of this series is shown in Table 10.1. Cases of post-operative and traumatic pancreatitis are not included in this review.

You will see that gallstones remain the commonest predisposing factor in Great Britain. With the current British surgical practice of removing gallstones on sight it was hoped that the incidence of acute pancreatitis might be falling, but careful analysis has not revealed any such trend (Trapnell and Duncan, 1975). This may perhaps be explained by the fact that in our study a quarter of the 316 cases with gallstone pancreatitis (81 patients) had no past history of any abdominal

Table 10.1 Aetiological factors in 590 cases of acute pancreatitis

Aetiological factors	No.	%
Biliary tract disease	316	54
Chronic alcoholism	26	4·5
Mumps	7	
Hyperparathyroidism	1	
Carcinoma	8	
Steroids	6	
Other	9	
Not stated	14	
Idiopathic	203	34·5

symptoms. The development of the acute pancreatitis was therefore the first indication that gallstones were present in this substantial percentage of cases.

The low incidence of chronic alcoholism will be noted and this is in marked contrast to experience in other parts of the world and in particular in Northern America, Europe and Australia, where alcoholic pancreatitis is a much greater problem. However, the British pattern appears to be changing, for our own studies have shown an increasing number of this type of case as the years have gone by (Trapnell and Duncan, 1975) and this trend is confirmed strongly by recent reports from London (James et al., 1974) and from Glasgow where Imrie (1975) is finding that over 20 per cent of his patients with pancreatitis are alcoholics.

Of the other smaller subgroups, mumps pancreatitis was of no great significance in our experience, for it is uncommon and mortality from this cause is virtually unknown. It is interesting, however, that of the 7 cases only 1 was in a child, 2 patients were in their teens and the eldest was a man of 48.

In spite of a careful check, either at autopsy or on follow-up, only 1 case of hyperparathyroidism was uncovered in this series. We therefore conclude that this is an uncommon cause of primary acute pancreatitis.

It is now well recognized that carcinoma of the head of the gland or of the ampulla may present as an acute pancreatitis. It was significant in analysis of these few cases that there was, in every instance, a gap of a year between the initial episode and a clear definition of the underlying malignant condition.

Steroid pancreatitis emerges as a definite entity from our study and it is likely to become increasingly important as more patients are placed on long-term therapy. While this will remain an uncommon complication of this form of treatment it is important, first because of the high mortality—5 of our 6 patients died—and secondly, because it is one of the causes of that rare condition, pancreatitis in children. This complication will also constitute a further hazard to patients undergoing organ transplantation who require long-term steroid therapy as part of their immunosuppressive regimen (Johnson and Nabseth, 1970).

Finally, you will see that the idiopathic group form the second largest subdivision in our experience and these cases also form a sizable proportion in other published series. The group represents an expression of our ignorance and it is therefore not surprising that attempts have been made to achieve a breakdown into smaller aetiological categories. Some writers have separated off a vascular subgroup (Mayday and Pheils, 1970). Certainly, vascular factors are largely responsible for the progression of the disease from its mild oedematous form to the severe haemorrhagic or necrotic state (Goodhead, 1969). Theoretically an acute ischaemia may well trigger the whole process in the first place. The difficulty really arises when one tries to formulate criteria upon which to incriminate this mechanism in the individual case. At the moment it would seem that more clarification must be achieved and more definite diagnostic criteria must be worked out before individual cases can be categorized into this particular subgroup.

Diagnosis

The diagnosis of acute pancreatitis can usually be made on clinical grounds with confirmation from a serum amylase level in excess of 1,000 Somogyi units/100 ml. However, at times it may be difficult to differentiate other abdominal disorders, especially as some of these, such as acute cholecystitis, perforated peptic ulcer, mesenteric infarction, strangulated intestinal obstruction and ruptured aneurysm, also show raised amylase levels. In addition to this problem our studies have shown that 5 per cent of patients with acute pancreatitis do not have any demonstrable elevation of amylase level and a further 5–8 per cent may present atypically without any pain. Obviously there will therefore be a diagnostic dilemma on occasions. Various alternative approaches to this diagnostic problem have been discussed elsewhere (Trapnell and Anderson, 1967), but basically the surgeon must decide whether or not a laparotomy should be performed in the dubious case. Traditional teaching has been that even a simple intervention is harmful, but in the last decade various studies have suggested that operation does not by itself increase mortality and our own series of cases certainly supports this view (Table 10.2). Let me, however, be quite specific on this point. Clearly operation must increase *morbidity*, for the patient has an incision which has to heal. Complications can arise, and stay in hospital will obviously be prolonged, but the evidence presently available shows that *mortality* is not increased. I would stress that I am not advocating a swing over to wholesale laparotomy in the diagnosis of acute pancreatitis, but it would seem that in a minority of patients, where the diagnosis is in doubt or where the patient fails to respond to rapid resuscitation, it would be safer to consider exploration than persist with conservative treatment. The argument runs as follows. All the alternative diagnoses which I have just mentioned—with the possible exception of acute cholecystitis—require surgical treatment if the patient is to be cured, and indeed if an aneurysm has ruptured it is obvious that operation must be undertaken very urgently if the patient's life is to be saved. If, therefore, laparotomy is performed in a doubtful case and the patient is found to have pancreatitis, usually no great harm will

Table 10.2 Immediate operation in acute pancreatitis

	Total	Died	%
Conservative treatment	442	89	20
Immediate operation	148	30	21

have been done, whereas if he is found to have something else a disaster may be averted.

The surgical management of acute pancreatitis

Diagnostic laparotomy

Whether or not the diagnostic procedure just outlined is carried out, from time to time an acute pancreatitis is uncovered at laparotomy and this will raise the old controversial question as to what further action, if any, should be taken at this time. We have looked at the records of our patients who underwent emergency laparotomy to see if they could provide any answers to this problem. Of the 148 cases, a number had a simple exploration and closure, but a considerable proportion also had some further procedure as well (Table 10.3). From an analysis of this clinical material some definite conclusions can be drawn, and first of all it is clear that the procedure to be adopted at this time really depends upon whether or not the patient has biliary tract disease.

Table 10.3 Operation in the acute state in 148 cases

Operation		
Laparotomy only	83	20
Cholecystostomy only	22	5
Cholescystoenterostomy	8	0
Cholecystectomy	25	1
with exploration of common bile duct	(11)	(1)
without exploration of common bile duct	(14)	(0)
Other operations	10	4

If gallstones are present then, provided that the patient is fit and the surgeon is sufficiently experienced and that the local conditions in the porta hepatis are satisfactory, cholecystectomy should be performed. What should be done about the common duct? First of all an operative cholangiogram should be performed with the precaution that bile should be aspirated from the common duct before dye is injected so as to prevent any rise in pressure in the hepatobiliary tree. If stones are demonstrated then, with the provisos already stated for cholecystectomy, the duct should be opened and these stones should be removed, but our experience has shown quite clearly that under no circumstances should the sphincter mechanism be tampered with at this time.

If there is no biliary tract disease present then cholecystectomy or indeed gall bladder drainage, whether external or internal, will not benefit the patient. Indeed, a study of our case material suggests that to operate on the biliary tract when it is not diseased may be positively harmful, but there were insufficient numbers to prove or disprove this particular point.

Can anything else be done for these cases in the 'acute laparotomy' situation— whether or not they have biliary tract disease? Three alternatives have been suggested: thoracic duct drainage, pancreatic resection and peritoneal dialysis.

We have already seen that in this condition a high concentration of damaging enzyme-rich fluid is produced in the vicinity of the pancreas. One of the routes by which this floods into the general circulation is through the thoracic duct, and Dumont et al. (1960) suggested that this might be diverted. Clinical experience of this form of treatment is very limited (Brzek and Bartos, 1969) and the method has not been taken up generally, so that no conslusions can be formed as to its value.

Pancreatic resection is also attractive theoretically, for this would remove not only the harmful fluid which has been produced but also the tissue from which it is being released. However, it is quite clear that near-total pancreatectomy is a major undertaking under any circumstances and in a patient with acute pancreatitis it must be regarded as distinctly hazardous. It is interesting, however, that this approach is being explored in various centres in different parts of the world at the present time (Hollender et al., 1971; Rives and Lardennois, 1974) and it seems likely that we shall hear more of the matter in the next few years.

Peritoneal dialysis has aroused considerable interest in the last few years and there have been a number of stimulating reports in the literature (Rosato et al., 1973). This is, so to speak, the 'halfway house' between heroic surgery and the pure conservative management with drugs alone. The method allows the washing out of the enzyme-rich broth.

When one is in the emergency laparotomy situation it is obviously important to know which patient is going to require some very major procedure such as subtotal pancreatectomy, for clearly it will only be indicated in the case that is likely to do badly. Because the whole matter of prognosis in the early stage of the illness presents considerable difficulties—and I will return to this problem again below—it would seem best at the present time, when one is faced with severe pancreatitis at operation, that dialysis catheters should be placed and that Trasylol should be added to the dialysate. Pancreatic resection should not be undertaken unless there are very special considerations and the surgeon is fully conversant with the handling of this operation.

Complications

While surgery may be required in the diagnosis of acute pancreatitis in the first 24–48 hours of the illness, operative intervention for the complications is rarely indicated until the second or third week or later. Fortunately, the complications of acute pancreatitis are not too common because when they do occur they lead to an increase in mortality. Seventy patients in our series (12 per cent) developed one or more problems and, of these, 27 (39 per cent) died. If the cases with abscess and pseudo-cyst formation, haematemesis and duodenal ileus are considered separately, then the mortality for this subgroup was 54 per cent and the seriousness of these major problems becomes fully apparent. In both abscess and pseudo-cyst the onset tends to be insidious so that the diagnosis can be extremely difficult. The management of all these complications has been discussed elsewhere (Trapnell, 1971) but in general terms it may be stated that surgical drainage is essential for the patient with a pancreatic or retroperitoneal abscess. The timing of operation is always difficult, but the patient will die unless drainage is effected. Laparotomy and gastrojejunostomy are also life-saving when duodenal ileus occurs. Surgery is less urgent for a pseudo-cyst and a conservative policy can be pursued because in a number of instances an upper abdominal swelling which may be thought to contain fluid is, in fact, simply a general inflammatory swelling around the pancreas with fat necrosis. Differentiation between such a swelling and a true pseudo-cyst is difficult clinically, but it appears that ultrasonic scanning is going to prove very useful in the differential diagnosis (Bradley and Clements, 1974). Surgical drainage is therefore only indicated either if the swelling persists or if it is enlarging, or if the patient develops signs of a spreading peritonitis suggestive of leakage. The other two major complications are haematemesis and renal failure. The former occurs usually as a terminal event and, unless immediate gastroscopy reveals some discrete lesion, operative intervention is probably best avoided. Renal failure may occasionally require dialysis, but with proper medical management it can be prevented in the majority of cases (see below, 'Medical treatment').

The final complication which requires mention is toxic psychosis, and in our experience these patients all presented in the same way. Each was admitted and then, 24–48 hours after the onset of their illness, they became confused, restless and hallucinated, so that restraint and heavy sedation were required. Within a further 48 hours the confusional state subsided and before the end of the first week all were normally orientated once again. A follow-up of these cases did not reveal any previous history of mental illness or any subsequent psychiatric disturbance. We have therefore concluded that this was just a manifestation of the severe illness. It is possible, however, that this confusional state was in a minor degree a manifestation of pancreatic encephalopathy. This has only been described in a few cases from autopsy findings and apparently it results from a lipolytic demyelinization of the central nervous system (Scharf and Bental, 1971).

Prevention of recurrent acute pancreatitis

Surgical intervention may be required, not only for the diagnosis or for the treatment of one of the complications of acute pancreatitis, but it may also be indicated after the patient has recovered from the acute episode. If the presence of gallstones is proved then cholecystectomy should be performed as an interval procedure—with operative cholangiography and exploration of the common bile duct if stones are shown to be present. In rare cases when a functioning para-thyroid adenoma is present, this should also be removed.

Clinical course and prognosis

Before the general aspects of the treatment of acute pancreatitis are discussed, it is pertinent for us to ask what is the likely outcome for a patient who suffers an attack. An analysis of our cases has shown that approximately one-fifth of the patients will die in their first attack, while half follow a mild uncomplicated course (Table 10.4). It would obviously therefore be most useful if one could

Table 10.4 Clinical course of acute pancreatitis

Course	%
Mild	46
Moderate	21
Severe	13
Died	20.2

Complications in 12%.

decide at the outset which path a particular patient is likely to follow. However, here one runs into another of the major problems which confront the clinician who is having to treat this condition. Acute pancreatitis is an unpredictable illness and it is difficult to give an immediate prognosis for an individual case. In the majority of patients the pattern is usually clear quite early on, but in a minority an unexpected deterioration or rapid improvement can occur, not only without warning but also as an apparent contradiction of the original clinical assessment. In particular, severe and most distressing pain can disappear rapidly, while even a shocked and apparently gravely ill patient often improves dramatically if adequate fluids are given intravenously. This unpredictable aspect of acute pancreatitis needs to be stressed at the present time for two reasons. First of all it makes the implementation of some major surgical procedure, such as pan-createctomy, very difficult, for one cannot predict at the outset which patient is going to require such radical treatment. Then secondly, this uncertainty makes the assessment of any form of treatment very difficult indeed. There is a real danger that improvement in the patient's condition may be attributed to some new drug when in fact it is just part of the natural history of the illness.

Medical treatment

The first and most important measure which must be taken in the treatment of all these cases is the massive replacement of lost fluid. Large amounts of saline, plasma and, in the later stages of the illness, blood will be required. In order that this fluid can be given rapidly it is now our practice to place a central venous pressure lead in all cases so that the rate of infusion can be carefully monitored. A nasogastric tube is also passed. This allows the stomach to be kept empty and lessens the vomiting and retching which will otherwise be so very distressing to the patient. Analgesics will obviously be required in nearly every patient and often in high dosage if the severe pain is to be controlled. Pethidine is the drug of choice, but if this is not effective morphine may be given.

Various forms of drug treatment have been advocated over the years, but in fact none is of any proven value. It has been traditional to give a full course of antibiotics and antispasmodics, but neither of these has ever been subjected to proper clinical assessment and there is no evidence that either is beneficial. In particular, it is worth stressing that if antibiotics are given they will not prevent abscess formation later on in the severe case where there has been tissue necrosis.

Steroids have also been advocated on the grounds that they may 'tide the patient over' during the initial phase of 'shock'. Once again, there is no evidence to support this hypothesis and I feel sure that group of drugs should not in fact be used. There is a real danger that, because they mask the clinical signs of hypovolaemia, the attending physician can be lulled into a false sense of security, for he will not be able to appreciate his patient's real need, which is for fluid.

In spite of the fact that these patients are hypovolaemic it has recently been recognized that the administration of a diuretic may be beneficial. In acute pancreatitis there is an alteration in renal blood flow and glomerular filtration rate (Werner et al., 1974) and it is this which predisposes to the renal failure which may complicate this condition. Frusemide is particularly indicated, not only because of its effect on the kidney but also because there is some evidence that it is beneficial in the shock lung state (Ranson et al., 1974). Obviously if this drug is to be used it becomes even more important that central venous pressure monitoring be maintained.

Studies in the last few years have clearly demonstrated that an alteration in pulmonary function is an important feature in this condition and it has been shown that in up to one-third of these cases there is a severe diminution in oxygen tension with Po_2 levels of less than 60 mm Hg. Not all patients with acute pancreatitis will require oxygen supplements, but it has become clear that all cases should have their arterial Po_2 measured, and if it is reduced then oxygen should be given by mask.

From the regimen which has just been outlined it is apparent that we now have a patient who is receiving large quantities of fluid, who has a central venous pressure lead in place, whose urinary output requires regular measurement and who may be receiving oxygen by mask. This type of case obviously requires high dependency nursing and it is therefore recommended that all these patients should be nursed in an intensive care unit, at least in the early stages. It may be argued that only a few patients really require this form of special care, but, as has already been stressed, because it is not possible at the outset of the illness to establish a firm prognosis it seems only reasonable to treat this potentially serious disease seriously in all cases.

In addition to the measures outlined, two further forms of treatment have received special attention in recent years.

Glucagon

Condon et al. (1973) have suggested that glucagon may be beneficial in the treatment of acute pancreatitis. They reported a small series of cases, but unfortunately their patients were uncontrolled and no valid assessment of this form of treatment has yet been published. Certainly glucagon does have a direct physiological effect, for it suppresses pancreatic secretion, but there are some theoretical objections to this very simple explanation if it should be proved to be effective in acute pancreatitis. Experimental work has clearly shown that the pancreas 'shuts down' at the onset of the acute attack (Dreiling, 1961) and there is also a considerable release of endogenous glucagon at this time (Paloyan et al., 1967). However, glucagon in addition to suppressing pancreatic secretion also increases coeliac blood flow and therefore tends to maintain the pancreatic micro-circulation. This in itself would be highly beneficial in a patient with acute pancreatitis (Goodhead, 1969) for it would tend to wash away and so dilute the vasoactive enzyme pool around and within the gland.

Aprotinin (Trasylol)

The proteolytic enzyme inhibitor, aprotinin, was introduced for the treatment of pancreatitis in 1958, and in the early 1960s there were many enthusiastic reports of its effectiveness. However, as time passed doubts began to creep in, conflicting findings were reported and, in Great Britain at least, its use has been largely discontinued until just recently. However, a further trial of this drug was begun in 1967 using a strict protocol. It was completed in 1973 and the results have been published recently (Trapnell et al., 1974). Time does not allow a full presentation of the results of this study, but in summary we took 105 patients who were suffering from their first attack of either gallstone or idiopathic pancreatitis. They were all treated in exactly the same way, except that one group received aprotinin A and the other aprotinin B. At the conclusion of the study it was found that the 52 cases receiving aprotinin A had a significantly lower mortality than the B group. There were 4 deaths in group A and 13 deaths in group B (Table 10.5). This difference was significant at the 5 per cent level. On breaking the code of the trial it was found that ampoule A had contained the active aprotinin, while group B had served as the controls. The effect of age was also studied (Table 10.6). It is well recognized that the mortality of acute pancreatitis rises with advancing age and our control group B conformed to this

Table 10.5 Results of aprotinin (Trasylol) trial

Grade	Group A		Group B	
	No.	Died	No.	Died
I	2	–	3	1
II	25	2	30	6
III	25	2	17	5
IV	1	–	2	1

pattern. However, in group A there was no such increase and when we came to compare the patients over 50 years of age in groups A and B there was now a highly significant difference in mortality in favour of the patients who had received aprotinin. This second analysis therefore confirmed not only that aprotinin was beneficial but that it appeared to minimize the usual effect of age on mortality.

Table 10.6 Effect of age on mortality

Age (years)	Group A		Group B	
	No.	Died	No.	Died
0–39	7	0	5	1
40–49	8	1	11	0
50–59	9	1	8	3
60–69	14	1	14	5
70+	15	1	14	4

The findings of this trial are clearly at variance with many other reports, but in the results of our study which we have reported we looked critically at the literature and concluded that most of the other trials did not provide sufficient data to merit some of the conclusions which had been drawn from them.

No drug should be finally accepted on the basis of just one report, but it would seem, in the light of this new evidence, that aprotinin should be reconsidered—that it should be thrown back into the ring for discussion rather than be thrown out of the window—and that while it is studied further it should now be used in the treatment of acute pancreatitis until it is proved to be ineffective.

Chronic relapsing pancreatitis

Space will only permit a few words about chronic relapsing pancreatitis. This is a difficult and nebulous condition, with ill defined diagnostic criteria. Indeed there is a danger that it may be used as a blanket diagnosis for all sorts of upper abdominal pain for which no other cause can be found. It has therefore tended to become a sort of upper abdominal ragbag. This has led to unnecessary confusion. There are in fact three fairly well defined syndromes which are produced by chronic pancreatic disease. First, a fibrotic gland may cause obstructive jaundice, although this is a rare finding in the United Kingdom at the present time. Obstructive jaundice due to a lesion in the head of the pancreas, whether painful or painless, is far more likely to be due to a carcinoma. Then secondly, the syndrome of pancreatic insufficiency both exocrine and endocrine, with steatorrhoea and diabetes, is well defined. These patients may also show calcification radiologically. When pain is present the condition should properly be categorized as chronic relapsing pancreatitis. Calcification is commonly, though not universally, present in this syndrome and as destruction of the gland progresses not only does the pain increase but, once again, diabetes and then steatorrhoea may develop so that there is overlap with the previous group.

The treatment of chronic pancreatitis is mainly medical. Replacement therapy will be required when the patient becomes diabetic and also for steatorrhoea, although the supplements presently available are not 100 per cent corrective. The only general indication for surgery is the presence of severe and intractable pain. Much more rarely, intervention may be required for jaundice and from time to time patients will be encountered who have suffered a haematemesis from a localized form of portal hypertension due to splenic vein thrombosis. In these cases splenectomy is a completely effective form of treatment.

However, as I have already stressed, the main indication for surgical intervention in these cases is the presence of severe pain. It is significant that a multitude of operations have been devised and this is an index of the unsatisfactory results which have been obtained. Various biliary tract procedures were advocated, including sphincterotomy, but these have not stood the test of time except in a very small group of patients where it can be shown that there is a dilated pancreatic duct with the dilatation extending right down to the sphincter of Oddi.

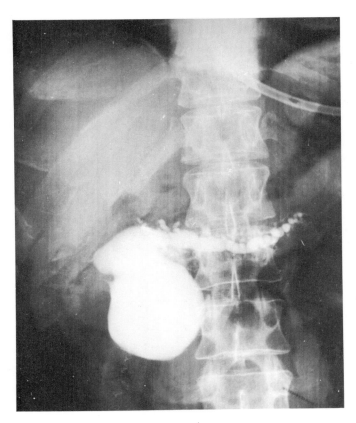

Fig. 10.1 Pancreatogram in chronic relapsing pancreatitis showing a 'chain of lakes' appearance and a pseudo-cyst.

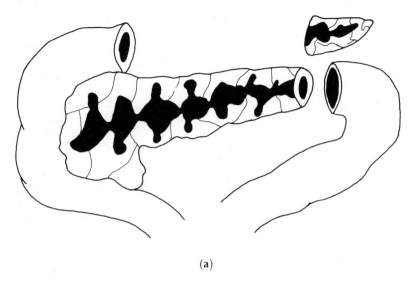

(a)

Fig. 10.2 (a) Surgical alternatives in treatment. Drainage by amputation and invagination.

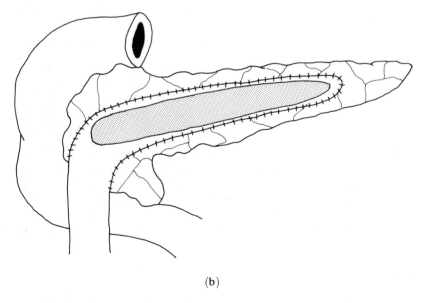

(b)

Fig. 10.2 (b) Surgical alternatives in treatment. Drainage by 'ductojejunostomy'.

Nerve cutting operations were popularized in France in the 1950s, but these, too, have fallen into disrepute. The two main alternatives in the treatment of this condition both involve a direct attack on the pancreas—the gland may either be drained or resected. Clearly the decision as to which type of operation is employed depends upon the state of the pancreatic duct. For this reason it should now be general practice that all patients who may require surgical treatment for chronic relapsing pancreatitis should have as part of their pre-operative work-up a peroral endoscopic retrograde pancreatogram. In expert hands this procedure is now achieving an 85–90 per cent success rate; the information it supplies is invaluable to the surgeon, not so much in providing him with a diagnosis of pancreatic disease as in guiding him as to what procedure he should perform once a decision has been taken that the patient has to be explored.

When the pancreatic duct can be shown to be grossly dilated (Fig. 10.1) then some form of drainage is advised. Originally, Duval and Enquist (1961) effected this merely by amputating the tail of the pancreas and anastomosing the stump of the body to a defunctional Roux loop. The results of this procedure were not too satisfactory and the operation was therefore modified by Puestow and Gillesby (1958) who advised that the main duct should be opened up and the gland 'filleted'. They mobilized the whole body of the pancreas and invaginated it into the Roux loop, thus promoting a much wider drainage of the dilated duct system (Fig. 10.2a). Further modification of the operative technique by White (1966), among others, now leaves the gland undisturbed; the duct is unroofed in situ and an opened Roux loop is patched over the surface so as to give an internal drainage (Fig. 10.2b). Up to the present time no long-term follow-up studies of any of these procedures have been published and it is therefore difficult to assess the results of this group of operations. They do, however, have the advantage that nearly all of the pancreas is left in situ and therefore there is a maximum preservation of both acinar and islet tissue.

Alternatively, in patients still with very severe pancreatitis the pancreatic duct may be compressed with no evidence of obstruction (Fig. 10.3) and indeed in our experience this is the commonest finding in this type of case in Britain. Clearly drainage would not be of any benefit and therefore resection must be considered. Most surgeons agree that a total removal of the pancreas is not justified for a benign condition and the operation most commonly employed at the present time is that devised by Dr Gardiner Child et al. of Ann Arbor University (1969). They described an 80–90 per cent resection of the gland with preservation of a strip of tissue in the head lying within the duodenal curve and protecting the common bile duct and the superior pancreaticoduodenal artery (Fig. 10.4). This operation involves sacrifice of islet cell tissue as well as of the general pancreatic gland substance, but it may be the only means of relieving pain in some of these chronic problem cases. The operation is technically quite difficult and in our experience there is a definite morbidity, though no mortality, associated with the procedure.

Conclusion

In this lecture it has only been possible to touch on some aspects of the complicated disease which we call pancreatitis. In both its acute and chronic forms many

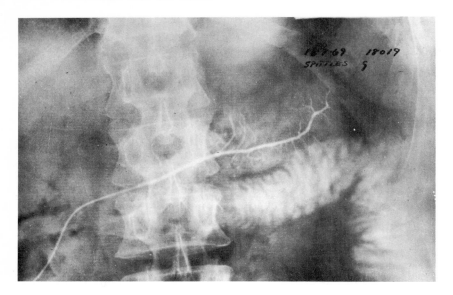

Fig. 10.3 Pancreatogram in a case of chronic relapsing pancreatitis showing a normal calibre duct.

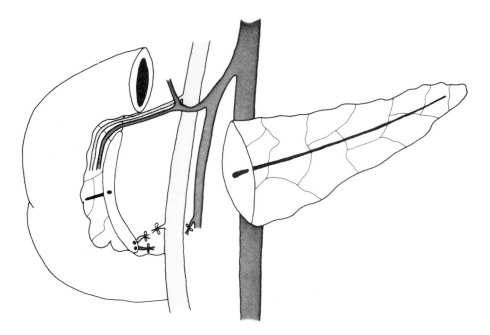

Fig. 10.4 Surgical alternatives in treatment. Resection.

problems remain, but it is encouraging to find that we are attaining a better understanding of the pathophysiology of the acute attack, that drugs are beginning to be tested properly, that mortality may be lowered with Trasylol, and that in the more chronic forms of the disease the indications for and selection of surgical procedures are becoming rationalized.

References

ANDERSON M. C., SCHOENFELD F. B., IAMS W. B. and SUWA M. (1967) Circulatory changes in acute pancreatitis. *Surg. Clin. N. Am.* **47**, 127–140.

BRADLEY E. L. and CLEMENTS J. L. (1974) Implications of diagnostic ultrasound in the surgical management of pancreatic pseudocysts. *Am. J. Surg.* **127**, 163–173.

BRZEK V. and BARTOS V. (1969) Therapeutic effect of the prolonged thoracic duct lymph fistula in patients with acute pancreatitis. *Digestion* **2**, 43–50.

CHILD C. G., FREY C. F. and FRY W. J. (1969) A reappraisal of removal of ninety-five per cent of the distal portion of the pancreas. *Surg. Gynecol. Obstet.* **129**, 49–56.

CONDON J. R., KNIGHT M. and DAY J. L. (1937) Glucagon therapy in acute pancreatitis. *Br. J. Surg.* **60**, 509–511.

DREILING D. A. (1961) The pathological physiology of pancreatic inflammation: current status 1960. *JAMA* **175**, 183–186.

DUMONT A. E., DOUBILET H. and MULHOLLAND J. M. (1960) Lymphatic pathway of pancreatic secretion in man. *Ann. Surg.* **152**, 403–409.

DUVAL M. K. and ENQUIST I. F. (1961). The surgical treatment of chronic pancreatitis by pancreaticojejunostomy: an 8-year reappraisal. *Surgery* **50**, 965–969.

GOODHEAD B. (1969) Vascular factors in the pathogenesis of acute haemorrhagic pancreatitis. *Ann. R. Coll. Surg. Engl.* **45**, 80–97.

GORDON D. and CALNE R. Y. (1972) Renal failure in acute pancreatitis. *Br. Med. J.* **3**, 801–802.

GUPTA, R. K. (1971) Immunohistochemical study of glomerular lesions in acute pancreatitis. *Arch. Pathol.* **92**, 267–272.

HOLLENDER L. F., GILLET M. and KOHLER J. J. (1971) Die dringliche Pankreatektomie bei der akuten Pankreatitis. Bericht uber 17 eigene Beobachtungen. *Langenbeck's Arch. Chir.* **328**, 314–327.

IMRIE C. W. (1974) Observations on acute pancreatitis. *Br. J. Surg.* **61**, 539–544.

IMRIE C. W. (1975) Personal communication.

JAMES O., AGNEW J. E. and BOUCHIER I. A. D. (1974) Chronic pancreatitis in England: a changing picture? *Br. Med. J.* **2**, 34–38.

JOHNSON W. C. and NABSETH D. C. (1970) Pancreatitis in renal transplantation. *Ann. Surg.* **171**, 309–314.

KWAAN H. C., ANDERSON M. C. and GRAMATICA L. (1971) A study of pancreatic enzymes as a factor in the pathogenesis of disseminated intravascular coagulation during acute pancreatitis. *Surgery* **69**, 663–672.

LEFER A. M., GLENN T. M., O'NEILL T. J., LOVETT W. M., GEISSINGER W. T. and WANGENSTEEN S. L. (1971) Inotropic influence of endogenous peptides in experimental hemorrhagic pancreatis. *Surgery* **69**, 220–228.

MAYDAY G. B. and PHEILS M. T. (1970) Pancreatitis: a clinical review. *Med. J. Aust.* **1**, 1142–1144.

NUGENT F. W., ATENDIDO W. A., BULAN M. B. and MACDONALD A. J. (1966) Kininase activity in experimental pancreatitis. *Nature* **211**, 207–208.

NUGENT F. W., ZUBERI S. and BULAN M. B. (1969) Kinin precursor in experimental pancreatitis. *Proc. Soc. Exp. Biol. Med.* **130**, 566–567.

PALOYAN E., PALOŸAN D., HAPER P. V. (1967) The role of glucagon hypersecretion in the relationship of pancreatitis and hyperparathyroidism. *Surgery* **62,** 167–173.

PUESTOW C. B. and GILLESBY W. J. (1958) Retrograde surgical drainage of pancreas for chronic relapsing pancreatitis. *AMA Arch. Surg.* **76,** 898–907.

RANSON J. H. C., TURNER J. W., ROSES D. F., RIFKIND K. M. and SPENCER F. C. (1974) Respiratory complications of acute pancreatitis. *Ann. Surg.* **179,** 557–566.

RIVES J. and LARDENNOIS B. (1974) La thérapeutique d'assèchement dans le traitment des pancréatites aiguës necrotico-hèmorragiques. (Aspiration gastro-duodénale pancréatectomie gauche d'assèchement et drainage externe contrôlé.) *J. Chir. (Paris)* **107,** 249–274.

ROSATO E. F., MULLIS W. F. and ROSATO F. E. (1973) Peritoneal lavage therapy in hemorrhagic pancreatitis. *Surgery* **74,** 106–115.

RYAN J. W., MOFFAT J. G. and THOMPSON A. G. (1965) Role of bradykinin system in acute hemorrhagic pancreatitis. *Arch. Surg.* **91,** 14–24.

SCHARF B. and BENTAL E. (1971) Pancreatic encephalopathy *J. Neurol. Neurosurg. Psychiatry* **34,** 359–361.

TRAPNELL J. E. (1971) Management of the complications of acute pancreatitis. *Ann. R. Coll. Surg. Engl.* **49,** 361–372.

TRAPNELL J. E. (1972) Acute pancreatitis. *Clin. Gastroent.* **1,** 147–166.

TRAPNELL J. E. and ANDERSON M. C. (1967) Role of early laparotomy in acute pancreatitis. *Ann. Surg.* **165,** 49–55.

TRAPNELL J. E. and DUNCAN E. H. L. (1975) Patterns of incidence in acute pancreatitis. *Brit. Med. J.* **2,** 179–183.

TRAPNELL J. E., RIGBY C. C., TALBOT C. M. and DUNCAN E. H. L. (1974) A controlled trial of Trasylol in the treatment of acute pancreatitis. *Brit. J. Surg.* **61,** 177–182.

WERNER M. H., HAYES D. F., LUCAS C. E. and ROSENBERG I. K. (1974) Renal vasoconstriction in association with acute pancreatitis. *Amer. J. Surg.* **127,** 185–190.

WHITE T. T. (1966) *Pancreatitis.* Baltimore, Williams and Wilkins. pp. 140–186.

11

Intestinal Obstruction in the Newborn

H. H. Nixon, FRCS

The many individually uncommon causes of intestinal obstruction in the new-born add up to a considerable clinical load in each region and account for about one-third of this specialized neonatal surgery. The units for treatment require the support of the surgeon by nurses, anaesthetists, physicians, pathologists and radiologists with experience in this field if satisfactory results are to be achieved.

The main grouping of causes of intestinal obstruction at this period is into the functional and organic causes. It is important to recognize that a considerable proportion of intestinal obstructions are caused by functional disorders which may not need surgery (about 20 per cent of our admissions) (Howat and Wilkinson, 1970), whereas those organic causes which do require surgery require it urgently to avoid complications. The cardinal presenting sign of obstruction is vomiting. This is green in all cases except obstructions above the ampulla of Vater. (Yellow vomits in the newborn are not uncommon and do not have the same significance. They are usually caused by concentration of carotene pigments from the colostrum and not really due to bile.) In obstruction above the ampulla of Vater significant vomiting of obstruction will be differentiated from the fairly common regurgitation of the normal, and particularly the premature newborn, by its persistence. The other classical signs of obstruction may be less helpful in this age group than in older patients. Distension, however, may precede vomiting in large bowel obstruction, whereas it will be virtually absent in duodenal obstruction. Constipation is not very helpful at the early stage when one hopes to make this diagnosis because the baby may pass normal meconium from below the obstruction for the first day or two.

Every green vomit merits a plain radiograph of the erect abdomen—an investigation which should confirm the presence of every complete obstruction. Only in cases suspected of incomplete or intermittent obstruction is it necessary to go on to the use of contrast examinations.

Fluid levels in the small intestine may be present in the normal newborn, particularly after a fit of crying. Only if the fluid levels are in dilated loops of gut are they significant of obstruction. In mechanical obstruction the dilatation will be progressive down to the level of the obstruction, and below this there will be a recognizably blank area in the abdomen (Fig. 11.1). In functional obstruction the distension is likely to be evenly distributed throughout the alimentary tract. Areas of calcification may be present, indicating pre-natal necrosis or

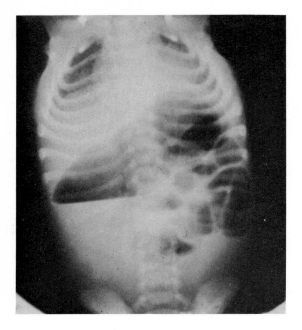

Fig. 11.1 Erect radiograph of mid small intestinal atresia.

perforation of gut with local or general intrauterine peritonitis. Clustering of the coils of bowel in one area of the abdomen, usually the upper left quadrant, also suggests adhesions caused by intrauterine peritonitis. Mottled meconium shadows in the area of the large bowel may be normal, but when they are visible in the area of the small intestine they suggest meconium ileus. In this condition the meconium may be so viscid that although the gut is visibly dilated no fluid levels are formed.

If the stomach has been aspirated and kept empty during transfer to the surgical unit as it should have been, then it is helpful to inject about 50 ml of air into the stomach as a safe contrast medium before taking this x-ray. Although the erect anteroposterior (AP) x-ray is the only essential one, it is useful to have a supine and lateral film in addition in some instances.

In perusing the film it is important to remember to look for evidence of gas under the diaphragm as an indication of perforation.

Functional obstruction

Neurogenic adynamic ileus may be a sequal to sepsis or to cerebral birth trauma or to a stressful birth without specific evidence of cerebral birth injury.

Adynamic ileus due to sepsis tends to occur later than the other forms of obstruction, towards the end of the first week of life, unless there has been prolonged rupture of the membranes before delivery. Hypotonia and poor peripheral circulation are common evidence of sepsis. The baby is often hypothermic rather than febrile. If frank peritonitis is present then the radiograph will show separation of the loops of intestine, but this form of obstruction will also occur with septicaemia in the absence of peritonitis.

The cerebral birth trauma may be recognizable from the jittery behaviour of the baby, who may have a tense fontanelle and a fluctuating temperature and other vital signs. In more severe cases, the baby may be flaccid and unresponsive.

In the absence of obvious cerebral birth trauma, stress caused by anoxia, prematurity, respiratory distress syndrome or exchange transfusion are all factors which seem to be related to the appearance of intestinal obstruction, which may imitate the low obstruction of Hirschsprung's disease. When such babies have been explored it has been observed that even at operation Hirschsprung's disease may be mimicked with the appearance of a cone from dilated to unexpanded colon, usually around the region of the splenic flexure. This has led to a number of unnecessary colostomies in the past. Immaturity of the ganglia has been suggested as being the cause of some of these functional obstructions. It seems to the author that this is probably a much less common cause than some perinatal stress.

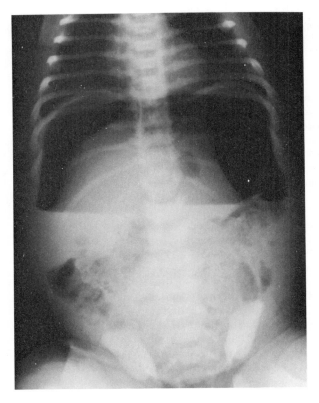

Fig. 11.2 Erect radiograph of perforation. 'Saddle bag' picture of gas under the diaphragm.

The majority of these settle on conservative management over a few days. There are some babies whose early symptoms are similar, and with a radiograph showing no more than a generalized gaseous distension of the gut, who progress to a much more serious condition of *necrotizing enterocolitis* (Touloukian et al., 1967). This condition seems to have the same aetiological factors. The primary reason appears to be a superficial ischaemia of the mucosa, suggesting a submucosal shunt of blood. No specific pathogenic infection has been incriminated. Following damage to the mucosa, secondary infections occur with the possibilities of pneumatosis intestinalis, septicaemia and perforation (Fig. 11.2). In surviving cases there may be late formation of fibrous strictures. It should be emphasized that in this age group pneumatosis intestinalis is evidence of a serious life-endangering lesion quite unlike the pneumatosis of the adult. The common practice of giving wide-spectrum antibiotics almost routinely to small premature babies with any symptomatology may mask the damage caused by this condition and delay the evidence of septic illness in the baby. The condition appears to be considerably commoner now than it was. This is probably in part due to the fact that improved neonatal care by the paediatricians allows babies who have had a severe anoxic insult to survive long enough to develop this bowel condition. It is also possible, as has been suggested by Barlow et al. (1974), that early feeding of cow's milk formulae and absence of the immunological support of breast milk is a factor.

Treatment

The treatment of functional intestinal obstruction will be primarily that of the underlying cause, such as cerebral birth trauma or septicaemia. The provision of a high oxygen concentration with constant positive airways pressure and correction of acidosis may be required in the respiratory distress syndrome. General measures will include nasogastric aspiration to avoid the risk of aspiration of vomit, which is the commonest complication of *any* obstruction in the newborn. Intravenous fluids will be required if the condition does not settle promptly. Barrier nursing in an incubator or radiant heat cot to preserve heat is mandatory.

Necrotizing enterocolitis is primarily treated conservatively by naso-gastric aspiration, wide-spectrum antibiotics, intravenous fluids and the usual general measures to preserve body heat. The abdominal x-ray is repeated 12-hourly, looking for evidence of perforation. A 'static loop' (that is, a fluid level which does not move) is also evidence of necrosis of that loop of bowel. Either of these factors or deterioration of the child's general condition are indications for operative intervention. The pneumatosis itself is probably not a definite indication for exploration. At operation the obviously necrotic bowel is excised and some difficulty may be found in deciding how much bowel it is necessary to resect. Primary enterostomy rather than anastomosis is wise. Intravenous feeding will then probably be required until the baby's condition and that of the bowel merits secondary anastomosis.

Organic intestinal obstruction in the newborn

Duodenal atresia and stenosis

In duodenal atresia the vomitus may not be bile-stained if the obstruction is above the ampulla of Vater, but its persistence will distinguish it from the occasional vomit of the healthy newborn. Abdominal distension will certainly be limited to the upper abdomen but is commonly not evident at all.

The x-ray shows the typical double bubble shadow of one fluid level in the stomach and one in the duodenum.

Unfortunately, about 30 per cent of duodenal atresias are related to Down's syndrome. In these the difficult ethical problem of whether or not to operate has to be faced.

Noblett (1970) and Gourevitch (1971) have independently made an interesting anatomical observation. In the past many cases of duodenal obstruction have been ascribed to an annular pancreas. This pancreatic abnormality, however, is unlike that seen in later life and consists more of an interposed pancreas. They have observed that in such cases the terminations of the biliary and pancreatic ducts may divaricate so that they enter the bowel above and below a complete atresia. Hence one has the paradoxical situation in which there may be complete intestinal obstruction and yet air is observed below the obstruction and bile may be seen in the vomitus of an obstruction above the pancreas. This may have accounted for an erroneous clinical impression that stenosis, as opposed to complete atresia, is much more common in the duodenum than elsewhere in the alimentary tract. The operation I prefer is an oblique end-to-end anastomosis rather than the classical duodenojejunostomy or gastrojejunostomy (Fig. 11.3). It avoids the persistence of a blind loop, and it is equally easy to perform. The right colon is gently mobilized to the left and the proximal duodenum is mobilized if necessary by the Kocher manoeuvre. The proximal and distal ends of the intestine at the site of the atresia are then easily approximated. The technique of suturing is much less important than the careful precise placement of each stitch.

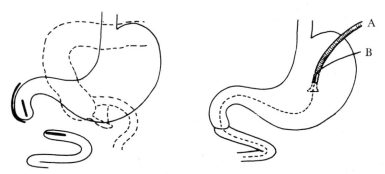

Fig. 11.3 Technique used in duodenal atresia. Colon reflected to left. Proximal duodenum mobilized by Kocher manoeuvre. Oblique end-to-end anastomosis. Gastrostomy tube (A) for aspiration. Silastic tube (B) for intrajejunal milk drip feeding. (Reproduced from Nixon, 1960, *Ann. R. Coll. Surg. Engl.* **27,** 105–124, by courtesy of the Editor.)

I usually use two stay-stitches to hold the pieces of bowel in apposition and then perform the anastomosis with interrupted invaginating sutures of 4–0 silk. A gastrotomy is made for placement of a 12-gauge French gastrostomy catheter. This is a much more effective means of maintaining post-operative gastric empty-ing than the tiny nasogastric tubes which can be placed in such small patients. A fine Silastic tube (such as that supplied for use with the Holter valve) is inserted through the same gastrotomy wound and is passed through the anastomosis and 5 or 6 cm down the jejunum before completing the anastomosis. This tube enables one to feed the baby by a milk drip from the day after operation. The gastrostomy is completed by suturing the catheter to the stomach wall with a catgut suture and then invaginating the stomach wall at right-angles to its long axis with two layers of black silk sutures on each side of the catheter. The tubes are brought out through a separate stab wound from the main incision and the stomach wall is held against the anterior peritoneum by two sutures. I believe this rather elab-orate form of gastrostomy is safer than simpler procedures.

Note that a mucosal diaphragmatic atresia or stenosis may not be externally recognizable. Gastrotomy and attempted passage of a 12F catheter may be neces-sary to confirm or exclude its presence.

A review of our experience at the Hospital for Sick Children, Great Ormond Street, demonstrated the value of early feeding as a general principle in neonatal surgery (Nixon and Tawes, 1971). Those mature babies who had duodenal atresia and no other abnormality all survived whether or not transanastomotic feeding was instituted. None of the babies who weighed less than 1.8 kg survived without transanastomotic feeding, but 40 per cent did when this was instituted.

In duodenal atresia, if one attempts early oral feeding vomiting tends to recur as the volume is increased because one still has an enlarged prominal duodenum and incompetent pylorus which may take about 2 weeks to recover function. In obstruction further down the intestine, feeding can usually be instituted within 48 hours of surgery, and if not then one now has of course the alternative of in-travenous feeding. Nevertheless, it remains a cardinal principle to use milk when-ever this is possible and human milk if this is available. Apart from the chemical suitability of human milk there is now evidence that it is also particularly bene-ficial in the first week or two of life for its immunological properties.

Jejunal ileal atresia and stenosis

Atresia of the mid-gut loop appears to be caused by a late fetal accident, unlike duodenal atresia which is probably developed at the organogenetic stage. In keeping with this, one finds that there is rarely any abnormality outside the ali-mentary tract. About 10 per cent occur as a complication of meconium obstruc-tion in cystic fibrosis. About 10 per cent are multiple. The classical clinical pre-sentation is by the development of green vomiting at about 24 hours of age, fol-lowed by progressive distension. (Most cases of stenosis present very similarly though perhaps rather later, but a few produce such mild obstruction that it is only recognized later in infancy or even in childhood due to persistent malnutri-tion and abdominal distension which has sometimes been mistaken for coeliac disease.)

The presence of distension at birth suggests pre-natal perforation with uterine peritonitis, or meconium ileus, as a cause of the obstruction. The x-ray typically shows progressively dilating loops down to the obstruction. Calcification may give evidence of intrauterine perforation, in which case one can anticipate troublesome adhesions.

Treatment

Treatment is by resection of the enlarged 15–25 cm of bowel proximal to the atresia with oblique end-to-end anastomosis to the collapsed distal bowel (Fig. 11.4). Even though the enlarged proximal bowel appears healthy it should be removed because it will not produce propulsive peristalsis at least for the next 14 days or so (Nixon, 1960). The acute dilatation of the gut may extend much further back but this, of course, is unimportant and collapses promptly after operation. What is important is to remove those last centimetres of bowel which are anatomically enlarged. It is technically important to take care in closing the mesenteric gap, adjusting this so as to shorten the lengthened proximal mesentery to the length of the distal mesentery. Otherwise the anastomosis is liable to be kinked at its outlet, causing obstruction.

The review of our series at the Hospital for Sick Children, Great Ormond Street, brought out some interesting points. Considering those babies weighing more than 1·8 kg and with no other life-endangering abnormality, the mortality of those occurring in the middle of the small intestinal loop was 20 per cent. Those in the terminal ileum had no mortality. However, those high in the jejunum (within 15 cm of the duodenojejunal flexure) had a 40 per cent mortality. It is my practice to resect these latter back to the duodenum and then to treat them just as for duodenal atresia. Howard and Otherson (1973), however, have recommended tapering the proximal bowel to a more normal calibre rather than excising it. Their results have been good, and the procedure is clearly preferable in the case where the bowel is unusually short.

Our series also demonstrated a 15 per cent occurrence of anastomotic complications, which had not diminished since 1949. These complications virtually all occurred in babies weighing less than 1.8 kg. It seems therefore that in such small babies primary anstomosis is unwise. My present policy in these is to carry out the Bishop–Koop type of vented anastomosis as described below for meconium ileus.

In babies of low birth weight a gastrostomy is added for ease of gastric emptying until peristalsis is resumed.

Another specific type of intestinal atresia is that which has been given the name of 'apple peel' atresia. The obstruction is at the duodenum or first few centimetres of jejunum. The distal bowel is unfixed by mesentery. It coils back and forth around the marginal vessel, receiving its blood supply from the inferior mesenteric artery. The appearances are apparently due to loss of the superior mesenteric vessel during development. The blood supply to the tip of the distal bowel is poor and primary anastomosis in my hands has broken down. It seems advisable to avoid it in these cases also by performing a primary jejunostomy or by some other means.

This condition is also unique amongst the atresias in appearing to have a strong

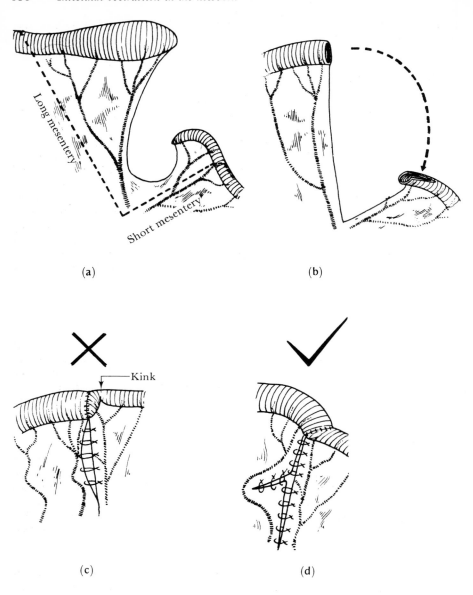

(a)   (b)

(c)   (d)

Fig. 11.4 Technique used in jejunoileal atresia. (**a**) Resection of enlarged 15–25 cm of bowel proximal to the atresia. (**b**) Incision of the anti-mesenteric border of distal bowel for 'end-to-back' anastomosis. (**c**) Hazard of kinking outlet when the proximal bowel distends. (**d**) Adjustment of the mesenteric suture to bring the proximal bowel down to the shorter mesentery of the distal bowel to avoid this. (Reproduced from Nixon and Tawes, 1971, Etiology and treatment of small intestinal atresia: analysis of a series of 127 jejunoileal atresias and comparison with 62 duodenal atresias. *Surgery* **69**, 41–51.

familial disposition to recurrence. (Blyth and Dickson, 1969; Mishalany and Najjar, 1968).

Multiple atresias

Frequently, the mutiple atresias are close together and can be resected *en bloc* so that a single anastomosis suffices. When they are more widely spaced the problem is more difficult. To perform two anastomoses in sequence invites trouble with the lower anastomosis. In general, it is considered that about 45 cm is the minimum length of small bowel in which one can expect normal function, but experience suggests that length is by no means the only factor. I have one child who was left with 27 cm of jejunum anastomosed to the ascending colon who is alive and well, having usually one stool a day and growing steadily along the 25th percentile at 9 years of age. It appears that if these children can be kept alive for the first 3 months of their life (a task made somewhat easier now by intravenous feeding) there is development of an increased absorptive area, allowing a positive balance to develop. The technique of narrowing rather than resecting the proximal bowel may be of particular value in such cases when the remaining gut is short.

Colonic atresia

Colonic atresia is rare, accounting for only about 5 per cent of all atresias. A primary colostomy is wise. Not only does it appear to be safer than attempted primary anastomosis but it also enables one to carry out a biopsy of the distal bowel to exclude the possibility of aganglionosis as an underlying cause of the pre-natal accident which has caused the atresia (I have treated two such cases).

Malrotation

The usual form of malrotation is in fact more correctly described as *incomplete rotation* (Fig. 11.5). The colon fails to complete the third stage of rotation so that the caecum remains in the upper abdomen with the colon proximal to it folded into a W loop. As a result the peritoneal bands which fix the caecum to the posterior abdominal wall cross the duodenum where they may obstruct it (Ladd's bands). In addition, this failure to complete the rotation leaves the mid-gut loop suspended from a narrow pedicle on the superior mesenteric vessels. The mid-gut loop is therefore prone to volvulus, which again presents clinically as a duodenal obstruction. Should the volvulus become tight enough the mesenteric circulation is interrupted and a closed loop strangulating obstruction may result, causing the onset of gangrene in virtually the entire mid-gut. It is for this reason that the diagnosis of malrotation is urgent even if the clinical condition at the time of presentation does not appear to be serious.

Whilst the majority of malrotations present in the newborn period, they may of course present later on in childhood and even in adult life either as the result of the progressive effects of a partial obstruction or of volvulus occurring later on.

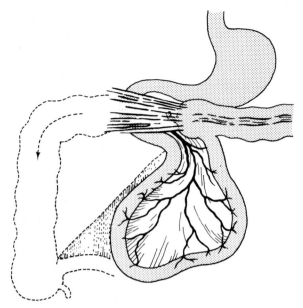

Fig. 11.5 Representation of the usual form of incomplete rotation. Bands cross duodenum and the mid-gut hangs from a narrow pedicle prone to volvulus. (Reproduced from Nixon and O'Donnell, 1966. *The Essentials of Paediatric Surgery*, 2nd edn. London, Heinemann Medical.)

Treatment

Treatment is by Ladd's ingenious procedure. He recognized that attempts to restore the normal anatomy were liable to be unsuccessful, but that if the intestine were returned to a completely unrotated state then this primitive position was nevertheless stable and compatible with a normal life, for it frees the duodenum from the obstructive bands and leaves the mid-gut hanging on a wider pedicle which is stable.

In volvulus neonatorum, when the abdomen is opened the first thing noticed is the absence of the transverse colon from its usual position across the abdomen. The intestines are brought out of the wound and the volvulus unwound. Attention is then given to the peritoneal bands which cross the duodenum from the undescended caecum. As these are divided the colon can be swept across to the left side of the abdomen. The misplaced ligament of Treitz is then divided so that the jejunum takes a straight course down from the duodenum on the right side of the vertebral column. This is usually all that is required except that it is usually wise to remove the appendix since it will be in an abnormal position following derotation. In babies in which the volvulus has taken place some time before birth, however, the loops of small intestine may be held together by shortened folds of peritoneum crossing from loop to loop and preventing the spread of the small intestine. In such cases it may be necessary to divide these peritoneal folds, leaving raw surfaces. This has not in my experience ever caused any trouble.

As long ago as 1955 I found that, of a series of 15 consecutive malrotations, 12 were alive and well; the 3 who had died had all done so as a result of diagnoses being delayed until mid-gut volvulus had proceeded to strangulation and hence loss of the mid-gut loop. It is therefore important to investigate further any baby with a history suggestive of incomplete or intermittent duodenal obstruction rather than continuing with further observations. A barium meal should be given, which will demonstrate duodenal obstruction by malrotation or any other cause. This is preferable to the traditional barium enema because the latter, although it does indicate the presence of incomplete rotation, does not give the essential information as to whether there is obstruction of the duodenum by this or some other cause. (There are many cases of incomplete colonic rotation which are quite symptomless and only discovered later *en passant*.) There are other less common forms of malrotation or malfixation which may cause obstruction.

1. Isolated malfixation of the duodenum by a misplaced ligament of Treitz may produce partial **obstruction** (including the 'accordion pleated duodenum'). It seems that some, if not all, of those cases described as mesenteric vascular duodenal ileus may be of this nature. The corrective operation is to divide the ligament of Treitz and move the duodeno-jejunal flexure to the right side, which would of course be corrective for either aetiology. Should mobilization be difficult due to shortness of the terminal vessels supplying the region of the flexure then a duodenojejunostomy around the area is a more elaborate but effective operation.

2. The so-called caecal volvulus is probably better described as volvulus of the mobile right colon. The defect here is malfixation of the right colon rather than malrotation. Suture of the caecum to the right iliac fossa is ineffective, but satisfactory fixation can be obtained by incising the parietal peritoneum and partially burying the caecum in the retroperitoneal space.

3. Reverse rotation of the mid-gut loop may occur, in which case the colon passes behind the duodenum. Relief is obtained by colostomy proximal to the retroduodenal loop. Continuity may then be re-established later by anastomosing the proximal colon to the distal part of the transverse colon. The retroduodenal colon may be left in situ if it is difficult to dissect out. It forms a blind diverticulum proximal to the anastomosis which empties satisfactorily into the distal bowel and hence no longer causes obstruction.

Incomplete rotation may occur in association with other forms of intestinal obstruction in the newborn such as a duodenal diaphragm. Such a diaphragm may not be recognizable externally; it is therefore important, if there is any doubt about filling of the distal bowel after relief of the malrotation, to perform a gastrotomy and pass a catheter several centimetres down the jejunum to be sure that there is no secondary cause of obstruction.

Meconium ileus

Meconium ileus is an obstruction caused by the abnormally viscid meconium in the condition of cystic fibrosis inspissating and blocking the lumen of the bowel. The obstruction is usually in the middle or lower ileum, though it sometimes occurs further proximally or more distally in the large bowel. It occurs in about

15 per cent of cases of cystic fibrosis. All will have to some extent the serious respiratory problems requiring prolonged care which are caused by the abnormally viscid bronchial mucus. They will also require pancreatin substitution for the lack of pancreatic secretion caused by the abnormal mucus in the ducts of that gland. However, the presence of meconium ileus does not mean that the pulmonary condition is more severe than in those cystic fibrotics who do not have meconium ileus. Indeed, the reverse may be the case and the fact that the condition is diagnosed at birth may enable the physician better to guard against the development of pulmonary infections (McPartlin et al., 1972). Clinically the baby presents with the onset of bile-stained vomiting, sometimes within a few hours of birth and sometimes delayed for 3 or 4 days. Abdominal distension may be present at birth or may develop later. On clinical examination it is usually possible to feel the firm masses of meconium in the dilated bowel. The x-ray appearance of mottled meconium shadows and failure to form fluid levels in the visibly dilated gut as described above may be quite typical.

However, as many as 50 per cent of cases of meconium ileus are complicated by pre-natal volvulus of the maximally dilated loop or perforation of the bowel or atresia, or combinations of these. Calcification may indicate these complications. Free gas under the diaphragm may indicate perforation, and clustering of the bowel shadows in one corner of the abdomen may also suggest pre-natal peritonitis. Frank distension of the abdomen at the time of birth is another indication of pre-natal peritonitis. Assessment of these indications of complication has become of more practical importance recently since Helen Noblett (1969) demonstrated that uncomplicated meconium ileus may be relieved by the use of a sodium diatrizoate (Gastrografin) enema without the need to resort to operation. Sodium diatrizoate (Gastrografin) acts both by its surface-acting agent and as a hygroscopic material to separate the viscid meconium from the bowel wall so that after the enema is given the meconium plugs are usually passed spontaneously (Fig. 11.6). She advises that a further enema should be given 48 hours later lest residual meconium re-inspissate and cause recurrent obstruction.

If the enema is unsuccessful, or if any of the factors described above suggest that this is a complicated case, then operation is required. The most effective operation has been found to be the Bishop–Koop (1957) procedure. The maximally dilated loop of ileum is resected, going far enough proximally to reach fluid bowel content. The proximal bowel is then anastomosed into the side of the bowel distal to the resected loop, leaving about 1·5 cm of this distal bowel proximal to the anastomosis to be drawn out through the abdominal wall through a small incision as a venting enterostomy. Bishop and Koop advised the insertion of a catheter into the bowel distal to the anastomosis so that irrigations could be given to clear the inspissated matter in the distal bowel. The use of sodium diatrizoate (Gastrografin) now facilitates this process, but it is not essential, for the ingress of intestinal flora soon liquefies the distal content. At first gas and bowel content are passed through the enterostomy; then as the distal bowel becomes clear, it ceases to act and the content passes on normally through the distal intestine. Bishop and Koop advised the formation of the enterostomy through a stab wound, expecting spontaneous closure. I have preferred to perform a formal enterostomy and to close this deliberately later by minor surgical procedure, having observed

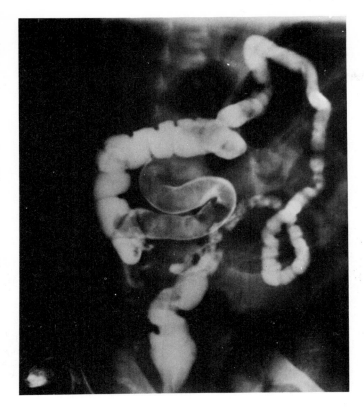

Fig. 11.6 Radiograph of Gastrografin enema in meconium ileus. Contrast passes through the empty colon to surround the mass of meconium in the ileum. This mass passed spontaneously.

leakage due to premature necrosis of the enterostomy drawn through a tight stab wound.

It is important to remember the hygroscopic effect of sodium diatrizoate (Gastrografin). If the baby is dehydrated this may be dangerously exacerbated unless intravenous replacement is instituted. This situation is particularly likely to occur in the small premature baby, and fortunately it is quite rare for meconium ileus babies to be of low birth weight.

Whilst about 75 per cent of babies with meconium ileus can be relieved of their obstruction, there is unfortunately a considerable mortality in infancy from the pulmonary effects of the underlying cystic fibrosis. The outlook for this condition, however, has been greatly improved recently by modern developments in their medical care.

Hirschsprung's disease

In Hirschsprung's disease or congenital intestinal aganglionosis the absence of the intramural plexuses always involves the distal bowel extending upwards from the anal canal for a varying distance. In the usual case the rectum and lower sigmoid only are involved. In short segment cases the entire aganglionic segment may be below the pelvic floor. In about 15 per cent of cases the aganglionosis may extend throughout the colon and even into the small intestine. Clinical presentation varies from a mere meconium retention relieved by an irrigation or even the passage of an examining finger per rectum up to a complete intestinal obstruction unrelieved by irrigation and requiring prompt laparotomy. The majority present with recurrent intermittent low intestinal obstructive symptoms. Abdominal distension will usually be recognizable before vomiting ensues. Although in general the longer segment cases present earlier than the short segment cases, the clinical severity does not regularly parallel the length of the segment though it is recognized that even in the milder cases there is almost invariably at least a history of delayed passage of meconium in the neonatal period. The mortality in infancy has been estimated to be at least 50 per cent without treatment; this is largely due to the complication of ischaemic enterocolitis which may complicate Hirschsprung's disease. Ischaemic enterocolitis produces a paradoxical picture of obstruction with apparent diarrhoea. The pathological appearance of the gut in this condition is very similar to that of the necrotizing enterocolitis which has already been discussed, and may lead similarly to death from septicaemia or 'endotoxic shock'. Some patients with Hirschsprung's disease appear to be prone to enterocolitis whereas others are not. The reason for this difference is not yet understood, but it is not dependent upon the length of the segment. The risk is present in short segment as well as long segment cases. Therefore the latter should not be considered as a less urgent problem. Even if transient obstructive symptoms appear to have relented in the newborn period, prompt investigation is still mandatory. Diagnosis is usually confirmed by barium enema (Fig. 11.7) which, even in the newborn period, is usually reliable in the hands of an experienced radiologist. It demonstrates the cone of transition from the unexpanded aganglionic segment to the dilated normally ganglionic bowel above. It is important that the investigation be carried out as a matter of urgency before any attempt is made to deflate the bowel by irrigation. Formal rectal biopsy can be a troublesome procedure in the newborn and requires general anaesthesia which may be ill withstood by a sick baby. Recently the technique of suction biopsy has been shown to be a reliable substitute in the hands of an expert pathologist (Campbell and Noblett, 1969). Histological examination reveals the absence of ganglia and the presence instead of massive nerve trunks in the submucosal region. Experience has shown that it can be accepted that the submucous and myenteric plexuses are present or absent to the same level in all cases. Full thickness rectal biopsy is therefore no longer necessary to confirm the diagnosis. When the diagnosis is confirmed the treatment is to perform a colostomy. It is always wise to attempt to deflate the bowel by saline irrigations before operation if possible.

This is particularly important in the presence of enterocolitis because sudden deflation by colostomy is sometimes followed several hours later by severe circulatory collapse even when care is taken to replace fluid lost into the third space (Fraser and Berry, 1967). In the presence of enterocolitis it is important to give wide-spectrum antibiotics, with blood, plasma or dextran as indicated to maintain the circulating volume. The value of massive doses of steroids is not proven, but many believe it is wise to give, say, 60–100 mg of hydrocortisone intravenously before fluid replacement, repeating this 6-hourly over the next 24 or 36 hours. In the newborn it is wise to site the colostomy immediately above the aganglionic

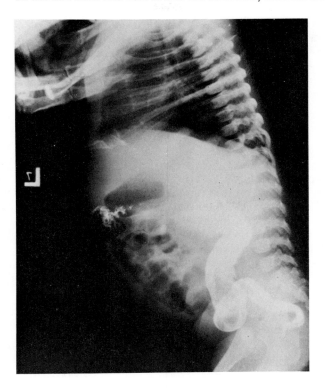

Fig. 11.7 Barium enema to demonstrate Hirschsprung's disease in a newborn: unexpanded (aganglionic) rectum 'coning' out into dilated (ganglionic) sigmoid.

segment so as to maintain all the ganglionic bowel in the functioning state so that it will develop and grow with the baby. Ideally, this level should be chosen with the help of frozen section biopsies at operation to confirm the presence of ganglia. In an emergency this may not always be practicable. Then the colostomy should be sited about 5 cm above the cone of transition from the distended but ganglionic bowel to the unexpanded aganglionic distal bowel. A sliver of bowel wall from the colostomy site is taken for prompt post-operative histological examination. Should the cone of transition be proximal to the splenic flexure then experience has shown that in the neonatal period it may be a considerable distance below the true zone of transition to aganglionosis. In such cases it would be wiser to perform a formal ileostomy, taking biopsies from selected sites on the colon at the same time if the child's condition allows. I prefer to perform an end colostomy, siting the opening as low in the abdomen as is practicable and bringing out the distal bowel as a suprapubic fistula. I find it more convenient to take down such a colostomy in a cleanly fashion at the time of the definitive resection than is the case with the usual loop colostomy.

If the standard right transverse colostomy is performed in the neonatal period for the usual length of segment, then the bowel distal to the colostomy fails to lengthen and, more important, its supplying mesenteric vessels fail to lengthen, so that it may be difficult to bring the ganglionic bowel down to the level of the anus without tension at the definitive operation. Such a right transverse colostomy is, of course, entirely suitable in infants and older children when the sigmoid loop has already developed and enlarged before the operation has been undertaken, and it can be left to protect the anastomosis at the definitive procedure.

Meconium plug

Some babies present an appearance of abdominal distension followed in due course by vomiting, which raises the clinical suspicion of Hirschsprung's disease. However, when a finger is passed into the rectum or perhaps when a rectal irrigation has been carried out, a long plug of inspissated meconium with a mucous tip is passed. This is followed by a gush of normal meconium. The child then remains well with no aftermath. Since the neonatal signs of Hirschsprung's disease can be equally transient and not recur for a matter of weeks or even months in the clinically milder cases, the diagnosis of meconium plug must only be made after barium enema and suction biopsy have excluded Hirschsprung's disease. It is also important to exclude the possibility of a forme frustre of meconium ileus by performing a sweat test to measure the level of chloride, which is abnormally raised in cystic fibrosis.

Rarities

Intestinal obstruction in the newborn can also be caused by a number of even less common conditions, such as mesenteric cysts. These may cause obstruction by stretching of the bowel over the periphery of the cyst or by volvulus of the loop containing the cyst. Similarly, a Meckel's diverticulum may form the axis of a volvulus causing neonatal intestinal obstruction. Another important group of conditions are those which are rare in the neonatal period but commoner later on in infancy. These include incarceration of an inguinal hernia, intussusception and pyloric stenosis. Delayed passage of meconium may also result from a generalized condition such as hypothyroidism. Milk bolus obstruction seems to be related to earlier feeding with roller-dried milks (Dickson et al., 1974).

Management

Management should begin in the obstetric unit, for it is unfortunately still not uncommon for unnecessary complications to arise from inadequate preparation for transfer to the paediatric surgical unit. Transport should be in an incubator to prevent heat loss to which the newborn, and particularly the premature, is very rapidly prone. Hypothermia is an important factor in the development of the potentially lethal condition of scleroedema. Even after rewarming, these babies seem to remain more vulnerable. A nasogastric tube should be passed to empty the stomach. The tube should be left open throughout transport and should be aspirated at quarter-hourly intervals. The baby should be nursed in the semi-prone 'coma' position, to avoid the risk of aspiration should vomiting occur. Unless diagnosis has been grossly delayed there will be no need for intravenous fluids before transfer, and increased oxygen in the incubator is unlikely to be necessary. With these precautions, the obstructed newborn can travel vast distances so that there is no justification for attempting surgery with inadequate facilities.

On arrival it is important that the clinical examination should include careful examination for associated anomalies and of the general condition of the baby as well as matters related to the obstruction. Confirmation of the latter will usually be achieved by an erect x-ray of the abdomen as discussed above. The serum electrolytes will be examined as a base line, although it is not usually necessary to correct losses before operation unless diagnosis has been late. If, however, a high obstruction has resulted in alkalosis, it is wise to correct this before surgery or the procedure appears to be ill tolerated. It is important to have blood cross-matched and a reliable intravenous infusion running before operation is started even though the actual blood loss in the majority of cases will not justify transfusion. The blood sugar should be estimated and the simple Dextrostix method is usually adequate. This is particularly important in the light-for-dates baby, who is especially prone to hypoglycaemia.

Dextrostix estimations should be repeated at least 12-hourly for the first day or two after operation. Should the baby become frankly jaundiced, it is important to estimate the bilirubin because of the hazard of kernicterus in the neonatal period caused by unconjugated hyperbilirubinaemia, especially in the premature baby. If the total bilirubin reaches 20 mg% exchange transfusion is indicated and in certain circumstances, again particularly in the premature, a lower level or a rapid rise on repeated estimation may justify exchange. Fits in the newborn may be caused by cerebral birth trauma or by metabolic disorders. The former usually occur in the first day of life and the latter a little later in the third or fourth day. Should they occur then alkalosis, calcium or magnesium deficiency should be suspected and treated according to the findings.

It is usual to keep the intravenous infusion running for the first day or two after operation lest it be required for any emergency situation such as hypoglycaemia. The actual fluid requirements, however, are very small and in general it is more important to avoid over-hydration than moderate dehydration. About 50 ml/kg/24 hours of 5% glucose will usually be sufficient. The electrolyte content of the infusion may be altered according to the state of the baby and serum electrolyte estimations. It should be remembered, however, that a moderate decrease in the serum sodium concentration after operation is common and is the result of a relatively greater water retention than sodium retention and not an indication of a true deficit requiring sodium infusion.

The nasogastric or gastrostomy tube will be left open after operation and aspirated at regular intervals. It must be remembered that the lumen of a nasogastric tube of a diameter which can safely be left in situ in the newborn is quite small and will block easily. It is important, therefore, that 1 ml of saline should be syringed through before each aspiration, to clear the tube. Oral feeding can usually begin about 48 hours after operation, ideally using expressed breast milk. This may not be obtainable, when a half-strength formula should be used and may be given at half strength for the first day. Small amounts are given hourly and gradually stepped up over the next 2–3 days to the baby's requirements. If there is delay in restoration of intestinal function for 4 days one should consider the use of intravenous feeding. If oral feeding is delayed for 7 days then one should almost certainly start an intravenous regimen. We have found the use of Vamin, 10% glucose, Intralipid 20%, electrolytes, trace elements and vitamins to be a satisfactory formula. It is given into peripheral veins, changing the site almost every 24 hours. This averts the more serious hazards of central line feeding.

Should the institution of milk feeds be followed by the development of diarrhoea and perhaps abdominal distension then carbohydrate intolerance must be suspected. The commonest form of intolerance is to lactose. Stool should be tested to see if it has become acid, and both stool and urine should be tested for abnormal sugars. Then oral feeding should be replaced by 5% glucose until the analyses are returned. Should the baby's general condition not have deteriorated it may be reasonable to go straight on to a glucose–galactamine milk which is suitable for lactase deficiency and is the one usually required. This disaccharide intolerance is of a temporary nature and tends to clear up in 6–12 weeks after intestinal surgery, unlike the congenital lactase deficiency which is persistent.

The anaesthetist may wish a high concentration of moisture in the incubator for the first day or so after anaesthesia, to reduce the risk of inspissation of mucus in the bronchi which can otherwise cause pulmonary collapse. The high humidity should not be continued longer without some specific indication because it does greatly encourage the development of *Pseudomonas pyocyanea* in the incubator. The incubator should be maintained at the thermoneutral temperature for the baby, which will be about 32–35°C. Since 'surgical babies' require much more handling than 'medical babies' the greatest care must be taken to avoid infection. Many believe that it is more easily attained by the use of a radiant heat crib, which is easier to clean. It has the added advantage that the baby can be nursed naked and observed in the closed crib whereas in the incubator it is necessary to cover the baby with Gamgee or alternatively with an internal Perspex shield to prevent heat loss by radiation.

References

BARLOW B., SANTULLI T. V., HEIRD W. C., PITT J., BLANC W. A., and SCHULLINGER J. N. (1974) An experimental study of acute neonatal enterocolitis. The importance of breast milk. *J. Pediatr. Surg.* **9,** 587–595.

BISHOP H. C., and KOOP C. E. (1957) Management of meconium ileus: resection Roux-en-Y anastomosis and ileostomy irrigation with panoreatic enzymes.

BLYTH H. and DICKSON J. A. S. (1969) Apple peel syndrome (congenital intestinal atresia): a family study of seven index patients. *J. Med. Genet.* **6,** 275–277.

BUGHAIGHIS A. G. and EMERY J. L. (1971) Functional obstruction of the intestine due to neurological immaturity. *Prog. Pediatr. Surg.* **3,** 37–52.

CAMPBELL P. G. and NOBLETT, H. R. (1969) Experience with rectal suction biopsy in the diagnosis of Hirschsprung's disease. *J. Pediatr. Surg.* **4,** 410–415.

DICKSON, J. A. S., LEWIS C. T. and SWAIN V. A. J. (1974) Milk bolus obstruction in the neonate. *Arch. Dis. Child* **49,** 825.

FRASER G. C. and BERRY C. (1967) Mortality in neonatal Hirschsprung's disease with particular reference to enterocolitis. *J. Pediatr. Surg.* **2,** 205–211.

GOUREVITCH A. (1971) Duodenal atresia in the newborn. *Ann. R. Coll. Surg. Engl.* **48,** 141–158.

HOWARD E. R. and OTHERSON H. B. JR (1973) Proximal jejunoplasty in the treatment of jejunal atresia. *J. Pediatr. Surg.* **8,** 685–690.

HOWAT J. M. and WILKINSON, A. W. (1970) Functional intestinal obstruction in the neonate. *Arch. Dis. Child.* **45,** 800–804.

MCPARTLIN J. F., DICKSON J. A. S. and SWAIN V. A. J. (1972) Meconium ileus. Immediate and long-term survival. *Arch. Dis. Child.* **47,** 207–210.

MISHALANY H. G. and NAJJAR F. B. (1968) Familial jejunal atresia: three cases in one family. *J. Pediat.* **73,** 753–755.

NIXON H. H. (1955) Intestinal obstruction in the newborn. *Arch. Dis. Child.* **30,** 13–22.

NIXON H. H. (1960) An experimental study of propulsion in isolated small intestine, and application to surgery in the newborn. *Ann. R. Coll. Surg. Engl.* **27,** 105–124.

NIXON H. H. and TAWES R. (1971) Etiology and treatment of small intestinal atresia: analysis of a series of 127 jejunoileal atresias and comparison with 62 duodenal atresias. *Surgery* **69,** 41–51.

NOBLETT H. R. (1969) Treatment of uncomplicated meconium ileus by Gastrografin enema: a preliminary report. *J. Pediatr. Surg.* **4,** 190–197.

NOBLETT H. R. (1970) Anatomical study of duodenal atresia. Proceedings of Centenary Meeting of Royal Children's Hospital, Melbourne (published privately).

TOULOUKIAN R. J., BERDON W. E., AMOURY R. A. and SANTULLI T. V. (1967) Surgical experience with necrotizing enterocolitis in the infant. *J. Pediatr. Surg.* **2,** 389–401.

12

Acute Intestinal Obstruction

L. P. Le Quesne, DM, MCh, FRCS, FRACS (Hon.)

Acute intestinal obstruction is a common condition which still carries a significant mortality. It can result from a variety of causes, and there is a tendency to concentrate on the features which differentiate one cause from another at the expense of the features of intestinal obstruction itself. This is unfortunate as patients do not present as cases of obstruction due to adhesions or sigmoid volvulus, but with the symptoms and signs of intestinal obstruction, and the factors common to all patients with acute intestinal obstruction are more important than the features which separate one cause from another. It is only by a consideration of these factors that we can properly understand the problems posed by a patient with acute intestinal obstruction. The purpose of this chapter is to review the main pathophysiological factors which constitute the illness of acute intestinal obstruction and which, unchecked, eventually lead to the death of the patient, and then to discuss the general principles of management.

Classification

As a preliminary, it is essential to have a logical foundation on which to base such a review, that is to say a meaningful classification of the condition as a whole. The traditional classification of intestinal obstruction as to whether the obstructing agent is intraluminal, in the wall of the bowel, or extramural is based on characteristics which are of little or no importance in relation to the essential consequences of intestinal obstruction. Such a classification is best abandoned, and replaced by one, as illustrated in Fig. 12.1, based on factors germane to the crucial pathophysiological changes occurring as a result of the obstruction. Acute obstruction is divided primarily (A) into two main categories; that in which the obstruction is due to *mechanical causes*, and that in which it is due to a disturbance of intestinal motility, so-called *adynamic obstruction*, of which the commonest example is paralytic ileus. This latter category will not be considered further here: its main features are reviewed by Le Quesne and Wilson (1974). Reverting to mechanical obstruction, the crucial subdivision (B) is into those patients with *simple intestinal obstruction* and those in which there is in addition interference with the blood supply of part of the intestines, namely, *strangulation obstruction*. Simple intestinal obstruction is further divided (C) into three groups according to the height of the obstruction, a consideration of importance in relation to the factors

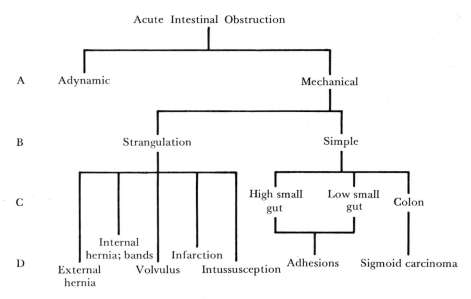

Fig. 12.1 Classification of acute intestinal obstruction. See text for discussion of this classification.

mainly responsible for the pathological disturbances. Finally (D), both simple and mechanical obstruction can be further broken down in relation to the common causative lesions.

The importance of this classification in relation to the clinical management of a patient with obstruction is emphasized in a later section, but it is also of importance in that it directs attention to the main pathophysiological disturbances which result from acute intestinal obstruction; in other words, the factors which make these patients ill and which will, if uncorrected, prove fatal.

Pathophysiological consequences of obstruction

Simple intestinal obstruction

Examining first the consequences of simple intestinal obstruction, the essential changes are those taking place above the site of obstruction, which are best considered under three headings:
1. Distension of the bowel with fluid and gas.
2. Multiplication of bacteria within the gut lumen.
3. Rise of intraluminal pressure.

Distension of the bowel

The bowel above the site of obstruction is distended with gas and fluid. Considering first the gas in the bowel, there are three possible sources: (a) it might accumulate as the result of diffusion of the blood gases into the bowel lumen; (b) it might result from bacterial fermentation; or (c) it might represent swallowed air. Analysis of the composition of the gas in the bowel lumen shows that it consists of a mixture of oxygen, carbon dioxide and nitrogen essentially in equilibrium with the blood gases, plus some water vapour and traces of gases such as methane formed by bacterial fermentation. In view of the fact that the intestinal mucosa is freely permeable to the blood gases it is in fact inevitable that the intestinal gases are in equilibrium with the blood gases, and hence the composition of the intestinal gases throws no light on their origin. There is, however, conclusive evidence from other sources that the major portion of the gas in the intestines represents swallowed air, with a small component produced by bacterial fermentation. The main evidence in support of this conclusion is provided by experiments on dogs showing that if at the same time as producing intestinal obstruction the oesophagus is divided, then no gas accumulates in the intestines above the site of the obstruction. This is reinforced by the common clinical observation that the gaseous distension can be controlled by keeping the stomach empty, and hence preventing the passage of further air down into the intestines.

The fluid in the intestine partly represents ingested liquids, but is largely due to the accumulation of gastrointestinal secretions. To appreciate the physiological consequences of the retention of these secretions in the lumen of the gut, where they are effectively lost to the body, two main facts must be borne in mind. First, their volume: in normal health some 8–10 litres of secretions (that is, a volume equal to over twice the average normal plasma volume) are poured into the intestine each 24 hours, and normally all but about 100–200 ml are reabsorbed back into the circulation, and thence into the extracellular space. Secondly, their composition: these fluids consist, not of water, but of a solution of electrolytes isotonic with plasma (see Fig. 12.2) and hence with the extracellular fluid, and further, save for gastric acid, they have a sodium concentration essentially equivalent to that of extracellular fluid. Bearing in mind the significance of sodium in the extracellular space, this means that the loss of these fluids constitutes a direct drain on the extracellular fluid volume. Furthermore, these figures actually under-estimate the extent of the fluid loss, for Shields (1965) has shown that obstruction produces, in the bowel above the obstruction, a marked alteration in the to-and-fro movement of water and electrolytes across the intestinal mucosa, resulting in a net increase in the loss of both into the bowel lumen. This net change is due to two factors. In the first instance, within 6 hours of the obstruction, there is an impairment of the rate at which water, sodium and potassium leave the bowel lumen, whilst at a later stage in addition the rate at which both water and electrolytes enter the bowel is increased, the two processes combining to produce a net increase in the loss of water, sodium and potassium into the bowel lumen, this loss being essentially isotonic with extracellular fluid.

The actual magnitude of the losses which can occur from the bowel is shown in Table 12.1, setting out the measured losses in 3 patients with acute intestinal obstruction. Note that in all 3 patients the sodium concentration in the intestinal loss is essentially equivalent to that in the extracellular fluid, and that whilst the fluid contains a modest potassium content, which can cause significant potassium depletion, the loss of this ion is insignificant in relation to that of sodium. It is of interest to note that in patient 3, who died some 12 hours after operation,

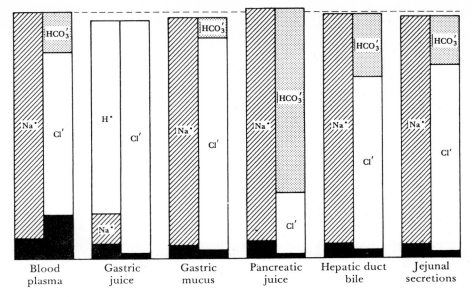

Fig. 12.2 Stick graph showing the composition of the gastrointestinal secretions. Note that they are all isotonic with plasma, and that, save for gastric acid, they have a sodium concentration essentially the same as that in plasma, i.e. in the extracellular fluid. (Reproduced from Gamble, 1964, *The Chemical Anatomy, Physiology and Pathology of the Extracellular Fluid.* Cambridge, Mass., Harvard University Press.)

Table 12.1 Actual measured fluid losses from the bowel in 3 patients with intestinal obstruction

Case	Source of gastrointestinal losses	Volume (ml)	Electrolyte concentration (mEq/l)			Electrolyte content (mEq)		
			Na+	K+	Cl−	Na+	K+	Cl−
1	Aspirated from intestine at operation	1,150	130	7·5	132	150	8·5	153
2	Vomited in 6 hours pre-operation; aspirated from intestine at operation	2,300	128	5·2	140	294	12	322
3	Aspirated from intestine at operation; gastric aspirate in 36 hours after operation; removed from intestine at autopsy	6,810	127	17	90	865	116	612

Note the uniformly high sodium concentration in the fluid lost. Note also that patient 3, in a period of 36 hours, lost into or from the intestine an amount of sodium approximately equal to that in 6 litres of extracellular fluid.

(Reproduced from Le Quesne, 1967, *Br. J. Surg.* **54,** 449–452, by kind permission of the Editorial Secretary.)

the amount of sodium recovered from the bowel in 36 hours equalled that in 6 litres of extracellular fluid.

Multiplication of bacteria

An important change in the bowel above the site of the obstruction is a great increase in the number of bacteria, the main organisms being coliforms, faecal streptococci and also certain anaerobes, such as Clostridia and Bacteroides. This increase in the bacterial content is of importance in the operative treatment of acute obstruction, particularly of the large bowel, but it is also of importance because it has been suggested that the absorption of bacterial toxins plays an important part in the illness of intestinal obstruction. Such toxins could be absorbed either via the blood-stream or via the lymphatics, or, having permeated the wall of the intestine from the peritoneal cavity. The available evidence suggests that only the latter route is of any importance, and then only in the later stages of obstruction when the permeability of the bowel is impaired by prolonged distension. Indeed, it is now clear that many, if not all, of the changes formerly ascribed to the absorption of toxins are in reality due to body fluid depletion, but the question of toxic absorption does draw attention to the third important change in the bowel, namely the rise in intraluminal pressure.

Raised intraluminal pressure

Above the site of the obstruction the pressure in the bowel rises from a normal of 2–4 mm Hg to 10 mm or more in the small bowel, and up to 25 mm Hg in the colon. The obvious effect of this raised pressure is to cause distension of the bowel, with initially increased peristalsis, giving rise to intestinal colic, though later this is replaced by paresis of the intestinal muscle. In addition, sustained increase in pressure in the bowel impairs the viability of the bowel wall, leading eventually to perforation. For any given pressure in the lumen of the bowel* the tension in the bowel wall is proportional to the diameter of the bowel, so that the greatest distension is seen in the caecum, which is also the commonest site of perforation of the bowel in intestinal obstruction. In addition, there is evidence, based on experiments on animals with Thiry–Vella fistulae, that distension of a loop of bowel is in itself deleterious to the animal as the result of nerve impulses set up in the distended loop.

Considering these three factors in relation to the cause of death in simple intestinal obstruction, there is no doubt that the factor of crucial importance is fluid loss, and this is particularly the case with high small gut obstruction. The main area for the absorption of water and electrolytes is in the lower small intestine, whereas most of the gastrointestinal secretions enter the upper reaches of the gut, with the result that in general the higher the obstruction the greater and the more rapid the fluid loss. As already indicated, the main loss is into the bowel lumen, but in addition the bowel above the obstruction becomes heavier as the result of venous engorgement and oedema formation, and there is some accumulation of fluid in the peritoneal cavity. All these forms of loss—into the lumen,

---

* The relationship between tension and pressure is governed by the law of Laplace, which states that $T = Pr$, where T = tension, P = pressure and r = radius.

into the bowel wall, into the peritoneal cavity—result in a diminution in the extracellular fluid space, leading to a diminution in the circulatory volume with, finally, death from peripheral circulatory failure. In obstruction lower in the bowel, the role of fluid loss becomes less obtrusive, the illness being altogether less acute and rapid in progression, and other factors, especially distension and its sequelae, play a more important role, until in low colonic obstruction they come to dominate the picture.

Strangulation obstruction

Important additional factors are involved in strangulation obstruction. In late strangulation obstruction with gangrene and perforation of the bowel, the most obvious is frank septic peritonitis, but before such advanced changes occur two other important factors are involved, namely blood loss and toxaemia.

Blood loss

In most instances strangulation does not cause immediate, complete interruption of the circulation to the affected loop. Usually in the first instance the strangulating agent (e.g. volvulus) obstructs the veins, leading to engorgement of the strangulated loop, and then rupture of small vessels with bleeding into the tissues, into the lumen and into the peritoneal cavity (hence the blood-stained effusion in strangulation obstruction), and it is only when the pressure in the tissues rises to that of the arterial inflow pressure that the circulation is completely arrested. If the strangulation loop is short the blood loss is small, but with long lengths of strangulated bowel it can be considerable, the most extreme example being mesenteric infarction from obstruction to the superior mesenteric artery. This loss of blood adds to and compounds the fluid loss already described as resulting from the obstruction itself.

Toxaemia

In strangulation obstruction, in contrast to simple obstruction, there is an undoubted and important toxic factor which is related to the bacterial content of the bowel. On the basis of animal experiments there is abundant evidence (Barnett, 1960; Yull et al., 1962; Barnett, et al., 1963; Barnett et al., 1968) to show that the peritoneal exudate which accumulates in strangulation obstruction is lethal when injected intraperitoneally into other animals, that the toxicity of the exudate is dependent upon the presence in it of *Escherichia coli* plus erythrocytes, and that the mortality of experimental strangulation obstruction is greatly reduced by the administration of suitable antibiotics at the time of strangulation, or by enclosing the strangulated loop in an impermeable Polythene bag. Interesting confirmation of the key role of bacterial infection in producing this toxaemia is provided by the observation that the peritoneal exudate following the production of strangulation obstruction in gnotobiotic (i.e. germ-free) animals is relatively non-toxic (Thomas et al., 1965). It is also of importance that Yull and his colleagues (1962) found that the peritoneal exudate from a patient with strangulation obstruction had the same properties as that from his experimental animal preparations.

In the early stages of strangulation obstruction, before the bowel wall becomes permeable to the bacteria in the lumen, this toxic process, which is in many respects similar to gram-negative septicaemia, is not active, but it comes to play an important part in the over-all disturbance in late cases of strangulation obstruction, particularly when a long loop is involved.

Summarizing the changes in their entirety, the essential factors leading to the death of a patient with acute intestinal obstruction are: in simple obstruction, body fluid, predominantly extracellular, depletion, with the consequences of distension of the bowel playing an important role in low bowel obstruction; and in strangulation obstruction, superimposed on these changes are the problems of blood loss and toxaemia, and in late cases frank peritonitis.

Clinical features

The three important clinical manifestations of acute intestinal obstruction are vomiting, intestinal colic, and distension. It is to be noted that constipation is not one of the essential features of intestinal obstruction; it is certainly a feature of late intestinal obstruction but, in that at the very least 24 hours must elapse before constipation can be said to exist, it is clear that to include constipation amongst the cardinal manifestations of acute obstruction is to invite delay in diagnosis.

The pattern of these main manifestations will vary from patient to patient according to the height of the obstruction, and according to the cause of the obstruction and its duration there may well be additional symptoms and physical signs. In addition, biochemical information plays an important part in the diagnostic assessment of most patients with acute intestinal obstruction. To catalogue all this information in relation to the common causes of obstruction causes confusion rather than clarity, and it is more helpful to analyse the whole problem in practical terms. Some 20 years ago Owen Wangensteen (1955) in his distinguished monograph set out a series of questions that have to be answered when faced by a patient with suspected intestinal obstruction. Somewhat modified, they still outline the essence of the diagnostic problem, and form an admirable approach to management of this situation.

The diagnostic approach

1. Has the patient got acute intestinal obstruction?

Clearly this is the first question to be faced, and it is answered in the first instance by a consideration of the clinical data—that is to say, does the patient display the manifestations of obstruction previously described? In that each of these features (namely, vomiting, colic and distension) can occur as the result of other conditions such as gastroenteritis or ascites, care is needed in the assessment of these features, and the presence or absence of others such as diarrhoea, dullness on abdominal percussion, etc., must be taken into account. To determine that abdominal pain is due to intestinal colic it is often useful to auscultate the

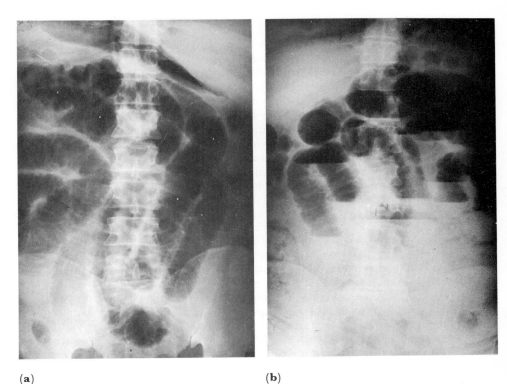

(a)   **(b)**

Fig. 12.3 Erect (**a**) and supine (**b**) films of the abdomen in a patient with acute obstruction of the small intestine. Note the many gas-filled loops of bowel, with multiple fluid levels. Note also the markings of the valvulae conniventes, passing right across the bowel, indicating that most of the distended loops are distended jejunum—i.e. fairly high intestinal obstruction.

abdomen during an attack of pain, when hearing increased bowel sounds will indicate that the pain is clearly due to increased bowel contractions.

On the basis of the clinical information it is usually possible to come to a fairly firm answer to this question, and this can be confirmed or refuted by plain x-ray films of the abdomen, taken in the erect and supine positions (Fig. 12.3). In the normal abdomen gas is seen only in the stomach and large bowel, and fluid levels are not normally seen, though occasionally there is a gas bubble with fluid level in the duodenal cap. The essential features of acute obstruction are the presence of gaseous distension of the bowel above the obstruction, with the presence of fluid levels, and the absence of gas in the bowel distal to the obstruction.

Considering together the clinical and radiological information, a decision must be made as to whether or not the patient is deemed to have intestinal obstruction: in most instances this decision can be made without great hesitation, and if the answer is 'yes', then the next question must be answered.

2. Has the patient got simple or strangulation obstruction?

Bearing in mind that most patients with intestinal obstruction are operated upon within a comparatively short time of admission to hospital, it may appear at first glance that it is unnecessary to face this question squarely, and hence it is important to consider why it is of such importance. If a patient is diagnosed as having a strangulation obstruction, this of necessity means that he has a condition which will prove fatal unless relieved by operation, and further that there is a real degree of urgency in performing the operation. This in its turn means that any fluid deficit must be replaced promptly, within a matter of a few hours at the most. In contrast, if a diagnosis of simple obstruction is made there is no compelling necessity to operate promptly, and indeed it may often be wise to treat the patient for 24 hours or more with intravenous fluids and nasogastric suction before the decision to operate is made. Clearly if a diagnosis of simple obstruction is made and the patient is treated for any length of time by conservative means he must be kept under close observation, so that if any signs occur suggesting that in fact strangulation is present then operation can be undertaken forthwith; none the less, at the time of the initial assessment a clear decision as to whether the patient is regarded as having simple or strangulation obstruction is an essential step in the diagnostic process.

The distinction between the two conditions can usually be made by consideration of three features in the clinical presentation. In the first place, patients with strangulation obstruction in general get iller quicker than patients with simple obstruction: a consideration of the pathophysiological consequences of strangulation obstruction makes the reasons for this apparent. Secondly, if the lesion causing the strangulation obstruction is within the peritoneal cavity (i.e. in all cases save for strangulated external hernia) the strangulated loop will give rise to local peritoneal irritation, which in its turn causes important symptoms and signs. The important symptom is continuous pain, upon which is superimposed the intermittent, colicky pain resulting from the obstruction. This is the basis of the classical surgical dictum that patients with acute obstruction with continuous pain require urgent operation. In addition, the localized peritonitis will give rise to the signs of localized tenderness and guarding, often with rebound tenderness. Accordingly, in all patients with acute obstruction the abdomen should be examined carefully with these considerations in mind.

Thirdly, one of the commonest causes of strangulation obstruction is a strangulated external hernia, a reminder that in all patients with intestinal obstruction (indeed, in all patients with an acute abdominal condition) the external hernial orifices *must* be examined carefully—all five of them: two inguinal, two femoral and one umbilical. The signs of a strangulated external hernia are so well known that it is almost superfluous to reiterate them; none the less, such is their importance that it cannot be out of place to recall that the crucial physical signs are: (a) a tense, tender mass situated over one of the external hernial orifices; (b) there is no cough impulse; and (c) the hernia is not (usually) reducible. In the interests of accuracy it is necessary to include the qualification about the reducibility of the lump, for in some circumstances (i.e. infants) the hernia may be treated by reduction, but in ordinary clinical circumstances the hernia is irreducible.

It goes without saying that if there is any doubt about the decision, then a diagnosis of strangulation obstruction must be made. It is wise to bear in mind a well authenticated clinical observation that if the patient has not previously had an abdominal operation then the obstruction is probably a strangulation, not a simple one. In fact, it is not infrequent in simple obstruction for there to be localized tenderness, perhaps with some guarding and rebound tenderness, over distended coils of intestine, with the result that if these signs are strictly interpreted then a diagnosis of strangulation obstruction will be made. As a consequence of this, provided that signs of localized peritoneal irritation are carefully sought and scrupulously interpreted, the overwhelming tendency is to diagnose strangulation in the presence of simple obstruction, rather than vice versa, a factor which greatly contributes to the safety of the management of patients with acute obstruction.

3. What is the height of the obstruction?

Previously, when discussing the pathophysiological consequences of intestinal obstruction, it was pointed out that the factors leading to death of the patient varied according to the height of the obstruction, with body fluid depletion predominantly in high intestinal obstruction and the consequences of distension playing an important role in obstruction of the distal bowel. A decision as to the height of the obstruction is, therefore, important as it will direct attention to the consequences of obstruction most likely to require prime attention. To cite an obvious example, if it is decided that the obstruction is in the sigmoid colon it immediately becomes apparent that relief of the distension is likely to be more important than replenishment of a body fluid deficit.

This question can be answered by a consideration of the clinical and radiological evidence. The clinical evidence depends upon the fact that the prominence of each of the three cardinal manifestations of acute obstruction (namely, vomiting, intestinal colic and distension) varies according to the height of the obstruction. The prominent symptom in high small gut obstruction is vomiting, colic is usually unobtrusive and distension absent. As the level of obstruction descends, colic becomes a more prominent, often the presenting, symptom and distension begins to become apparent. In low small gut obstruction, colic and distension are the outstanding symptoms with significant vomiting developing later. In colonic obstruction, vomiting may be absent, and finally in obstruction in the sigmoid colon, distension may be the presenting symptom with colic an unimportant feature.

In addition to this clinical assessment, valuable evidence is provided by the plain films of the abdomen, from a consideration of the pattern of the distended loop. In the small intestine this pattern depends upon the arrangement of the mucous membrane, and in the colon upon the haustrations of the bowel. Figure 12.4 shows the radiological appearances of three segments of small intestine removed at autopsy and then distended with air. The upper segment is from the proximal jejunum, showing the typical, parallel striations, running right across the bowel, caused by the close mucosal folds of the upper jejunum. Lower in the jejunum, these folds, as shown in the middle segment, become sparser and wider apart, until finally, in the distal ileum (lower segment), they disappear

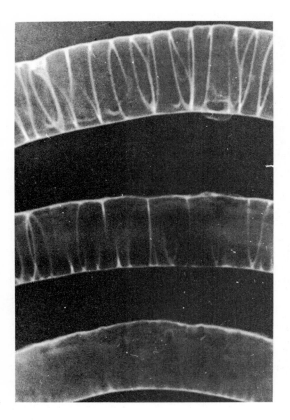

Fig. 12.4 Radiograph of three segments of small intestine removed at autopsy and distended with air. The upper segment comes from the upper jejunum: note the frequent transverse markings, running right across the bowel, caused by the valvulae conniventes. In the middle segment, from the middle of the small intestine, these markings are fewer, and they are absent from the terminal ileum, as shown in the lower segment.

altogether, giving the characteristically featureless appearance of distended low small intestine. In contrast, the features of distended colon are shown in Fig. 12.5; at first glance the markings of the haustra resemble those of the jejunum, but they differ in an important respect in that the haustrations rarely run completely across the bowel, and in addition the colon can usually be distinguished by its greater calibre. In plain films of the abdomen, particularly in the supine film, careful examination of the features of the distended bowel will usually give evidence as to the height of the obstruction. A further important point to look for is the presence or absence of a distended caecum, for a characteristic feature of the films in large gut obstruction is the presence of a large fluid level, in the erect film, in the caecum (Fig. 12.6, see p. 180).

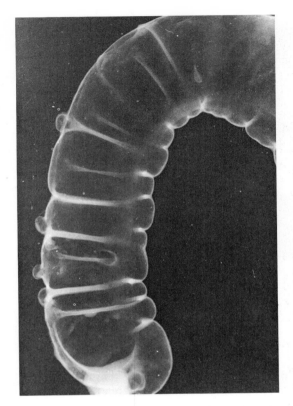

Fig. 12.5 Radiography of a portion of large intestine removed at autopsy and distended with air. Note that the haustral markings do not go right across the bowel, in contrast to those in the jejunum (see Fig. 12.4).

4. Has the patient got significant body fluid depletion?

Regardless of the height of the obstruction, an essential part of the initial assessment of any patient with acute obstruction is an examination directed to discovering whether or not the patient has a body fluid deficit and, if so, its magnitude. Such an examination is a standard clinical exercise; a detailed analysis of this problem is beyond the scope of this chapter and it must suffice to consider only its main features.

As discussed previously, acute intestinal obstruction gives rise to a fluid deficit which mainly affects the extracellular space and, most importantly, the intravascular component of that space, that is to say the circulating volume. The assessment of the size of any deficit is based on clinical and biochemical evidence. Clinically, the important signs to elicit are as follows. First, the state of skin elasticity or turgor; this sign is best elicited over the flexor surface of the elbow or at the root of the neck, a diminished skin elasticity indicating depletion of the interstitial compartment, always bearing in mind that skin elasticity can also be

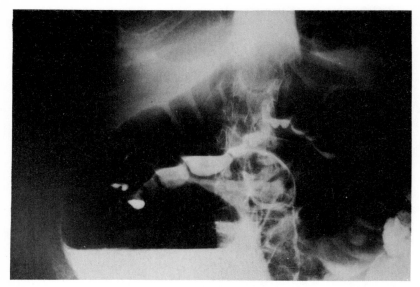

Fig. 12.6 Erect, plain film of the abdomen in a patient with acute large gut abstruction, due to a carcinoma of the sigmoid. Note the greatly distended caecum, with a large fluid level. This fluid level is particularly pronounced as the patient had received some barium by mouth 3 days previously. Note also the typical haustral markings in the transverse colon.

diminished by old age or weight loss. Secondly, the peripheral circulation must be assessed for signs of a diminished circulating volume. The obvious signs of a severe fall in the circulating volume are a raised pulse rate and lowered blood pressure, but before such a state is reached important evidence that the plasma volume is lowered is provided by the evidence of peripheral vasoconstriction; namely, pale, cool extremities and empty peripheral veins. It cannot be emphasized too strongly that, particularly in otherwise healthy, relatively young subjects, such signs develop long before there are obvious changes in the pulse rate and blood pressure, and if reliance is placed only on these gross changes then important depletion of the intravascular volume can easily be overlooked.

Biochemical information can be obtained from two sources: the blood and the urine. Considering first the information to be obtained from the blood, it is important to recall that the fluid lost, whether it be blood, plasma or intestinal secretions, has an electrolyte content essentially the same as extracellular fluid. As a result, there may well be no important changes in the electrolyte concentrations in the plasma, save possibly that of potassium, and the important evidence to look for is that indicative of a diminished circulating volume, especially a fall in the plasma volume. Such evidence is provided by measurement of the haemoglobin or haematocrit, which will give a direct indication of haemoconcentration, and by an estimation of the blood urea concentration, which will reflect the effect of a lowered circulating volume on renal function. It is true that these measurements can be affected by either pre-existing anaemia or pre-existing renal disease, but provided due attention is paid to these possibilities these two observations are the most important to be made on a blood sample. These measurements should be made in all patients with acute obstruction, as apart from their immediate significance they may be of great importance if complications develop in the post-operative period. Measurement of the serum electrolyte concentrations is commonly performed, and probably the most important figure is that of the potassium concentration, a lowered potassium concentration being indicative of potassium depletion. Considering the urine, again the concentration of the various electrolytes can be measured, but again the most useful information can be obtained from two simple observations: the urine volume, always bearing in mind that the volume is only significant when related to time; and the urine concentration as indicated by the specific gravity.

Based on these two sources of information, an assessment can be made of the extent of any fluid depletion. The absence of any of the physical signs described, together with normal haemoglobin and blood urea figures, indicates the absence of any significant depletion, whereas deviations from normality give an indication of the size of the deficit. The information obtained will not allow the deficit to be quantified accurately, but it will enable a working estimate to be made, bearing in mind that if there is obvious clinical and biochemical evidence of depletion then there is probably a deficit of at least 3 litres. But probably of more importance than giving a predictive assessment of the deficit, these initial observations give essential information against which to control replacement of the deficit and to judge of its completeness, and at the same time they give essential base-line information should the patient develop any body fluid disturbance in the post-operative period.

Bearing in mind the pathophysiological consequences of acute obstruction outlined earlier, the correction of which mainly determines the outcome of the illness, it is apparent that the answers to these first four questions indicate the main priorities of treatment. Thus if it is decided that the patient has a strangulation obstruction, it is clear that urgent operation is required. Further, if the obstruction is high in the intestine and there are signs of extracellular depletion, then replenishment of the deficit is of major importance, whilst if the obstruction is in the distal colon it may well be that there is little or no fluid deficit and the urgent therapeutic requirement is to relieve the distension. All of these strategic decisions can be reached regardless of the exact cause of the obstruction, but important tactical decisions about the operative approach and technique and many details of the actual management of the patient depend upon the answer to the fifth, and final, question.

5. What is the cause of the obstruction?

The answer to this question clearly depends upon a consideration of all the features of the patient's history and examination. In many instances, as for instance a strangulated femoral hernia, the answer is clear; in others, for example obstruction to the sigmoid colon by a carcinoma, the evidence may be strong but not conclusive; and in others a clear diagnosis may be impossible and treatment must be planned on the basis of the evidence pertinent to the earlier questions. This, however, is rarely of great consequence, for if these questions are clearly answered, it should be possible to plan a rational course of treatment.

Principles of management

In any patient with intestinal obstruction the ultimate object of treatment is to relieve the obstruction and restore unimpeded progress of the intestinal contents throughout the entire length of the alimentary canal. Frequently this is achieved by the initial, definitive treatment, but, as previously indicated, the patient's life is threatened not so much by the obstruction as by its consequences, and accordingly to save the patient's life the prime therapeutic requirement may be to correct these consequences, leaving the definitive treatment of the obstructing lesion to a later date. An obvious example of this is seen in the management of acute large bowel obstruction by a carcinoma of the sigmoid colon, where the standard primary treatment is relief of the distension by a proximal vent, usually a colostomy, leaving the obstructing lesion initially untouched and for excision at an appropriate time later.

In considering the treatment of acute intestinal obstruction, a clear distinction must be drawn between strangulation and simple obstruction. In patients with strangulation obstruction, the urgent requirement is to relieve the strangulation by operation, but if there is a significant body fluid deficit the operation should not be undertaken without restoring at least the circulatory volume. The importance of this is underlined by the fact that general anaesthesia causes vasodilatation, so that if operation is undertaken without prior restoration of the circulating volume a precipitous fall in blood pressure is likely to occur. In these patients rapid restoration of the fluid deficit is required, and it is in these circumstances that measurement of the central venous pressure may be of great value, enabling considerable volumes of fluid to be given rapidly without danger of overloading the circulation: in this process repeated estimation of the haematocrit is also helpful. It is, in addition, of importance to check the serum potassium level because, if it is significantly lowered, this may interfere with the action of muscle-relaxant drugs (Vaughan and Lunn, 1973) and it may be wise to give some potassium prior to the operation. However, it must be emphasized that such treatment is never as important as restoration of the volume of the extracellular fluid.

In simple intestinal obstruction the problem is in many ways less straightforward. Rigid analysis of the problem indicates that the logical treatment is to replace the body fluid deficit and relieve the intestinal distension, and then to operate at leisure on a fit patient. It was this reasoning that led to the development of the Miller–Abbott tube, and the primary treatment of simple obstruction by intestinal intubation and intravenous fluids. There is no doubt that this treatment can be successful, but it is not without its dangers, is certainly not an easy alternative to operation, and in general is not commonly used these days. However, the experience gained with this technique has clearly shown the benefits that can accrue from a period devoted to the control of distension and correction of any body fluid deficit, and that it is often wise to delay operation 24 hours or more.

In the management of simple small bowel obstruction, if the distension is not marked it is, in general, wise to operate as soon as the body fluid deficit is replaced. If, however, there is much distension it is often wise to delay operation for at least 24 hours whilst attempts are made to relieve the distension by nasogastric suction. By keeping the stomach empty and aspirating fluid and gas as it regurgitates back from the intestine, marked decompression may be achieved; this not only relieves the patient from the consequences of distension but also makes easier any operation that has to be performed. Such so-called conservative treatment of this sort (i.e. 'drip and suck') is of particular value in patients with obstruction due to adhesions, as in these circumstances emptying of the distended intestine often relieves the obstruction (probably by allowing a kink, at a point fixed by adhesions, to straighten out) and so saves the patient from a further operation. In large gut obstruction, the essential requirement of treatment is to relieve the distension. Even if the ileocaecal valve is incompetent this cannot be done effectively by nasogastric suction, and if, as may well be the case, the obstruction cannot be relieved by an enema then no time should be lost in relieving the distension by construction of a proximal vent, either a colostomy or caecostomy.

The details of the operative and post-operative care of patients with acute obstruction are beyond the scope of this chapter, but two further general points require emphasis. Earlier it was pointed out that one of the consequences of obstruction is an increase in the bacterial content of the intestine. As a result, contamination of the peritoneal cavity with the contents of the distended bowel, especially large bowel, is more dangerous than with those of normal bowel. Every effort should be made to avoid such contamination, particularly if the bowel is opened to evacuate its contents: distended small intestine is preferably emptied by milking the contents back into the stomach, whence they are aspirated via the nasogastric tube. Secondly, peripheral circulatory inadequacy with a falling blood pressure and rising pulse rate (so-called 'shock') may well develop in the first 48–72 hours after operation. By far the commonest causes of this situation are uncontrolled sepsis, and unrecognized, and hence unreplaced, fluid losses resulting in a diminished circulatory volume. The possibility of a serious infection after a strangulation obstruction is obvious. Fluid losses may result from exactly the same causes as prior to the operation, for if there is an ileus fluid will accumulate in the intestinal lumen and if, as a result of a strangulation obstruction, there is an area of peritonitis, an exudate of fluid (i.e. essentially plasma) into the inflamed tissues and into the peritoneal cavity may well continue for 24 hours or more: these losses, which have precisely the same effect as those already described as occurring as the result of the obstruction, are easily overlooked. Whilst the majority of patients with intestinal obstruction have an uneventful post-operative course, these problems are mentioned to emphasize that the successful management of such patients involves a continuity of care from the initial assessment, through the operation and post-operative period, to final recovery.

References

BARNETT W. O. (1960) Experimental strangulated intestinal obstruction—a review. *Gastroenterology* **39,** 34–40.

BARNETT W. O., OLIVER R. I. and ELLIOTT R. L. (1968) Elimination of the lethal properties of gangrenous bowel segments. *Ann. Surg.* **167,** 912–919.

BARNETT W. O., TRUETT G., WILLIAMS R. and CROWELL J. (1963) Shock in strangulation obstruction. Mechanisms and management. *Ann. Surg.* **157,** 747–758.

GAMBLE J. L. (1964) *Chemical Anatomy, Physiology and Pathology of the Extracellular Fluid*, 6th edn. Cambridge, Mass., Harvard University Press.

LE QUESNE L. P. and WILSON J. P. (1974) Intestinal obstruction. In: WELLS C., KYLE J. and DUNPHY J. E. (ed.), *Scientific Foundations of Surgery*, 2nd edn. London, William Heinemann Medical.

SHIELDS R. (1965) The absorption and secretion of fluid and electrolytes by the obstructed bowel. *Br. J. Surg.* **52,** 774–779.

THOMAS, M. A., HENEGHAN J. B., MATHIEU F. J., STIRLING C. T., DI VICENTI F. C., WEILBAECHER D. A., BORNSIDE G. H. and COHN I. (1965) Strangulation obstruction in germ-free dogs. *Surgery* **58,** 37–46.

VAUGHAN R. S. and LUNN J. N. (1973) Potassium and the anaesthetist. A review. *Anaesthesia* **28,** 118–131.

WANGENSTEEN O. (1955) *Intestinal Obstruction*, 3rd edn. Springfield, Illinois, Charles C. Thomas.

YULL A. B., ABRAMS J. S. and DAVIS J. H. (1962) The peritoneal fluid in strangulation obstruction. *J. Surg. Res.* **2,** 223–232.

13

Ulcerative Colitis

J. E. Lennard-Jones, MD, FRCP

This chapter deals with practical aspects of the management of colitis. The term management is used because the patient is likely to need advice, encouragement and different types of treatment over a long period. Typical clinical situations requiring decision may be summarized as follows:

Acute symptoms
  1. Assess severity
  2. Choice of treatment
       very severe attack
       severe attack
       moderately severe attack
       mild distal disease

Colitis in remission
  1. Consider prognosis
  2. Reduce relapse rate
  3. Early treatment of relapse
  4. Prevent cancer

Chronic colitis
  Review current treatment. Can medical treatment be improved or should surgical treatment be advised?

Acute colitis

1. Assess severity

The severity of an acute attack of colitis is often under-estimated and depends on the following factors:

  the extent of the inflammation
  the depth of the mucosal ulceration
  the systemic response
  metabolic depletion
  the age and physique of the patient

Inflammation confined to the rectum and sigmoid colon rarely causes severe illness. When the whole or a substantial proportion of the colon is involved the attack is likely to be more severe with some systemic upset. Even though much of the colon is inflamed the illness can still be mild if ulceration is absent or superficial. On the other hand, deep ulceration, especially if the deep muscle layer is exposed over a large area, causes severe illness. Systemic manifestations of colitis such as erythema nodosum, arthritis or pyoderma do not bear a direct relation to the extent and severity of the mucosal inflammation, but they are more common when the disease is extensive. Depletion of protein with a low serum albumin, loss of muscle bulk and loss of body weight are common features of severe colitis. Colitis in the elderly tends to be much more dangerous than in younger patients, and the post-operative mortality after colectomy for acute disease is usually very high.

2. Choice of treatment

Very severe colitis requiring immediate colectomy

The indications for immediate surgical treatment without preliminary drug therapy at St. Mark's Hospital are:

perforation
dilatation of the colon with mucosal islands

Both these complications may be diagnosed from a plain abdominal x-ray which should be performed in all cases of severe colitis. The combination of dilatation *and* marked mucosal irregularity suggests that there is partial denudation of mucosa with spread of inflammation into the deep muscle layers.

Severe colitis requiring potent drug therapy and collaboration between physician and surgeon

The following features, particularly when more than one is present, suggest that the attack of colitis is severe and that urgent surgical treatment may become necessary (Lennard-Jones et al., 1975):

maximum fever $> 38°C$
observed bowel frequency greater than 8 in 24 hours
severe abdominal tenderness
serum albumin $< 30\,g/litre$
prostration and malaise
age over 60 years

Such patients should be seen by physician and surgeon in consultation at the earliest opportunity and observed carefully during the first few days after admission to hospital. Energetic medical therapy includes:

Replacement therapy:
blood, fluids, electrolytes (particularly potassium) and, possibly, parenteral nutrition

Anti-inflammatory drugs:
a corticosteroid such as prednisolone 21-phosphate, 60 mg in 24 hours, or

hydrocortisone hemisuccinate, 400 mg in 24 hours, given by intravenous infusion

or

corticotrophin gel, 80 units daily I.M.

Other drugs:
    Sulphasalazine, 1 g t.d.s., may be given if it does not cause or increase nausea. An antibiotic may be given parenterally for coincidental infection. Nystatin suspension or amphotericin B lozenges may be required for moniliasis.
    Codeine phosphate and similar drugs are not usually helpful

The indication for urgent surgical treatment is failure to respond to a regimen of this type. Useful indications of failure to respond are the development or persistence of:

high fever (or pulse rate)
anorexia and malaise
severe abdominal tenderness
and/or falling body weight, haemoglobin and serum albumin

The timing of operation varies according to the clinical condition of the patient. If there is no improvement a decision is usually reached between 4 and 8 days after admission to hospital. If there is partial or transitory improvement decision may be delayed for 1–3 weeks. Since the post-operative mortality in elderly patients is particularly high, early, rather than late, surgical treatment for those over 60 years should be the rule.

Moderately severe colitis usually responsive to drug therapy

Many patients with colitis are admitted with some systemic upset in the form of fever, weight loss or associated features, but who are not severely ill. Such patients usually require:

Replacement therapy:
    blood, iron, potassium, a high protein diet

Systemic corticosteroid:
    such as prednisolone, 10 mg q.i.d. daily by mouth

Other drugs:
    Sulphasalazine, 1 g t.d.s., should be started provided that nausea is absent. The drug should be stopped, the dose reduced or enteric-coated tablets used if it causes nausea or dyspepsia. A few patients develop malaise, headache or other symptoms, in which case the drug should be stopped.
    Corticosteroid retention enemas may be started once the diarrhoea decreases and the enemas can be retained. Usually patients with colitis of this severity have disease involving at least the distal half of the colon. The enema volume should begin with 50–100 ml and then be increased slowly and progressively to the maximum easily tolerated by the patient, usually 200–300 ml. An abdominal x-ray taken after a little barium has been added to a therapeutic enema will then show if the enema solution is coming into contact with all the diseased mucosa (Swarbrick et al., 1974).

Psychotrophic drugs are indicated only if anxiety or depression is a feature of the illness.

Codeine phosphate and diphenoxylate (Lomotil) are of little help and can cause trouble by causing the collection of hard stool in the normal colon proximal to the diseased area.

Mild distal colitis

These patients rarely require surgical treatment. Most can be treated as outpatients, without restriction of activities. The main lines of treatment are:

Replacement:
iron, sometimes needed parenterally

Drug:
Sulphasalazine, 1 g t.d.s. alone, or in combination with a topical corticosteroid preparation, is usually successful. Steroid suppositories are useful if the upper limit to the disease can be seen on sigmoidoscopy. A useful preparation contains 5 mg of prednisolone 21-phosphate in each suppository (Predsol).

Corticosteroid retention enemas can be administered by the patient at night if the disease extends proximal to the rectum. The prepared enema packs containing 100 ml of fluid are suitable when the disease is confined to the rectum and sigmoid colon.

If the disease is more extensive a larger volume of fluid may be needed and, if the disease fails to respond as expected, it may be necessary to see how far the enema travels by arranging an x-ray after administration of a therapeutic enema containing barium.

Colitis in remission

A patient who has recovered from an acute attack of colitis is not cured; he is liable to further attacks and, in some cases, he is liable to a greater risk of colonic cancer than the general population The prognosis for each patient should be considered as some patients should be advised to accept elective colectomy. In most cases, medical treatment and observation will be continued with the aims of decreasing the relapse rate and treating recurrent attacks early and vigorously. Patients with extensive colitis need careful follow-up because of the cancer risk and prophylactic colectomy may have to be advised because of the length of history or because dysplastic changes are found in colonic or rectal mucosal biopsies.

Consider prognosis

Severe acute colitis is a dangerous illness and the post-operative mortality after urgent colectomy undertaken because of failed medical treatment is rarely less than 10 per cent and is often greater (Ritchie, 1974). The mortality of elective colectomy, on the other hand, is low, usually less than 2 per cent and the post-operative morbidity is less than after operation on all ill patient. It is therefore advisable to recommend surgical treatment during a phase of remission for a patient who has suffered recurrent severe attacks of colitis.

The risk of cancer complicating colitis appears to be confined to those patients who have had extensive disease and whose symptoms began 10 or more years previously. It is arguable as to whether or not all such patients should be advised to undergo surgical treatment. Where meticulous supervision is possible, supported by facilities for regular rectal mucosal biopsy, colonoscopy with multiple colonic biopsies and double contrast barium enema, results suggest that it is safe to allow a proportion of such patients to continue without operation (Lennard-Jones et al., 1974). Where regular follow-up is not possible, where there is chronic disability or where there is evidence of dysplasia in mucosal biopsies, colectomy should be advised.

Diminish the risk of relapse

Experience suggests that relapse can be precipitated by minor intestinal infections, by broad-spectrum antibiotics given orally for coincidental illness and by emotional upsets. A few patients appear to remain well as long as they exclude milk from their diet. These factors should be discussed with the patient and appropriate advice given about such matters as holidays abroad.

The only drug known to diminish the relapse rate is sulphasalazine in a dose of 2 or 3 g daily (Misiewicz et al., 1965; Dissanayake and Truelove, 1973). There is evidence that this drug still exerts an effect 5 years after the last attack and it is difficult to know how long treatment should be continued. There are good grounds for advising continuous treatment for at least a year after an attack of colitis and many patients continue treatment, apparently with benefit and without side-effects, for many years. Patients should be encouraged to persist taking the drug and general practitioners should be encouraged to prescribe it on a long-term basis in the same way as they prescribe drugs for chronic illnesses such as hypertension and diabetes.

The role, if any, of azathioprine or other immunosuppressive drugs in treatment is not at present clear. Azathioprine may be tried as a maintenance treatment for the occasional patient who cannot take sulphasalazine, or in whom this drug is unsuccessful in preventing relapse and in whom surgical treatment is contraindicated, provided that the disease is severe enough to warrant this treatment and that close supervision is maintained (Jewell and Truelove, 1974).

Prepare for relapse

It is important that the patient should understand that colitis tends to be a relapsing disorder and that recurrent symptoms require early and energetic treatment. It is useful for the patient to have a reserve supply of corticosteroid retention enemas to use for a week or two before seeking medical advice. Letters to general practitioners should include suggestions about possible action to be taken if the patient consults him about recurrent symptoms. Where appropriate the patient's own doctor should be encouraged to start a course of systemic prednisolone in an adequate dose. Special arrangements should be available for urgent outpatient appointments and a patient whose illness exhibits the warning features already discussed should be admitted to hospital as an emergency.

Prevent cancer

Fortunately, the cancer risk appears to be confined to a relatively small proportion of the colitic population. Patients with distal colitis and those with a short history can be managed without worry about this aspect of the illness. The patients at risk are those with extensive colitis, a history of 10 years or more, and especially those who developed extensive colitis in childhood.

This group of patients is well recognized and requires careful management as already discussed. Some patients do not obviously fall into the high-risk group and these are in particular danger. Examples are the patient who had a severe attack of colitis involving the whole colon many years ago and who has been well since with reversion of the x-ray appearance to normal or near-normal, the patient in whom the extent of colitis has never been recognized, or the patient with extensive colitis who has been treated by a diverting ileostomy, partial colectomy or colectomy with retention of the rectum.

Our own practice is to follow indefinitely all patients with extensive colitis and all patients with an ileorectal anastomosis. We place considerable reliance on the appearance of dysplastic epithelial changes in biopsy specimens obtained from the rectum at sigmoidoscopy and the colon at colonoscopy, but recognize that this change may involve only part of the colon and can therefore be missed. We are therefore guided also by the statistical factors already described, the health of the patient and the disability from his disease.

A physician's attitude to surgical treatment of colitis

Colectomy is an effective and satisfactory treatment for colitis when the indications are appropriate. It must, however, be recognized that the majority of patients with colitis have distal disease of slight or moderate severity and that for them the need for colectomy is uncommon.

Proctocolectomy cures colitis, but at the cost of a permanent ileostomy. The operation is not trouble-free as there is a considerable early post-operative morbidity and a late morbidity associated with complications such as intestinal obstruction. There is a risk of sexual dysfunction, particularly in men. The majority of patients adapt extremely well to the ileostomy and live normal, healthy lives. There are, however, patients who find an ileostomy a great disability either because of their fastidious personality or because the stoma is technically unsatisfactory.

Colectomy with ileorectal anastomosis is an attractive alternative to proctocolectomy and ileostomy, but this operation also has problems. Since colitis almost always involves the rectum, this operation tends to remove the inflamed colon but leaves an inflamed rectum. Persisting or recurrent proctitis is common in my experience after this operation and medical treatment of this proctitis is often helpful. Thus, while the patient's general health is restored by removal of the colon, symptoms of diarrhoea and urgency may persist due to liquid or semi-formed ileal effluent entering an inflamed, and sometimes narrowed, rectum.

There is an increased risk of cancer in the diseased rectum, and careful follow-up with regular mucosal biopsy is therefore necessary. The avoidance of a stoma and the preservation of sexual function may outweigh these disadvantages of the procedure.

My own attitude, therefore, is to regard colectomy and ileorectal anastomosis as particularly suitable for younger patients provided that there is no severe rectal or perianal disease. It is also to be recommended for patients of all ages when the rectum is normal or only slightly diseased, a situation which may be found after emergency subtotal colectomy in a patient with a short history of colitis. Before recommending a patient to accept ileorectal anastomosis it is important that he should understand the arguments for and against the operation. He should be warned that a perfect functional result is not to be expected and that some bowel frequency may persist, that some treatment for diarrhoea or rectal inflammation may be needed, and that indefinite outpatient supervision will be advisable. The possibility that ileostomy could eventually be required should also be mentioned. A patient who accepts these possibilities will be delighted with an excellent result, accept an average result and not be dismayed by a poor result. If a patient wants a certain cure of colitis by one operation, if the patient is in an older age group so that cure by one operation is clinically indicated, if the rectum or anus is severely diseased, or if there appears to be a major cancer risk in the rectum, then proctocolectomy is to be preferred.

References

DISSANAYAKE A. S. and TRUELOVE S. C. (1973) A controlled therapeutic trial of long-term maintenance treatment of ulcerative colitis with sulphasalazine (Salazopyrin). *Gut* **14,** 923–926.

JEWELL D. P. and TRUELOVE S. C. (1974) Azathioprine in ulcerative colitis: final report on controlled therapeutic trial. *Br. Med. J.* **4,** 627–630.

LENNARD-JONES J. E., MISIEWICZ J. J., PARRISH J. A., RITCHIE J. K., SWARBRICK E. T. and WILLIAMS C. B. (1974) Prospective study of out-patients with extensive colitis. *Lancet* **1,** 1065–1067.

LENNARD-JONES J. E., RITCHIE J. K., SPICER C. C. and HILDER W. (1975) The assessment of severity in colitis: a preliminary study. *Gut* **16,** 579–584.

MISIEWICZ J. J., LENNARD-JONES J. E., CONNELL A. M., BARON J. H. and JONES F. AVERY (1965) Controlled trial of sulphasalazine in maintenance therapy for ulcerative colitis. *Lancet* **1,** 185–188.

RITCHIE J. K. (1974) Results of surgery for inflammatory bowel disease: a further survey of one hospital region. *Br. Med. J.* **1,** 264–268.

SWARBRICK E. T., LOOSE H. and LENNARD-JONES J. E. (1974) Enema volume as an important factor in successful topical corticosteroid treatment of colitis. *Proc. R. Soc. Med.* **67,** 753–754.

14

Crohn's Disease and the Surgeon

J. Alexander-Williams, MD, ChM, FRCS

The surgeon cannot cure Crohn's disease by excision. To believe so is almost as naïve as thinking that a plastic surgeon can cure flexural eczema by excising the affected flexure. Crohn's disease is a pan-enteric disease. In some patients with apparent localized disease in the terminal ileum, it is possible to demonstrate characteristic histological abnormalities in the mucosa from the mouth, upper small bowel, colon and anal canal. What the surgeon is called upon to treat is a local complication of the florid areas of disease where the mucosal ulceration has penetrated the bowel wall, bled or healed with fibrosis and stenosis. In many patients complications occur often, particularly when the disease process continues in an active phase.

The analogy of the disease with that of eczema of the skin is reasonably apt since both are diseases of unknown aetiology with a hereditary tendency and probably a local hypersensitivity to a local antigenic substance. The primary pathological lesion results in a breach of the epithelial surface and secondary infection is inevitable, particularly in the bowel. The eczema analogy should not be pressed too far, but the concept is useful if it induces in the physician and, particularly, the surgeon a sense of therapeutic humility.

The surgeon must recognize that recurrence is common; if follow-up is long enough it is virtually inevitable. He should realize that recurrence of the disease does not mean that his original resection was inadequate. There is no evidence to show that wider excision carries a lesser risk of recurrence than limited excision. After resection of a segment of small bowel, recurrence, when it occurs, usually does so immediately proximal to the anastomosis; this does not necessarily mean that if that segment containing the recurrence had originally been resected there would now be no recurrence. It could be that the risk of recurrence is determined by local exposure to an antigenic agent in the gut lumen and that proximal to an anastomosis there is an area of relative stasis leading to prolongation of contact between exciting agent and mucosa. There are so many possible explanations for the site and frequency of recurrence that the policy of wide primary excision cannot be advocated solely on theoretical grounds. The question warrants investigation by a prospective planned study. However, such a study would be extremely difficult to conduct due to the large number of variable factors and so it is not surprising that in the literature there is no evidence, only opinions.

Pathology

The pathological feature of Crohn's disease that is of particular importance to the surgeon, because it predisposes to complications requiring surgical treatment, is the tendency to develop penetrating ulcers. The ulcers, penetrating deep into the muscle layers of the gut, distinguish Crohn's disease from other inflammatory diseases of the bowel such as ulcerative or ischaemic colitis. It is probably infection, gaining access to the muscle layers, that is responsible for the transmural inflammatory reaction that gives rise to the characteristic gross thickening of the wall of the gut and the later fibrotic stenosis. It is the ulceration penetrating through the muscle to the serosal layer of the gut that is responsible for the complications of perforation, abscess and fistula.

Although histological changes characteristic of Crohn's disease can be found in any part of the alimentary tract from the mouth to the anus, some sites are particularly common and some have particular surgical significance. Two of the commonest sites to be affected are the terminal ileum and the anal canal. The particular predisposing factors at these sites are not known with certainty, but could be related to the distribution of lymphoid tissue or to the relative stasis of the bowel contents that could occur at the end of the small and large bowel. Stenosis is likely to manifest as an obstruction particularly in areas where the bowel is narrow, such as the terminal ileum, the site of end-to-end anastomoses or, more rarely, the pylorus and duodenum.

External fistulae through surgical wounds are more likely to occur from mobile parts of the gut, which, if inflamed, may become adherent to the peritoneal surface of an abdominal wound.

Indications for surgical intervention

The surgeon may be required in the management of Crohn's disease for either an emergency or an elective operation.

Emergency operations

The three classical alimentary tract emergencies can all occur in Crohn's disease: perforation, bleeding and stenosis. To these should be added a fourth indication for emergency surgical treatment: abscess.

Free perforation

Free perforation is a rare complication, probably because the ulceration of Crohn's disease is a chronic process; the deepening ulcer is preceded by a zone of inflammatory reaction that causes the serosa of the affected gut to become attached to adjacent structure before the ulcer penetrates right through the bowel wall. Thus abscess and fistula are common but free perforation rare. We have encountered free perforation only 8 times in a series of 500 patients with Crohn's disease (Steinberg et al., 1973a). Perforation is almost always of the small bowel; once in our series and once in the series of Waye and Lithgoe (1967) it occurred in a bypassed ileal segment. The situation that predisposes to free perforation is the presence of a chronic stenotic lesion and a sudden acute exacerbation of florid disease extending proximally. The scarred area becomes oedematous, the obstruction acute or subacute, and an area of acute ulceration proximal to the obstruction perforates before the gut can become firmly adherent to adjacent structures. It is useless to attempt to close the perforation. The best treatment is to excise the perforated segment and all obstructing distal disease. In most cases continuity can be restored by anastomosis, but it may be safer in some cases to exteriorize the ends of the bowel as an ileostomy for later closure (Steinberg et al., 1973a).

Bleeding

Bleeding is rarely a dramatic event in Crohn's disease. Because active disease is always associated with mucosal ulceration, occult blood loss is very common and most patients at some time show evidence of iron deficiency. In our series overt blood loss has occurred in colonic disease and in the remaining small bowel after proctocolectomy. In 4 patients it has been one of the principal indications for early elective surgery. In only 3 patients has intestinal blood loss been the indication for emergency operation, twice due to an acute exacerbation of extensive colonic disease and once from a bleeding duodenal ulcer possibly the consequence of extensive small bowel resection for Crohn's disease (Fielding and Cooke, 1970).

Acute obstruction

Acute obstruction rarely occurs in Crohn's disease although subacute obstruction is common. The mechanism of the obstruction is usually the supervention of acute inflammatory oedema in an area already scarred and thickened from chronic disease. The attack is sometimes precipitated by a bolus of undigested food lodging proximally. Treatment is bed rest, no food by mouth, intravenous replacement therapy and, sometimes, nasogastric suction. This usually results in rapid subsidence of the inflammatory oedema and relief of the obstruction. In one of our patients the obstruction would not resolve because an enterolith had formed between two strictured areas, but even in this instance the indication for operation was not as acute as in a strangulation obstruction.

Although it is a useful management rule that obstruction in Crohn's disease always resolves with rest and replacement therapy, it must not be forgotten that adhesion and strangulation obstruction can occur in patients who have had operations for Crohn's disease. One patient in our series lost many centimetres of previously normal small bowel from strangulation obstruction due to a simple adhesion because of persistence of conservative management of an obstructive episode. If the signs of peritonism can be elicited it is safer to explore the abdomen than to wait and see.

Abscess

Abscess formation is a very common complication of Crohn's disease. Perianal abscesses will be considered in a later section. Abdominal wall abscesses occur most commonly after operations; either early, due to septic complications of the intestinal operation, or late, due to further disease activity with ulceration penetrating the bowel wall. Rarely, an abscess presents spontaneously in the abdominal wall or the groin without any previous operation. Sometimes post-operative sepsis will remain dormant for months or years before presenting as an abscess in the absence of any recurrent activity in adjacent bowel. Superficial abscesses require emergency surgical treatment. This should be simple external drainage; there is no need to perform wide saucerization or to break down deep loculi. A fistula will almost inevitably follow simple drainage if there is underlying active bowel disease.

Deep abscesses may be encountered during elective operations; these are rarely an indication for emergency operation. They are usually found in elective operations in patients with chronic ill health not responding to medical therapy. The abscesses are usually small, between adjacent loops of bowel, and represent a stage in the development of enteroenteric fistulae. These abscesses are usually resected en bloc with the adjacent affected bowel. If the bowel from which they are arising is resected there is no need to drain the deep abscess cavity even if part of its wall is left behind. Occasionally, a very large deep abscess is encountered in the retroperitoneal area. This is usually a psoas abscess, of which we have treated four. Treatment should be excision of the bowel from which the abscess is arising, with simple tube drainage of the cavity to the exterior by the most direct dependent route.

Elective operations

The indications for elective operation in Crohn's disease are local complications such as abscess or fistula, chronic blood and protein loss from continued active mucosal ulceration, persistent urgent diarrhoea, chronic obstructive symptoms and severe or recurrent perianal symptoms. The indications for elective surgical treatment are rarely single. For example, in most patients with fistula or chronic obstructive symptoms, there is also chronic ill health from continued blood and protein loss. Few patients with colonic Crohn's disease have socially inconvenient diarrhoea without also suffering from chronic blood and protein loss. I have attempted to assess the relative frequency of the principal indication for elective operations in our series. The figures in Table 14.1 must be considered in the

Table 14.1 Relative indications for elective operation

	Principally or wholly small bowel disease	Principally or wholly large bowel disease
Abscess or fistula	25%	2%
Chronic ill health (blood and protein loss, diarrhoea)	15%	70%
Obstructive symptoms	60%	12%
Gross perianal disease	0·5%	15%

knowledge that the indications are almost always multiple. I have not listed diarrhoea as a principal indication because, unlike ulcerative colitis, Crohn's disease rarely requires surgical treatment merely for the symptom of diarrhoea.

Fistula

Fistula is a common complication of Crohn's disease. Anal fistulae are the commonest and will be discussed later under the heading of perianal disease.

Apart from anal fistulae, almost all fistulae arise from disease of the small bowel. Fistulae occasionally arise between the sigmoid colon and an abdominal scar or the bladder but, in our experience, fistulae are relatively less common from the large than the small bowel (Steinberg et al., 1973b).

External fistula to the skin usually occurs in the scar of a laparotomy wound, and appears to complicate from 10 to 50 per cent of all abdominal operations for Crohn's disease. The incidence is highest after operations that bypass an active area of Crohn's disease of the ileum or when a laparotomy without resection is performed for an exacerbation of Crohn's disease erroneously diagnosed as an abdominal emergency. In many such operations the erroneous diagnosis is appendicitis and often the appendix is removed. The subsequent fistula is blamed on the appendicectomy, and on the basis of this observation some surgeons condemn appendicectomy. However, I believe that the fistula is as likely to arise even if the appendix is not removed. Experience of operations on many patients with such fistulae has convinced me that the fistula usually arises from the active ileal disease rather than the appendix stump. I do not feel that appendicectomy can be condemned in Crohn's disease on the grounds that it predisposes to the complication of fistula. However, it may be reasonable to criticize the surgeon who is misled into the diagnosis of appendicitis in a patient who gives a long history of weight loss, borborygmi and diarrhoea.

External fistulae may discharge only small quantities of pus and intestinal content and only inconvenience the patient because of smell or skin excoriation and require only frequent changes of dressing. However, if in addition to the fistula there is also a stenosis of the bowel distal to the fistula then the fluid output may amount to several litres per day and cause serious disturbances of electrolyte and nitrogen balance. Such a profuse discharge necessitates the fitting of an adhesive appliance to collect the fluid. The temporary management of skin excoriation from a profusely discharging fistula has been revolutionized by the development of a non-permeable, adhesive, malleable dressing such as Stomahesive. The sheet of impervious material adheres to the skin and granulation around the fistula and allows the fluid to come through a central hole into an appliance stuck on to the surface.

Small fistulae may cause so little trouble that it is not necessary to treat them actively, but fistulae in Crohn's disease rarely close spontaneously. Many fistulae that begin in a small way eventually cause so much trouble that active treatment is essential. In our series we have experienced the greatest success with radical resection of the segment involved by active disease from which the fistula arose. The operation often appears to present a formidable technical problem but is rarely difficult once the tissue plane is entered between the gut and the adherent abdominal wall. The oedematous tissues separate readily and the mass of involved gut can often be 'cracked' off the parietes. Our earlier experience of operations that bypassed the fistula, or attempted to close the fistula or reimplant the track, has been uniformly disappointing. Radical operations were successful in 84 per cent of patients with a mortality of 6 per cent (Steinberg et al., 1973b).

Most of the deaths in the series occurred many years ago in seriously ill patients. Our recent experience indicates that with proper pre-operative preparation the mortality for operations on Crohn's disease fistulae should be less than 2 per cent.

Internal fistulae may occur into the genitourinary tract or between different parts of the gut. A fistula from rectum to vagina should be treated as an anal fistula (see below).

Fistulae into the bladder are uncommon, usually arising from ileal disease. The effect on the urinary tract is often remarkably slight, causing only intermittent cystitis. I have seen one patient who had intermittent pneumaturia for over 10 years as the result of a Crohn's disease fistula from sigmoid colon to bladder. Her general health remained good and her renal function was unaffected.

When surgical treatment is required, often because of the added factors of active or stenosing ileal disease, the principles are the same as described for cutaneous fistula; the attached bowel is 'cracked' off the bladder and resected. I have done this on three occasions and have been surprised to find no sign of the hole in the bladder (even if it was distended with fluid) despite the patient having pneumaturia immediately before operation. No special manœuvres are employed to cover the bladder with peritoneum. The affected small gut is removed and the bladder drained by catheter for 1 week.

Internal fistula between loops of gut are often not suspected or detected until the pathologist unravels the resected mass. This is particularly so with the commonest form of internal fistula: ileoileal. We have encountered patients with ileotransverse fistulae who have remarkably little disturbance and who did not need surgical treatment merely because a fistula was present. On the other hand, ileosigmoid fistulae have been associated with severe diarrhoea and metabolic disturbances. The sudden onset of deterioration and diarrhoea in a patient with relatively quiescent Crohn's disease should raise the suspicion of the development of a fistula between the upper and lower parts of the alimentary tract. We have seen similar sudden deterioration due to the development of fistulae between duodenum and colon, or between duodenum and ileum.

When treating a patient surgically with a fistula between widely different parts of the bowel such as ileum and sigmoid colon or ileum and duodenum, it is important to prepare adequately with elemental diet or parenteral nutrition and mineral replacement. It is usually apparent which segment of gut is primarily affected; that is, from which segment the deep ulceration arises causing the local abscess that then ruptured into the adjacent viscus giving rise to a fistula. This is commonly the ileum. It is necessary only to resect the primarily affected bowel, merely closing the hole in the secondarily affected gut. Unfortunately, sometimes it is difficult to determine which is the primarily affected gut. In some patients I have found a fistula between sigmoid colon and ileum with a small intervening abscess cavity when both segments of bowel were thickened and oedematous. It has been difficult in these cases to know whether to resect the sigmoid as well as the ileum. It is helpful in such a case to have an accurate pre-operative radiological and endoscopic assessment of the sigmoid colon. However, the presence of inflammatory oedema often makes the sigmoid appear to be more severely affected than it is. My policy is to attempt to avoid resection of the sigmoid unless there is a definite fibrotic stricture. In 2 patients I have resected the ileum, closed the hole in the sigmoid and performed a temporary bypass loop ileostomy (Alexander-Williams, 1974). In 1 patient in whom I did not temporarily divert the bowel contents, a free perforation of the sigmoid colon occurred 5 days later: the only free perforation of the colon in our series.

In recent years our experience with the surgical management of fistulae in Crohn's disease has been so satisfactory that we feel it is the optimum method of treatment, associated with a smaller risk than the use of immunosuppressive drugs. Azathioprine has certainly had some success in causing the temporary healing of enterocutaneous fistulae, but we have found that the fistulae recur when the drug is stopped and sometimes recur even during therapy. We feel that the possible long-term effects of immunosuppressive therapy preclude its continuous use, but it may have a place in the temporary control of a fistula while a patient is prepared for definitive surgical treatment (Cooke, 1972).

Blood and protein loss, and obstruction

Chronic blood and protein loss from mucosal ulceration and obstruction from oedema and fibrosis are complications that often co-exist. Surgical treatment is required when the disability or symptoms cannot be controlled by replacement or symptomatic therapy. The technical problems presented to the surgeon are similar with both complications. The questions that he has to consider are: (1) should the affected gut be excised or bypassed; and, if excised, (2) how much gut should be removed?

Bypass of an area of Crohn's disease that is the cause of blood and protein loss is not advisable because disease activity and ulceration can continue in a bypassed segment (Burman et al., 1971).

Bypass of an obstructing segment of bowel may seem an attractive and less difficult manœuvre than excision of a matted area of bowel. However, the long-term results of bypass are less good than those after excision, a second operation often being required after bypass to treat abscesses or fistulae (Alexander-Williams, 1971).

In my opinion there is rarely any reason for preferring bypass to excision and anastomosis for localized Crohn's disease.

How much bowel to excise is another question that has exercised surgeons treating Crohn's disease. Recognizing that the disease is diffuse and therefore incurable by operation, I tend to limit excision to the length of bowel giving rise to the particular complication that is the indication for operation. I am prepared to leave macroscopically abnormal lengths of bowel provided that they are producing no complications, a view supported by the experience at the Mayo Clinic (Barber et al., 1962).

However, other surgeons believe that limited excision leads to early recurrence (Wallensten, 1971) and that leaving large mesenteric nodes predisposes to recurrence (Stahlgren and Ferguson, 1961).

The surgical policy followed by Professor Goligher and his colleagues in Leeds has been based on the premise that it is best to perform a wide excision, taking a margin of 25 cm of apparently normal bowel on either side of the affected length and removing all the enlarged nodes (de Dombal, 1972).

A comparison of the results of the surgical treatment of Crohn's disease in Leeds and in Birmingham is shown in Table 14.2. Too many conclusions should not be drawn from this comparison because the patients are not necessarily compar-

Table 14.2 Comparison of rates of re-operation and mortality in Leeds and in Birmingham: Crohn's disease of large and small bowel

	Leeds (radical surgical policy)	Birmingham (conservative surgical policy)
Number of patients treated surgically	295	254
Number of operations	415	677
Mean number of operations/patient	1·4	2·7
Surgical deaths	24	15
Surgical mortality	8·1%	5·9%
Operative mortality	5·8%	2·2%

After Alexander-Williams (1972).

able, most of the patients in the Leeds series being referred first to a surgical clinic and in Birmingham first to a medical clinic. However, I am prepared to accept a higher rate of surgical intervention during the lifetime of a patient with Crohn's disease provided that there is a low cumulative life risk from the repeated operations.

Perianal disease

Perianal disease is a remarkably common complication of Crohn's disease anywhere in the alimentary tract and is almost universal in patients with colonic Crohn's disease. The lesions are characteristically multiple, indurated and remarkably asymptomatic. It is the fact that they produce few symptoms that leads to their being overlooked. In many reported series of Crohn's disease the incidence of perianal disease is reported as about 25 per cent if the primary disease affects the small bowel alone and about 75 per cent if the main Crohn's disease is in the large bowel (Lockhart-Mummary, 1972).

In 1968 a survey of patients attending our Unit by Fielding (1970) included a detailed study of perianal lesions. He found an incidence of perianal lesions (including oedematous skin tags) of 85 per cent associated with small bowel disease and over 70 per cent associated with large bowel disease. A group of 109 patients were documented with perianal abscesses, fissures or fistulae. These patients were then followed for 5 years and reassessed in 1973 (Steinberg et al., 1975). In the majority of patients (78 per cent) the state of the perianal disease was unchanged after 5 years despite a transient local flare-up of inflammation, requiring drainage, in 7 (8 per cent). In a few patients (6 per cent) the disease appeared to have resolved completely, sometimes without any treatment.

As the disease produces few symptoms and, untreated, tends to run a benign course, it seems to be advisable to pursue a very conservative course of management. The mere presence of a fissure or fistula-in-ano in Crohn's disease is not an indication for surgical treatment.

When the disease causes symptoms, it is usually due to the pain of an abscess under tension. Simple drainage relieves the pain and is all that should be done.

The serious complications of perianal Crohn's disease are stenosis and incontinence; both of these usually follow aggressive surgical treatment.

Stenosis has presented as a major problem in 14 of our cases. Four followed the operations of fissurectomy, wide excision of a fistula or haemorrhoidectomy; 6 followed laying open of a fistula track. All operations were performed either many years ago or before referral to our Unit. In only 4 patients did the stenosis appear to arise spontaneously from the effects of the disease itself unaided by surgical treatment.

Faecal incontinence is an even more serious complication occurring in 16 patients, 6 having permanent loss of control and 10 intermittent only when they have severe diarrhoea. The 6 with permanent incontinence had been treated either by a wide excision of a fistula or extensive drainage of an ischiorectal abscess. In our experience incontinence has been the result of aggressive surgery rather than progressive disease.

If radical treatment is to be condemned how then can we treat the complications of perianal Crohn's disease?

Pain indicates pus under tension and should be drained in the simplest way. Fissures *per se* do not cause pain and should not be treated.

Stenosis should be treated conservatively by gentle anal dilatation with one finger, under general anaesthesia if necessary, followed by the provision of a small plastic dilator or finger cots for the patient to practice self-dilatation. Under no circumstances should forcible four-finger dilatation be employed. I have seen patients with a tight anal canal stenosis of only 2–3 mm in diameter gradually improve and become asymptomatic over the course of years.

Incontinence is difficult to treat, and complete incontinence is usually an indication for a proctectomy. There may be a place for considering sphincter reconstruction operations in patients with inactive anal disease who have been damaged by ill-advised operations.

The surgeon whose experience of anal fissures, abscesses or fistulae is confined to patients without Crohn's disease is often horrified by the appearance of the perineum affected by perianal Crohn's disease. He usually feels that something drastic must be done for the patient. He should be restrained. The essential in treatment of perianal Crohn's disease is conservatism.

References

ALEXANDER-WILLIAMS J. (1971) The place of surgery in Crohn's disease. *Gut* **12,** 739–749.
ALEXANDER-WILLIAMS J. (1972) Surgery and the management of Crohn's disease. *Clin. Gastroenterol,* **1,** 469–491.

ALEXANDER-WILLIAMS J. (1974) Loop ileostomy and colostomy for faecal diversion. *Ann. R. Coll. Surg. Engl.* **54,** 141–148.

BARBER K. W. JR, WAUGH J. M., BEAHRS O. H. and SAUER W. G. (1962) Indications for and the results of the surgical treatment of regional enteritis. *Ann. Surg.* **156,** 472–482.

BURMAN J. H., THOMPSON H., COOKE W. T. and ALEXANDER-WILLIAMS J. (1971) The effects of diversion of intestinal contents on the progress of Crohn's disease of the large bowel. *Gut.* **12,** 11–15.

COOKE W. T. (1972) Survey of results of treatment of Crohn's disease. *Clin. Gastroenterol.* **1,** 521–531.

DE DOMBAL F. T. (1972) Results of surgery for Crohn's disease. *Clin. Gastroenterol.* **1,** 493–506.

FIELDING J. F. (1970) Crohn's Disease. MD Thesis, University of Cork.

FIELDING J. F. and COOKE W. T. (1970) Peptic ulceration in Crohn's disease (regional enteritis). *Gut* **11,** 998–1000.

LOCKHART-MUMMARY H. E. (1972) Anal lesions of Crohn's disease. *Clin. Gastroenterol.* **1,** 377–382.

STALGREN L. H. and FERGUSON L. K. (1961) The results of surgical treatment of chronic regional enteritis. *JAMA* **175,** 986–989.

STEINBERG D. M., ALLEN R. A., COOKE W. T. and ALEXANDER-WILLIAMS J. (1975) Unpublished data.

STEINBERG D. M., COOKE W. T. and ALEXANDER-WILLIAMS J. (1973a) Free perforation in Crohn's disease. *Gut* **14,** 187–190.

STEINBERG D. M., COOKE W. T. and ALEXANDER-WILLIAMS J. (1973b) Abscess and fistulae in Crohn's disease. *Gut* **14,** 865–869.

WALLENSTEN S. (1971) Results of surgical treatment in Sweden. In: *Skandia International Symposium on Crohn's Disease.* Stockholm, Nordiska Bokhandelns Forlag.

WAYNE J. D. and LITHGOE C. (1967) Small bowel perforation in regional enteritis. *Gastroenterology* **53,** 625–629.

15

Gynaecological Problems and the General Surgeon*

M. D. Cameron, FRCS, FRCOG

Introduction

Surgeons who specialized in the treatment of disorders of the female genital tract were among the first to form a group separate from surgeons in general. Special women's hospitals were founded at which techniques were developed, notably by the school of Victor Bonney, which are still the basis of gynaecological surgery. However, the resultant isolation impeded the exchange of ideas; many gynaecologists were poorly trained in general surgery and general surgeons ignored gynaecology.

A discussion of gynaecology in relation to general surgery may be considered under four headings:

1. The acute abdomen.
2. Gynaecological disorders discovered unexpectedly at laparotomy.
3. Abdominal pain in pregnancy.
4. Pregnancy and cancer.

The acute abdomen

It is salutary to remember that the diagnosis of acute abdominal symptoms is more difficult in the female than in the male. In a recent series (Gilmore et al., 1975), the clinical diagnosis of acute appendicitis proved at laparotomy to be wrong twice as often in females as in males.

Ectopic pregnancy

Implantation of the fertilized ovum in the fallopian tube occurs when its descent into the uterus is obstructed, usually by mucosal adhesions, a legacy of past salpingitis. Alternatively, Iffy (1961) suggests that the ovum may be held back in the tube by retrograde menstruation if fertilization takes place late in the cycle.

The site of implantation is commonly in the ampulla, less often in the isthmus, and rarely in the intramural part of the tube. The chorionic villi rapidly erode

* Reprinted, with additional text, from Annals of the Royal College of Surgeons of England, 1975, Vol. 56, pp. 115–123.

the mucosal and muscular layers of the tube where their invasion is not limited, as it is in the endometrium, by a decidual reaction. When the walls of blood vessels are penetrated the extravasated blood separates the ovum from its attachment. Complete separation produces a *tubal mole* which may undergo abortion into the peritoneal cavity. Continued survival and growth of trophoblastic tissue produces repeated episodes of haemorrhage and ends in *tubal rupture.*

Blood from the implantation site passes through the fimbriated end of the tube to collect in the pouch of Douglas, forming a pelvic haematocele, though tubal rupture results in free intraperitoneal bleeding. Blood also flows down the fallopian tube into the uterus, from which it passes into the vagina and sometimes into the other tube.

A tubal mole, commonly seen in ampullary implantations, accounts for 65 per cent of cases, and tubal rupture from isthmic implantations accounts for 35 per cent of cases (Llewellyn-Jones, 1970).

Diagnosis

The diagnosis of ectopic gestation is made primarily on the patient's history and demands a high level of awareness on the part of the surgeon.

Acute tubal rupture causes little difficulty. A young woman in a state of shock complains of sudden severe abdominal pain. She usually but not invariably gives a history of a short period of amenorrhoea and vaginal bleeding, though common, is not always present.

The subacute picture of tubal mole is a more difficult diagnostic problem. Amenorrhoea, usually of less than 6 weeks' duration, is followed by lower abdominal pain which precedes vaginal bleeding. Pain is the most important symptom; amenorrhoea may be absent or there may be a history of prolonged bleeding.

The pain which is characteristically severe and episodic is caused initially by distension of the tube and later by blood in the peritoneal cavity. In each attack the severe pain persists for about 30 minutes, subsequently diminishing to leave residual tenderness which is exacerbated by sudden movement. Even a small quantity of blood in the peritoneal cavity causes reflex fainting and when blood irritates the diaphragm, pain is felt in the shoulder tip. Urinary and gastrointestinal symptoms are unusual unless a pelvic haemotocele is present.

The blood passed per vaginam is initially dark in colour and originates at the implantation site; later, bright red blood is passed when the decidua is shed following the decline of the pregnancy hormones on the death of the ovum. Occasionally the entire decidua is shed as a decidual cast. Histological examination of such material, which contains no chorionic villi, may be helpful in differentiation from an abortion.

On examination the woman is shocked if profuse intraperitoneal bleeding has occurred. Otherwise her condition is good. Pyrexia above 37·2°C is unusual. Lower abdominal tenderness, especially when pressure is suddenly released, is usual and sometimes a mass of blood clot may be palpable. On vaginal examination dark blood may be seen escaping from the external os; the uterus is normal or a little enlarged in size. Extreme tenderness which is elicited by movement of the cervix makes palpation of any tubal swelling difficult, though a pelvic haematocele is readily identified.

Investigations include estimation of the haemoglobin level and white blood cell count, both of which are likely to be normal. However, during normal pregnancy the haemoglobin level is often no more than 11 g/dl, the white cell count may be as high as $15 \times 10^9/1$ (15,000/mm^3), and the erythrocyte sedimentation rate may be elevated to 80 mm in 1 hour. The blood group is identified and serum is retained for cross-matching.

The pregnancy test proves negative in 20 per cent of cases either because the ovum is already dead or because implantation is too recent for sufficient chorionic gonadotrophin to have been produced.

Laparoscopy which is the one certain method of diagnosis is used in all difficult cases but should be avoided if the woman is in a state of shock. Its widespread use marks a major advance in gynaecological surgery.

Differential diagnosis

This is usually from:

Abortion, in which the duration of amenorrhoea is generally 8–12 weeks; bleeding precedes pain; uterine enlargement is consistent with the duration of pregnancy; the cervical os may be open; and pelvic tenderness is not remarkable unless the abortion is septic.

Salpingitis is associated with a purulent discharge and pyrexia usually above 38°C.

Appendicitis nearly always causes anorexia, nausea or vomiting, which are rarely present with a tubal pregnancy.

Cystitis may be ruled out by microscopic examination of the urine.

An ovarian cyst complicated by haemorrhage or torsion may be impossible to differentiate from a tubal pregnancy. In particular a haemorrhagic corpus luteum, causing a delayed period, abdominal pain, and a tender swelling in the pelvis, may mimic ectopic gestation.

Treatment

This consists of laparotomy and, when necessary, simultaneous blood transfusion. Through a small transverse suprapubic incision blood in the pelvis is cleared away to allow inspection of the uterus, tubes and ovaries. No organ is removed and no clamp is applied before such an inspection. The site of the tubal pregnancy is carefully identified and differentiated from a possible haematosalpinx in the other tube.

Subtotal salpingectomy is performed provided the other tube appears normal; the ovary must not be removed unless it is disrupted by haematoma. If the other tube is diseased or has already been removed the affected tube may be preserved. For example, in Fig. 15.1, where right salpingectomy was indicated for a pyosalpinx, the ectopic pregnancy in the left tube was evacuated through a longitudinal incision which was then repaired.

Acute salpingitis

Salpingitis is caused by infection which may either ascend the genital tract from

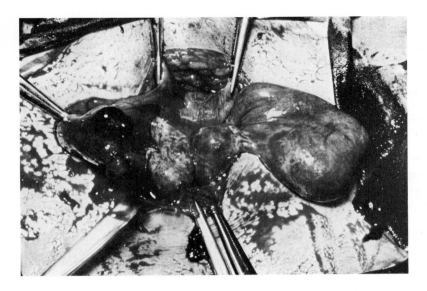

Fig. 15.1 Left tubal pregnancy; right pyosalpinx.

the cervix via the endometrium as in a gonococcal infection or be part of a generalized infection of the pelvis following childbirth, abortion or an operation on the cervix.

The inflammation generally affects both tubes, which initially appear red and oedematous, with pus exuding from the abdominal ostia. At a later stage each ostium becomes blocked by adhesions of fibrin and a pyosalpinx forms (Fig. 15.1). Involvement of the ovary results in a tubo-ovarian abscess and is accompanied by pelvic peritonitis. The fallopian tube, unlike the appendix, has a double blood supply so that gangrene occurs only in the presence of a clostridial infection. For the same reason, rupture of a pyosalpinx is rare.

Early resolution of the inflammatory process allows the tube to return to normal. If an abscess forms the tube is permanently damaged and the woman is likely to experience recurrent attacks of subacute salpingitis.

The symptoms of acute salpingitis include lower abdominal pain, malaise and a purulent vaginal discharge from which the infecting organisms sometimes can be isolated. An initial rigor with fever of 39–40°C is common. Vomiting and other gastrointestinal symptoms are unusual.

Examination of the abdomen reveals tenderness, especially marked on release, and guarding in both iliac fossae. Bowel sounds are present. Extreme pelvic tenderness prevents palpation of the pelvic organs and a purulent vaginal discharge is seen coming through the external cervical os.

Investigations include haemoglobin estimation, white cell count, and blood grouping. The urine is examined for evidence of infection and a pregnancy test is performed. Specimens of the discharge should be obtained from the endocervix, urethra and rectum to culture for *Neisseria gonorrhoeae* and from the vagina for other organisms. Differential diagnosis from ectopic gestation, appendicitis or an accident to an ovarian cyst must be made.

Treatment

The treatment of acute salpingitis is conservative, as the infection usually responds to antibiotics, but if the diagnosis is in any doubt laparotomy must be undertaken. No harm is done and no blame attaches to a surgeon who operates on a woman with acute salpingitis. Indeed, Sünden (1950) has shown that permanent tubal damage causing sterility is less likely to follow salpingitis when surgery is combined with chemotherapy. At such an operation pus is expressed from the abdominal ostia and any exudate in the pouch of Douglas is mopped out, a specimen being obtained for bacterial culture. Should the ostia be occluded, an opening is made to ensure drainage.

Accidents to ovarian cysts

An ovarian cyst causes abdominal pain only in the presence of some complication.

Torsion of an ovarian cyst, like that of a testis, results in severe pain of sudden onset and sustained character. The pain is unrelieved by any measure and is often accompanied by vomiting. Guarding of the abdominal wall together with extreme pelvic tenderness, though obscuring the presence of the cyst, indicates clearly the need for laparotomy. Provided the ovary is viable ovarian cystectomy is performed; otherwise oöphorectomy is indicated. The other ovary must always be inspected to make sure that it also does not contain a cyst.

Sometimes torsion is less acute and then attacks of lower abdominal pain may recur over weeks or months.

Haemorrhage is most likely to occur into an endometriomatous or a malignant cyst or into a corpus luteum. Each condition will be considered under the appropriate heading.

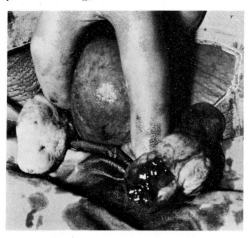

Fig. 15.2 Corpus luteum haematoma of right ovary.

Rupture of an ovarian cyst is an uncommon event and often indicates malignancy. Rupture of a mucinous cyst causes myxoma peritonei.

Ovulation pain is a common symptom, particularly in women aged between 25 and 35 years, and may be severe enough to raise the question of a surgical emergency. The diagnosis is made on a history of mid-cycle pain recurring over several months and may be confirmed by laparoscopy at which blood is seen in the peritoneal cavity arising from a corpus luteum. Very rarely such bleeding may be profuse. Figure 15.2 shows a corpus luteum haematoma of the right ovary.

A *corpus luteum cyst* may cause pain throughout the second half of the menstrual cycle, and the ensuing period is often delayed by the high level of ovarian hormones. The presence of a tender cystic swelling in the pelvis makes such a syndrome clinically indistinguishable from tubal gestation.

Abortion

Complications of abortion may cause acute abdominal emergencies. Pelvic peritonitis from septic abortion commonly follows criminal interference with pregnancy, and clostridial gangrene of the uterus is seen on rare occasions. Surgical damage to the cervix or uterus may result in a broad-ligament haematoma or uterine perforation. Air embolism leading to sudden collapse and even death may follow vaginal douching in attempts to procure criminal abortion. Douching may also lead to intravasation of chemicals, causing hypofibrinogenaemia and sometimes renal damage and anuria. Septic abortion is the commonest cause of endotoxin shock which, despite modern therapy, causes a high mortality.

Although the general surgeon is unlikely often to encounter these conditions, his opinion may be sought when the woman conceals the history of a recent pregnancy.

Unsuspected gynaecological disorders found at laparotomy

Under this heading I have included gynaecological conditions which the general surgeon may encounter unexpectedly at laparotomy. To avoid making serious mistakes in treatment I offer the following advice.

1. The uterus, both ovaries, and both tubes should be inspected before any structure is removed.

2. Ovarian disease is frequently bilateral; each ovary should be regarded as one-half of a single structure.

3. Removal of an ovarian cyst, preserving the rest of the ovary—that is, ovarian cystectomy—is usually a simple procedure (Fig. 15.3).

4. When a surgeon operates on a young woman to remove the appendix and this is found to be normal he must resist the temptation to remove the ovary even though it appears cystic. The left ovary is fortunate in being out of reach of the surgeon using a McBurney's incision.

5. The general surgeon should realize that the ovary is as important to a woman as is the testis to a man.

208

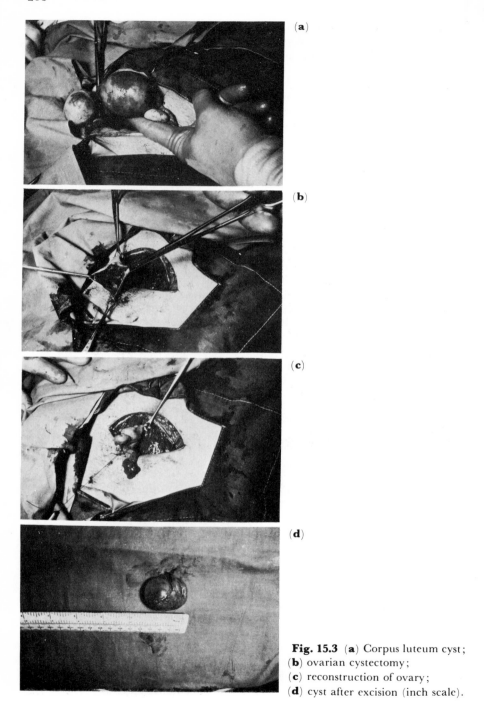

Fig. 15.3 (**a**) Corpus luteum cyst;
(**b**) ovarian cystectomy;
(**c**) reconstruction of ovary;
(**d**) cyst after excision (inch scale).

6. The opinion of an experienced gynaecologist should be sought when the nature of a lesion is doubtful or its surgical treatment is uncertain.

7. A woman should cease the use of oral contraceptives a month before elective major surgery.

8. Diagnostic x-rays of abdominal or pelvic organs should not be taken during the second half of the menstrual cycle lest an early pregnancy be irradiated.

Endometriosis

The ectopic endometrial tissue which characterizes this condition is usually found in the ovary, uterosacral ligaments and pouch of Douglas. The bowel may be affected, especially in the rectosigmoid and ileocaecal parts. Less common sites include the scar following a gynaecological operation, the bladder, the umbilicus and the inguinal canal.

At operation endometriosis is recognized by the presence of endometrial cysts

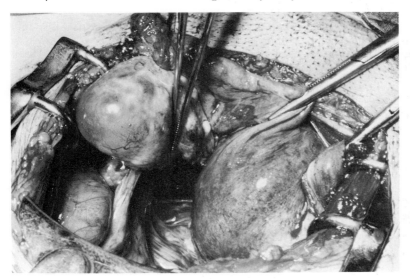

Fig. 15.4 Endometriosis with adhesions in pouch of Douglas; follicular cyst of left ovary and small chocolate cyst on medial side of forceps.

and fibrosis. The cysts vary in size from a pin's head to an orange and are filled with altered blood forming 'chocolate cysts'. The surrounding fibrous reaction produces dense pelvic adhesions which make dissection very difficult. Figure 15.4 shows adhesions due to endometriosis between the uterus and rectum obliterating the pouch of Douglas. Endometriosis of the gut may mimic carcinoma.

Endometriosis is limited to the years of menstrual activity and is commonest in women over the age of 30 who have not borne children. The most important symptom is lower abdominal pain which is worse before periods, when the endometrium becomes secretory and then haemorrhagic. Rupture of an endometrioma—which, because of surrounding fibrosis, is rare—causes extreme pain and collapse. Other symptoms, which more concern the gynaecologist, include dyspareunia, infertility and menstrual disorders. On examination the characteristic finding is of tender nodules in the pouch of Douglas.

Laparoscopy is the most satisfactory method of confirming the diagnosis.

Treatment

The best treatment for endometriosis is pregnancy. When for any reason this is not possible and the patient's symptoms are severe, laparotomy is advised in a young woman to remove all deposits of endometriosis, in an older woman to perform hysterectomy. Should symptoms recur after a conservative operation medical treatment with hormones may be tried, but the results are not encouraging.

The general surgeon may rarely encounter extensive pelvic endometriosis at laparotomy. In the absence of a gynaecological opinion his approach should be conservative. After mobilization and inspection of the pelvic organs all deposits of endometriosis are either excised or destroyed by diathermy. The uterus should be anteverted by shortening the round ligaments. Hysterectomy or removal of all ovarian tissue should never be performed without the woman's previous consent.

Table 15.1 *Classification of ovarian tumours*

Cysts

Non-neoplastic

Follicular	Diameter 2·5–5 cm; thin-walled; translucent; smooth lining (Fig. 15.4)
Luteal	Diameter 2·5–5 cm; haemorrhagic or yellow; smooth lining (Figs. 15.2 and 15.3)
Endometrial	Variable size; contains 'chocolate' material; adherent to surrounding structures

Benign neoplastic

Dermoid (benign teratoma)	Variable size; waxy appearance (Fig. 15.5)
Mucinous cyst	Multilocular; blue appearance; smooth lining
Serous cyst	Multilocular; blue appearance; papillary ingrowths

Malignant

Malignant teratoma	
Mucinous cystadenocarcinoma	Malignant counterparts of benign cysts and often impossible to differentiate clinically
Serous cystadenocarcinoma	

Solid tumours

Benign

Fibroma and similar tumours	Hard white lobulated tumours; may be associated with ascites

Malignant

Primary adenocarcinoma	Early development of multiple peritoneal metastases
Metastatic carcinoma	Primary growths in breasts, stomach, colon or endometrium
Rare tumours	Some secrete sex hormones

Ovarian tumours

Ovarian tumours may be simply classified as in Table 15.1. All types of ovarian tumour are slow to cause symptoms unless complications arise; herein lies their danger. Novak and Novak (1958) found that 15 per cent are malignant and in middle-aged women the proportion is much higher. In malignant tumours

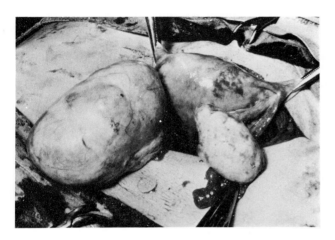

Fig. 15.5 Benign teratoma of left ovary.

metastatic spread throughout the peritoneal cavity is often found at operation. As the prognosis is then very bad, any ovarian cyst should be explored as urgently as one would explore a lump in the breast.

The type of operation is determined by the nature of the tumour and the patient's age, the surgeon aiming always to be conservative and remove no organ unless it is absolutely necessary to do so. A benign cyst is treated by ovarian cystectomy, though if the woman is of menopausal age total hysterectomy and bilateral salpingo-oöphorectomy may be preferable. When a cyst of doubtful nature is found in a woman of child-bearing age histological examination of a frozen section may be helpful. In such a woman, unless the cyst is malignant, some ovarian tissue should be retained.

Although most ovarian carcinomata are relatively radioresistant, post-operative treatment with deep x-ray therapy is indicated when the disease appears limited to the pelvic cavity. More widespread abdominal metastases render the treatment impracticable.

Many women with these tumours respond favourably to chemotherapy, the initial choice of drug usually being chlorambucil. Reduction in the rate of formation of ascites and an improved feeling of well-being are the main benefits, which often continue for many months or even years.

Myomata (fibroids)

A fibroid is a benign smooth-muscle tumour arising from the myometrium.

Fibroids vary in diameter from a few millimetres to several centimetres and are often multiple. The general surgeon will most often encounter fibroids by chance at laparotomy when their presence should merely be noted. Occasionally a fibroid may undergo infarction (often known as red degeneration), which causes severe pain and is particularly common in pregnancy. Generally such a fibroid should not be removed as the pain settles within a few days. At a later date calcification is likely to occur in such a fibroid and this can be seen on x-ray as a round stippled opacity which may have to be differentiated from other causes of calcification in the pelvis. These include calcification in an ovarian teratoma, an ovarian adenocarcinoma and, rarely, tuberculous salpingitis or lithopaedion.

The general surgeon should not forget that at myomectomy haemostasis may be difficult to achieve and the post-operative recovery is more likely to be complicated by haematoma formation than is hysterectomy.

Abdominal pain in pregnancy

Abdominal pain in pregnancy may result from complications of the pregnancy or from unrelated conditions, some of which are much more common in pregnancy. The causes of the pain tend to differ in each trimester, as shown below.

1st trimester	2nd trimester	3rd trimester
Ectopic pregnancy	Red degeneration in fibromyomata	Premature labour
Abortion	Pyelonephritis	Abruptio placentae
Corpus luteum haematoma	Cholestasis	Uterine rupture
(these are described under 'Acute abdomen')	Gastro-oesophageal reflux	

Pain caused by conditions unconnected with pregnancy include accidents to ovarian cysts and appendicitis. Other general surgical conditions are rare and will not be considered further. Musculoskeletal pain which arises from an increased mobility of joints and altered body posture is common and may be severe. Gastro-oesophageal reflux results in upper abdominal burning pain and cholestasis may cause pain in the right hypochondrium.

Red degeneration in fibromyomata

Women, especially those who delay childbearing until the age of 30 years or more, often have uterine fibromyomata. These seldom prevent conception or cause abortion but, during pregnancy, generally enlarge. Sometimes, especially in the second trimester, they undergo red degeneration. An initial venous thrombosis causes intense engorgement of the fibroid and eventual obstruction to its arterial blood supply. On histological section the appearance is of a typical red infarct, with the necrosed myoma cells interspersed with many red blood cells.

The patient experiences abdominal pain, the severity of which depends on the size of the fibroid and the degrees of its engorgement. If the pain is intense and associated with vomiting and shock, the clinical picture is one of an acute surgical emergency. A less severe condition causes localized pain and an area of abdominal tenderness limited to the fibroid.

If a woman who is pregnant and who has abdominal pain is known to have fibroids, the diagnosis should not be difficult; a tender, firm swelling is felt arising from the uterus. However, when pain and tenderness are severe it may not be possible to identify the swelling though tenderness is maximum over the uterus. Vaginal bleeding does not occur, but there is often a low grade pyrexia.

Treatment is conservative and consists of bed rest with the administration of analgesic drugs until the acute pain has subsided. Surgery is avoided, but even if laparotomy is mistakenly performed myomectomy is contraindicated because of the risk of profuse and uncontrollable bleeding from the pregnant uterus. Red degeneration does not prevent the pregnancy proceeding to term and fibroids rarely cause mechanical difficulty in labour.

Pyelonephritis

It has been shown that 7 per cent of pregnant women have symptomless bacteriuria, and 35 per cent of these will develop acute pyelonephritis during pregnancy unless prophylactic chemotherapy is given. The infection results from urinary stasis brought about by relaxation and dilation of the muscular wall of the ureter in response to the high level of progesterone produced by the placenta. Because the uterus is rotated to the right, the right ureter is subjected to more pressure at the pelvic brim than the left ureter. Acute pyelonephritis is therefore much commoner in the right than in the left kidney. The illness generally has an abrupt onset during the second trimester. Loin pain, usually right-sided, occasionally bilateral and rarely left-sided, is associated with a rigor and often with vomiting. Urinary frequency and dysuria are usual, but these symptoms are of course not uncommon in normal pregnancy. The diagnosis can best be confirmed by finding white blood cells and organisms on microscopic examination of the urine.

Acute appendicitis in pregnancy

Pregnancy renders a woman no more and no less likely to develop acute appendicitis. However, the symptoms and signs are likely to be modified, leading to delay in diagnosis and treatment. Finch and Lee (1974) found that acute appendicitis occurred in 0·6 per 1,000 pregnancies, but was less common in its latter weeks, possibly as the result of diagnostic mistakes. It is prudent always to suspect acute appendicitis in a pregnant woman who has right-sided abdominal pain.

The increasing size of the uterus in pregnancy displaces the caecum and appendix to a progressively higher and more lateral position in the abdominal cavity. Pain and tenderness should therefore be expected in the flank where the pain may be mistaken for one of renal origin. The uterine enlargement disguises the signs of guarding and rigidity. Abdominal palpation may be facilitated by tilting the patient 30 degrees on to her left side. The uterus is then displaced to the left, allowing deeper palpation of the right side of the abdomen. Furthermore, tenderness resulting from a uterine lesion shifts to the left, whereas that of an extrauterine source remains fixed. Rectal tenderness is absent. It should be remembered that the white cell count is elevated in normal pregnancy. The presence of white blood cells in the urine indicates the probability of urinary tract infection. If, after careful assessment, the differential diagnosis from acute pyelonephritis is in doubt, observation of the patient for a few hours in hospital will establish the correct diagnosis; in Finch and Lee's series the accuracy of diagnosis was 75 per cent. Surgery, however, should not be delayed because the dangers of acute appendicitis are increased in pregnancy for the following reasons:

1. Delayed diagnosis.
2. The appendix lies not in the pelvis but in the upper abdomen, into which generalized spread may more readily occur.
3. The omentum is prevented from reaching the inflamed organ by the bulk of the uterus.
4. The normal contractions of the uterus, which are exacerbated by a nearby inflammatory process, prevent the formation of adhesions. Should abortion suddenly reduce the uterine bulk, the risk of generalized peritonitis is much increased.

Appendicectomy is performed through a muscle-splitting incision, which is sited at a higher level and more laterally in the abdominal wall than usual. Exposure may be improved by tilting the patient partly on to her left side. Mortality figures for acute appendicitis in pregnancy quoted by the Mount Sinai Hospital (Rovinsky and Guttmacher, 1965) are as follows:

1st trimester	0	Fetal loss	12%
2nd trimester	3·9%	Fetal loss	16%
3rd trimester	9·0%	Fetal loss	20%

However, Finch and Lee (1974) at Oxford had no death in 75 cases, though the post-operative morbidity was considerable and the fetal loss was 8 per cent.

Laparotomy in pregnancy

The need for laparotomy in early pregnancy usually arises because of a suspected ectopic pregnancy, a subject which has already been considered. Laparotomy is otherwise performed in pregnancy most commonly for an ovarian cyst which is found at routine antenatal examination. The operation is ideally performed at about the 14th week, when the risk of abortion is minimal but before the size of the uterus greatly impairs access to the cyst. Less often, laparotomy is required for an acute surgical condition such as torsion of a cyst or acute appendicitis.

The operation seldom presents great technical difficulty. The risk of post-operative abortion is minimized by giving progestational agents.

Saunders and Milton (1973) at St Thomas' Hospital recorded abortion or neonatal death from prematurity in 23 per cent of 74 women who had laparotomy performed in pregnancy. However, the risk of post-operative abortion should not deter the surgeon from laparotomy for suspected appendicitis or prevent him from then removing the appendix even if it proves to be normal.

Third trimester

Premature labour

Colicky abdominal pain in pregnancy may be due to contractions of the genital, alimentary or urinary tract. The diagnosis of premature labour is made by observing the patient carefully and continuously for 30 minutes or more. Only pain which is coincident with palpable uterine contractions indicates labour. However, some women in the latter weeks of pregnancy experience painful contractions which are not those of true labour; such contractions, which are usually irregular, do not cause dilatation of the cervix.

Abruptio placentae

If the placenta becomes partly or wholly detached (abrupted) from the uterine wall bleeding, which is often profuse, ensues. Sometimes the blood forms a retroplacental clot without any bleeding per vaginam. Such a concealed haemorrhage is associated with severe, continuous abdominal pain and a variable degree of shock. The uterus, which is in a state of continuous and sustained contraction, feels hard and is tender to palpation. Fetal parts cannot be identified and the fetal heart cannot be heard. After a few hours the continuous contraction relaxes and labour supervenes.

Abruption is often associated with failure of blood coagulation due to defibrination and may cause renal damage, which is either temporary or permanent. Treatment requires the energetic replacement of blood volume with intravenous fluid and blood. Failure of clot formation is corrected by intravenous infusion of fibrinogen or of plasma, while excessive fibrinolysis may be treated with epsilon aminocaproic acid. Induction of labour is then encouraged by artificial rupture of the membranes and the use of intravenous oxytocin. Caesarean section is contraindicated because of the risk of excessive bleeding.

Uterine rupture

Rupture of the uterus may be complete, i.e. through all its layers including the peritoneum, or incomplete, in which case the peritoneum remains intact.

Complete rupture, which is particularly common after a previous classical caesarean section, involves the upper segment and usually takes place before the onset of labour, sometimes as early as the 20th week of pregnancy. Incomplete rupture involves the lower segment and is associated with labour.

Complete rupture occurring during pregnancy causes severe continuous abdominal pain and shock, but not necessarily any vaginal bleeding. Often the condition is unsuspected and the diagnosis is correspondingly delayed. Laparotomy reveals the-dead fetus in its sac lying free within the peritoneal cavity. After removal of the fetus and placenta, the uterus may either be repaired if future child-bearing is desired, or hysterectomy is performed. Incomplete rupture generally results in profuse vaginal bleeding during labour or immediately after delivery; repair of the rupture of hysterectomy is required.

Surgical emergencies in the puerperium have recently been reviewed by Munro and Jones (1975).

Cancer and pregnancy

The overall incidence of malignancy in pregnancy was recorded as 0·07 per cent by Nieminen and Remes (1970). The rarity of the association prevents the collection of reliable statistics and precludes dogmatic statements.

The surgical aspects of cancer and pregnancy may be considered under the following headings:

1. What is the effect of pregnancy on the incidence of the tumour?
2. What is the effect of the pregnancy on the course and prognosis of the disease?
3. How is treatment of the tumour modified by pregnancy?
4. What effect has a future pregnancy on the treated disease?

Carcinoma of the breast

Lowe and MacMahon (1970) found that childbearing early in life tends to protect a woman against the later development of breast cancer and this seems to be unrelated to lactation.

White and White (1956), from a survey of the world literature, found the incidence of breast cancer to be 1 in 3,200 pregnancies. Applewhite et al. (1973) analysed 2,689 cases with carcinoma of the breast and found 55 associated with pregnancy, 48 of which were treated during pregnancy or lactation. The 5-year survival rate was 25 per cent compared with 36 per cent for patients treated when not pregnant. The poor prognosis was ascribed largely to delay in treatment.

All authorities agree that breast cancer in pregnancy should be treated immediately by the method most appropriate to the nature and stage of the lesion. The question of termination of pregnancy is not fully settled; Lewison (1954) favoured termination whereas White (1955) held the contrary opinion. As the evidence does not strongly support either view, the wishes of the woman should be paramount. However, the surgeon must remember that whereas termination of pregnancy in the first trimester is a straightforward procedure, abortion at a later date is more complicated and likely to distress the patient, and that in the last trimester the fetus is legally viable.

The effect of a future pregnancy on the woman who has been treated for cancer of the breast depends on the presence or absence of dormant metastases. The woman with lymph node metastases at the time of primary treatment must be advised against pregnancy, and in the event of pregnancy termination should be recommended. The woman whose lymph nodes were not involved should be advised to avoid a pregnancy for at least 3 years and warned that even then a risk still remains that dormant metastases may be reactivated.

Malignant melanoma

In 1,000 cases of malignant melanoma reviewed by Pack and Scharnagel (1951), 12 were associated with pregnancy. The 5-year survival of the pregnant patients did not differ from those who were not pregnant, though the numbers are too small for a definitive statement.

A malignant melanoma occurring during pregnancy should be treated surgically in the appropriate manner. The evidence indicates that no medical grounds exist for termination of pregnancy, which should be performed only at the patient's request. A woman who has been treated for malignant melanoma should be advised to avoid pregnancy for at least 3 years, during which time most recurrences will have become manifest.

Carcinoma of other organs

Pregnancy is thought not to influence carcinoma arising in other organs, apart from those of the genital tract, and this subject will not now be considered. However, the climate of medical opinion with regard to termination of pregnancy has greatly changed in recent years; most gynaecologists would be prepared, at the woman's request, to terminate an early pregnancy in the presence of any malignant condition.

References

APPLEWHITE R. R., SMITH L. R., DiVINCENTI F. (1973) Carcinoma of the breast associated with pregnancy and lactation. *Am. Surg.* **39,** 101–104.

FINCH R. A. and LEE E. (1974) Acute appendicitis complicating pregnancy in the Oxford region. *Br. J. Surg.* **61,** 129–132.

GILMORE O. J. A., BRODRIBB A. J. M., BROWETT J. P., COOKE T. J. C., GRIFFIN P. H., HIGGS M. J., ROSS I. K. and WILLIAMSON C. N. (1975) Appendicitis and mimicking conditions. *Lancet* **2,** 421–424.

IFFY L. J. (1961) Contribution to the aetiology of ectopic pregnancy. *J. Obst. Gynaec. Br. Emp.* **68,** 441–450.

LEWISON E. F. (1954) Collective review: breast cancer and pregnancy or lactation. *Internat. Abstr. Surg.* **99,** 417–424.

LLEWELLYN-JONES D. (1970) *Fundamentals of Obstetrics and Gynaecology.* London, Faber & Faber, Vol. 2, p. 212.

LOWE C. R. and MACMAHON, B. (1970) Breast cancer and reproductive history of women in South Wales. *Br. Med. J.* **1,** 153–156.

MUNRO A. and JONES P. F. (1975) Abdominal surgical emergencies in the puerperium. *Br. Med. J.* **4,** 691–694.

NIEMINEN V. and REMES N. (1970) Malignancy during pregnancy. *Acta Obstet. Gynecol. Scand.* **49,** 315–349.

NOVAK E. and NOVAK E. R. (1958) *Gynaecological and Obstetric Pathology,* 4th edn. Philadelphia and London, W. B. Saunders, p. 362.

PACK G. T. and SCHARNAGEL I. M. (1951) The prognosis for malignant melanoma in the pregnant woman. *Cancer* **4,** 324–334.

ROVINSKY J. J. and GUTTMACHER A. F. (1965) *Medical, Surgical and Gynaecological Complications of Pregnancy.* Baltimore, Md., Williams & Williams; Edinburgh and London, Churchill Livingstone, p. 238.

SAUNDERS P. and MILTON P. J. D. (1973) Laparotomy during pregnancy: an assessment of diagnostic accuracy and fetal wastage. *Br. Med. J.* **3,** 165–167.

SUNDEN B. (1950) The results of conservative treatment of salpingitis diagnosed at laparotomy and laparoscopy. *Acta Obstet. Gynecol. Scand.* **38,** 286–296.

WHITE T. T. (1955) Prognosis of breast cancer for pregnant and nursing women. Analysis of 1,413 cases. *Surg. Gynecol. Obstet.* **100,** 661–666.

WHITE T. T. and WHITE W. C. (1956) Breast cancer and pregnancy: report of 49 cases followed 5 years. *Ann. Surg.* **144,** 384–393.

16

Infantile Urinary Infection, Obstruction and Reflux

D. Innes Williams, MD, MChir, FRCS

Urinary obstruction and reflux, usually complicated by infection, are the two important causes of progressive renal destruction in infants and are the areas in which the urologist has most to offer in the correction of the primary disorder with improvement, or at least prevention of further deterioration, in renal function. At no period in life does the damage due to these causes progress more rapidly than during the first six months of life, and although this can be a difficult time for surgical treatment, it is here of the greatest importance. The population of nephrons in the kidney is determined and complete some months before birth, but the DNA content continues to increase until some 6 months after birth, indicating that there is still multiplication of cells up till that time. The later growth of the kidney is due to increasing size of cells rather than increasing number. It follows from these facts that the greatest effect on development will result from a pathological process present before birth, though that is unfortunately beyond our ability to influence. Similar processes occurring during the first 6 months of life will, however, still prevent the multiplication of cells, and therefore permanently limit the size and functional capacity of the kidney. It can, in fact, often be observed that infective process which is controlled very early in life, so that there is no continuing inflammatory process, may leave the child with a kidney which fails to grow.

Quite apart from the possible long-term nephron loss, the infantile kidney is most susceptible to immediate and life-threatening functional disturbances. The function of the neonatal kidney, by whatever standard, is poor in comparison with the adult, and the infant is more liable to exhibit vascular, glomerular and tubular function disorders. There appears to be a high renal vascular resistance at birth, with resulting low renal plasma flow, a fact which perhaps accounts for the liability to thrombosis in the neonatal kidney. Glomerular filtration in the neonate, as measured against body surface area, is only 5 per cent of the mature value, and proximal tubular function is characterized by diminished reabsorption of sodium and water. Even normal infants have, by adult standards, a mild acidosis, and are very rapidly precipitated into a severe acidosis by the pathological conditions which we are to consider (Rickham and Johnston, 1969).

Urinary infection

The problems of recurrent urinary infection with reflux and pyelonephritis have been very fully discussed in the medical literature of the past decade, but it is important to point out here the difference between the neonate and the older child. In the newborn, boys are more often infected than girls: this is certainly true of the overt and symptomatic infections, and probably also of symptomless bacteriuria (Lincoln and Winberg, 1964). In the serious cases, urinary infection is almost always accompanied by bacteraemia or septicaemia, and not infrequently by meningitis. The signs in such examples do not clearly indicate a urinary tract origin for the infection, though some micturition disorder is almost certainly present. The child is evidently ill, often with a subnormal temperature, sometimes jaundiced; diagnosis is reached by urinary examination and blood culture. The treatment required is immediate resuscitation and parenteral antibiotics. Curiously enough, in many boys with this type of disease, the kidneys remain entirely healthy, and years later the pyelogram may be indistinguishable from normal. However, the same type of septicaemic infection may well complicate a urinary tract disorder with progressive renal disease; the severe urinary tract obstructions often present to the doctor for the first time with such an infection, and in these destruction of the kidney can progress rapidly. Similarly, infection complicating congenital bilateral reflux, often with gross ureteric dilatation, can lead to rapid nephron loss. It is therefore evident that immediate recognition and vigorous treatment are the most urgent requirements, but in a neonatal urinary infection a full investigation is still essential to determine the state of the urinary tract. Later in the first year of life the pattern of urinary infections comes to approximate to that of the older child, but still at this stage is frequently overlooked. There are many girls with severe bilateral pyelonephritis and reflux who have a long history of unexplained feverish episodes during the first year of life: they clearly represent an opportunity for early surgical correction, which has been missed through inadequate investigation.

The pathological change seen in infective damage is chronic pyelonephritic scarring with blunting of the calices, indentation of the renal outline, fibrosis and colloid change in the renal parenchyma. The pathogenesis of such changes is, however, as much concerned with reflux as with infection.

Reflux

The older child with reflux has been exhaustively investigated, and it is now well recognized that reflux is potentially a serious complication of the child with infected urine, that it predisposes to recurrent infection and facilitates the ascent of infection to the kidney. It carries with it the danger of chronic pyelonephritis, leading on to renal failure and hypertension. Nevertheless, minor degrees of reflux are extremely common and may well cease spontaneously with the growing maturity of the child. Others, even with more severe reflux, may preserve normal kidneys in spite of an occasional infection. Discussion therefore continues as to the relative importance of reflux and of infection, and therefore of the need for surgical treatment. There are those paediatricians for whom chemoprophylaxis is sufficient for all but a tiny minority of children with reflux, and may be carried on for many years to puberty. At the other extreme, some urologists believe that almost all cases of total reflux should be operated upon without delay. Between these extremes a reasonable compromise appears to be that operative correction of reflux is appropriate for those children in whom there is, for anatomical reasons, virtually no chance of spontaneous cessation, and for those in whom its persistence through the years has shown that such a cure is not to be attained; for those where chemoprophylaxis proves unacceptable or ineffective in preventing disease; and for those in whom there is already some evidence of progression of scarring (Scott, 1969).

Turning to the problem of infancy, however, we find that less information is available concerning the frequency and course of the disorder, and that opinions are less crystallized concerning its treatment. However, increasing attention is now paid to the problems it creates at this stage, for it is recognized that where severe renal scarring is seen later in childhood, it has almost always commenced, at least in some minor degree, during the first few months of life. At this age, too, there is increasing evidence that reflux can be damaging, even in the absence of complicating urinary infection. In assessing these cases we find it essential first to distinguish not only those cases where reflux complicates some other bladder abnormality from the so-called 'primary disorder', but also within the latter

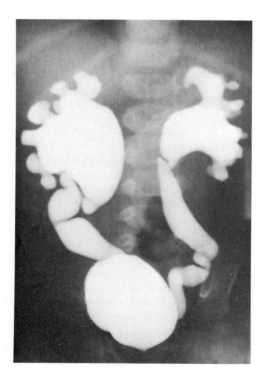

Fig. 16.1 Infantile reflux. Cystogram showing typical bilateral severe reflux with ureteric dilatation in infancy.

group between the severe and mild cases. The routine investigation of infants who have suffered a urinary infection will reveal a number in whom the bladder is normal but who have free reflux, usually bilaterally, without significant dilatation of the ureters or deformity of the kidneys. These mild examples have a good prognosis: in many, the reflux will cease spontaneously, and even if it does not, the proper control of infection allows normal renal growth. By contrast, there is a group in whom bilateral reflux occurs with considerable ureteric dilatation (Fig. 16.1); the degree of dilatation may be hard to judge since it varies with the state of the contraction of the bladder, but the group with which we are now concerned has evident dilatation in intravenous urographic series, even where the bladder is relaxed and relatively empty. Although reflux is bilateral the changes are often asymmetrical, and it is common to find that although the infection can be controlled by careful medication, the more severely affected kidney fails to grow, so that as the years go by the disparity between the two kidneys becomes more and more evident. This could, of course, be due to continuing disease, but it seems more likely that the initial episode has resulted in a permanent restriction of growth.

It is in this infantile group that we must suspect that sterile reflux may be damaging, and Hodson (1975) has drawn attention to the possibility that intrarenal reflux may be the factor responsible for such damage. By intrarenal reflux we mean that the opaque medium introduced into the bladder not only fills the pelvis and calices, but also spreads outwards to opacify the renal parenchyma (Fig. 16.2), first of all within the collecting tubules, but later throughout the nephron as far as the capsule. Such intrarenal reflux is not very commonly observed in routine cystograms; when it is, we often find that the reflux has occurred under high pressure, as when the child has a severe bladder contraction while the filling catheter is still within the urethra. However, it is only when a sufficient volume of opaque medium enters the renal tubules that we can detect intrarenal reflux radiologically, and it may well occur in a lesser degree under ordinary circumstances. Hodson's (1975) experiments on piglets seemed to indicate that sterile intrarenal reflux can be responsible for a scar in the kidney, indistinguishable from that of pyelonephritis, and Rolleston and his colleagues (1974) have correlated the observation of intrarenal reflux with the progressive contraction of the kidney in infants. If these observations are confirmed, and there are certainly many points which will require clarification and confirmation, then it would seem that we have a surgical obligation to prevent reflux in the moderate or severe cases of infancy without delaying to see whether medication controls the infection. Urologists have, in the past, fought shy of operating on very young infants in whom considerable dilatation of the ureters and a relatively thin-walled bladder seem to pose some technical problems. However, most of the severe bilateral reflux cases in infancy have also a degree of megacystis, which renders the operation somewhat easier, and the advancement technique of Cohen can be performed with relative safety (Williams, 1975) It may be, of course, that remodelling of the lower ends of the dilated ureters will be required, and this is something which can never be undertaken without an element of risk, but the younger the infant, the more likely are the ureters to be supple and elastic with a good muscular contraction, and the more likely they are to be restored to normal calibre by reflux prevention.

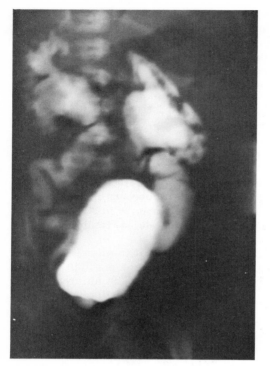

Fig. 16.2 Intrarenal reflux. Cystogram in an infant with severe bilateral reflux and opacification of the renal parenchyma, particularly in the upper pole of the left kidney.

Renal dysplasia

In all infantile urinary disorders we are faced with the problem of deciding what is congenital and what is acquired disease. Many cases of reflux, with or without urinary infection, prove to have one or both kidneys which are small and deformed in a manner which suggests that they have failed to develop, rather than having contracted as a result of pyelonephritis. The term 'dysplasia' should indicate a histological abnormality of the kidney in which, for instance, there are embryonic rests of cartilaginous and other inappropriate tissues, cysts, and a number of straight tubules lined by cuboidal cells extending out to the capsular area. It has been demonstrated by Bernstein (1968) that ureteric obstruction in utero is capable of causing such dysplastic changes, and we occasionally see examples in urethral valve obstruction. More commonly, we find a small deformed kidney with a cluster of closely packed clubbed calices lying above a vertically disposed and somewhat dilated renal pelvis with reflux, but no obstruction (Fig. 16.3). It is, of course, possible that a primary reflux in utero may be responsible for such changes, but clinically, even in the newborn, we are concerned with the progress rather than the pathogenesis. A unilateral dysplastic kidney may, of course, be better removed, particularly if there is any question of hypertension. In bilateral examples we may find in early infancy that there is a salt-losing type of renal failure which, unless carefully controlled, may be fatal within a few months. If, however, expert medical treatment brings the child through this dangerous period, somewhat to our surprise we may find that renal

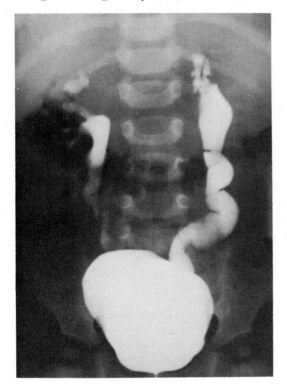

Fig. 16.3 Renal dysplasia. Cystogram in a child with severe renal failure, showing reflux into dilated ureters but minute dysplastic kidneys.

function is picking up, and the blood urea falling to figures only slightly above normal. Later on, however, such children are liable to recurrent infection, which will reverse this tendency to improvement. At this stage, or perhaps earlier, they may well require reflux prevention, and the fact that the dysplasia is present should not inhibit us from undertaking this type of reconstructive surgery. Unfortunately, a number of such children will inevitably develop irreversible renal failure in adolescence or early adult life, when they will be candidates for renal transplantation.

We sometimes extend the concept of dysplasia, applying it to a deformity of the ureters, or even of the entire urinary tract. This is particularly the case in the prune belly syndrome, where there is a combination of dysplastic kidneys, grossly dilated and tortuous ureters, a large-capacity bladder with umbilical fixation, a relaxed bladder neck, a utricular diverticulum and relative narrowing in the membranous area. In such children we must recognize that it will never be possible to make a normal urinary tract, yet we can prevent deterioration of the existing abnormality by surgery at various levels, particularly by urethrotomy of the membranous urethra.

Urinary obstruction

Congenital urinary obstructions may occur at almost any level in the urinary tract, but there are certain characteristic forms which are apt to present in infancy; the commonest of these is the obstructive valve in the posterior urethra. There are, however, comments to be made on the infantile forms of disease at various levels, and it seems logical to start at the upper end.

Pelviureteric obstruction

Pelviureteric obstruction causing hydronephrosis is common throughout childhood, but in cases presenting during the first 3 months of life a characteristic form is that of an enormously ballooned extrarenal pelvis, with a cap of relatively good renal parenchyma pushed far laterally. The calices are only moderately dilated, and renal function is often surprisingly good in spite of the enormous volume of the renal pelvis. In such examples a palpable kidney is the usual mode of presentation, and bilaterality is more common in infancy than in later childhood. Pyeloplasty is successful in preserving renal function in these cases, though the appearance of the kidney scarcely ever returns to normal. In another neonatal type of hydronephrosis the renal pelvis is relatively small, but there is below it a 3 or 4 cm stretch of ureter which is extremely narrow, and exhibits multiple kinks of mucosa and muscularis within the adventitia. This form is particularly associated with urinary infection, and it may be more difficult to secure satisfactory pyeloplasty because of the length of the narrow segment. Cystic dysplasia may complicate pelviureteric obstruction, and only where this form of parenchymal disorder is present will there be a danger of renal failure.

Atresia of the ureter

Atretic sections of the ureter are rarely seen outside the infantile period. In their most extreme form they are associated with the multi-cystic kidney; that is to say, an organ which is entirely replaced by a loose agglomeration of cysts without any patent collecting system. However, less severe forms of atresia may be encountered, and in one characteristic form the mid-ureter is obstructed by such a segment, leading to hydronephrosis on the one side, whereas on the other there is a more severe atresia with mutli-cystic kidney. Renal deterioration in these circumstances may be rapid, and it is of vital importance to recognize the nature of the disease. Its mechanical correction may be relatively easy, but there is one problem which must be recognized and dealt with. Atretic sections may be multiple, one higher and one lower in the ureter, and whereas there is well marked dilatation above the higher obstruction, the segment of ureter between the two may look apparently normal, so that the lower one is apt to be overlooked.

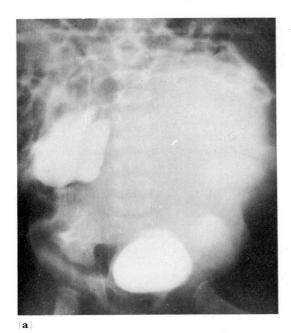

(a)

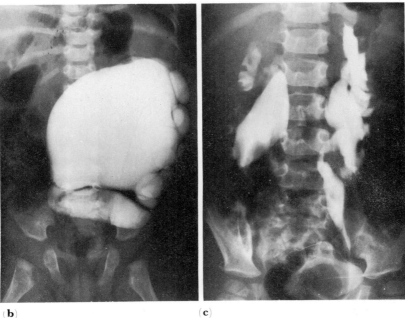

(b)   (c)

Fig. 16.4 Obstructive megaureter in infancy. (a) Intravenous pyelogram showing huge hydronephrosis in a newborn child. (b) Antegrade pyelogram showing ureteric dilatation. (c) Intravenous pyelogram 2 years after correction, showing good recovery.

Primary obstructive megaureter

Primary obstructive megaureter is an abnormality more commonly presenting in later childhood with pain and recurrent infection. Nevertheless, neonatal cases are seen from time to time, and often exhibit, as in the pelviureteric obstructions, an enormously ballooned renal pelvis with, nevertheless, some preservation of renal function (Fig. 16.4). Thus a palpable abdominal swelling is likely to be the feature drawing attention to the disorder. Bilateral cases in early infancy may well be a cause of renal failure. As with megaureter, the ectopic ureterocele may present as an abdominal swelling in early infancy, often showing a grotesque radiological appearance for which interpretation is difficult.

Urethral obstruction

In the urethra, several forms of congenital obstruction are found, taking the form of simple stenosis, urethral diverticula and valves, but it is the posterior urethral valve which is the common cause of the serious obstruction in male infants, and requires full discussion.

The classical description of the pathological anatomy was given by Young et al. (1919) and this has influenced all further discussion, although it is clear that his type I is the only important variety. This is usually depicted as a pair of valvular folds springing from the lower end of the verumontanum and passing outwards to the lateral walls of the urethra. However, this appearance in the dissected specimen is partly due to the mode of preparation in that the urinary tract is

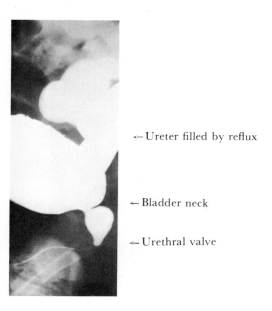

←Ureter filled by reflux

←Bladder neck

←Urethral valve

Fig. 16.5 Micturating cystogram in a case of urethral valves, showing dilatation of the posterior urethra and a sharp cut-off in the membranous area. Reflux is also present.

laid open anteriorly. The valvular flap would be better described as a fold of mucosal and fibrous tissue based on the anterior wall of the urethra and having a small slit in it posteriorly immediately below the verumontanum. This is clearly shown in specimens prepared by sagittal section and by urethrograms in the lateral plane (Fig. 16.5). Nevertheless, it is not so easily appreciated endoscopically, as the urethroscope is passed through the posteriorly placed slit and the portions of the valve most easily observed are the lateral margins of the slit.

The degree of obstruction produced by the valve is variable, but in any case presenting in early infancy there will be severe changes. Mild cases of obstruction due to valves may present later in childhood with incontinence or difficulty in micturition, but the infant will always have some degree of hydronephrosis. Above the valve the urethra is grossly dilated, leaving the bladder neck relatively narrow, and the detrusor hypertrophy which accompanies the obstruction often renders this bladder neck very prominent in a way which might be thought to constitute an obstruction. Experience has shown, in fact, that this bladder neck ring is not obstructive and its resection only increases later incontinence. The bladder is trabeculated and there is not infrequently a para-ureteric saccule, which may be productive of either obstruction or reflux. There are, in fact, a few cases where there is a relatively mild urethral obstruction but a severe ureteric obstruction due to the saccule formation. The ureters are dilated and frequently tortuous with some fibrous replacement of muscle tissue as time goes on. The degree of renal damage is curiously variable, and it is possible to consider the infantile cases in two groups. In one there appears to be something approaching acute retention during the first few days after birth. In such infants the damage to the kidney may be still largely reversible (Fig. 16.6), and the condition is in some ways comparable with a prostatic case whose acute retention has been precipitated by a drinking session. There is, in fact, some analogy here since the urinary output almost certainly increases quite rapidly after birth, although some urine has been formed throughout the last month of fetal life and regularly evacuated into the amniotic fluid. In the other group, we have cases more akin to the chronic retention of adults in which there is a less tense overflowing bladder, but severe damage to the kidney which has been sustained during fetal life. These two groups illustrate something of the difference between acute and chronic obstruction which merits some general discussion. Experimentally, it can be shown that an acute obstruction causes a rise of intrarenal pressure with dilatation of the upper urinary tract and swelling of the whole kidney. Functionally there is an increased fractional reabsorption of filtered sodium by the proximal tubule, accompanied, of course, by an almost complete cessation of urine flow. This produces a characteristic radiological picture during intravenous urography. The opaque medium will remain within the lumen of the renal tubule, its concentration being increased by the reabsorption of water. Thus the nephrographic phase of urography, instead of disappearing after the first minute or two, will persist and increase in density for some hours, leaving the renal passages radiolucent. If with this form of obstruction drainage is secured, there will be a rapid return to normal, the dilatation will disappear and the kidney will resume its normal size and normal function. There is a hazard in that the immediate post-obstructive period may be complicated by a sudden loss of salt and water, a natriuresis, which can lead to very serious electrolyte imbalance.

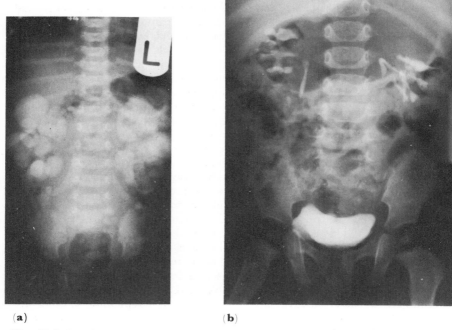

(a)   **(b)**

Fig. 16.6. Urethral valvular obstruction in the neonate. (**a**) Intravenous pyelogram during acute retention phase. (**b**) Intravenous pyelogram a year later showing good recovery.

If the obstruction persists, a change gradually takes place: the intrarenal pressure falls to something like normal values, though it can be raised again during an episode of polyuria. The nephrons are gradually destroyed. The factors concerned in this selective but progressive nephron loss are not altogether clear, but it results in a situation where the surviving nephrons operate under conditions of relative diuresis with a decreased fractional reabsorption of filtered sodium by the proximal tubules. In these circumstances there will be no prolongation of the nephrographic phase of urography. Opacification of the dilated calices will appear relatively early, if at all. It is in some ways difficult to explain why the chronic form of obstruction, in which the pressure is low, is progressive; perhaps it is because there are episodes of acute high pressure obstruction in the course of the chronic process, but at least it is evident that nephron loss and shrinkage of the parenchyma are continuing hazards. Such infants already have considerable electrolyte problems, but curiously enough are not so liable to be precipitated into a major disturbance by the sudden natriuresis consequent upon decompression of the bladder.

As an aside we may mention here a further radiological picture of some importance, where a relatively acute obstruction supervenes upon a chronic process. Here we consider a hydronephrotic kidney with dilated calices, but without gross impairment of function. An acute obstruction supervening in such a case will lead to concentration of opaque medium in the collecting tubules and ducts of **Bellini, which because of the dilatation of the calices are now lying tangential** to the spherical calix. This concentration gives a shell or soap-bubble appearance to the kidney in the early phase of the urography, but later films will demonstrate opacification of the dilated calices.

Returning then to the clinical problem of infants with urethral valves, we must note that, in addition to the acute and chronic forms of retention, some infants with severe renal damage present with generalized abdominal distension which is often attributed to a bowel disorder, and the bladder may not, in fact, be palpable. This arises from the fact that the detrusor muscle in these infants is massively hypertrophied so that the bladder is able to empty itself completely in spite of the obstruction, but the very high pressure within the system leads to severe dilatation of the ureters and damage to the kidneys. Thus, a good urinary stream is not necessarily a feature which eliminates the possibility of valvular obstruction. Other infants again present with a septicaemic urinary infection, and in these, too, the bladder distension may not be so marked as the renal swelling.

The diagnosis of urethral valves is made by urography and micturating cystourethrography. An intravenous pyelogram will show bilateral hydronephrosis provided there is sufficient renal function still present, and is always well worth performing, even when the child is uraemic. The only danger involved is in giving a large dose of contrast medium to a dehydrated infant: provided the fluid balance has been restored, many such pyelograms, although not showing clear definition, will give very valuable information as to the state of the kidneys and to the difference between one side and the other. The cystourethrography must include films taken during micturition or during manual expression of the bladder contents. A simple filling cystogram will by itself fail to outline the dilated posterior urethra, which makes evident the presence of valves. Usually with infants there is very little difficulty in filling the bladder up through a urethral catheter until micturition becomes inevitable, possibly even while the catheter is still in place. The films will show the sacculated bladder, a relatively narrow bladder neck, a wide dilatation of the posterior urethra and a sharp cut-off in the membranous area, which bulges forward over the bulb of the urethra.

It will be evident that a flimsy obstructing valve will not present any major surgical problem in ablation, provided a very small urethroscope (9–11F) is available. It is easily possible to visualize the valve and to destroy its obstructive edge with a diathermy electrode, if necessary simply using the metal stilette within a ureteric catheter. Older children may require actual loop resection of the valve, but in the baby coagulation is sufficent. The ablation can, in fact, be accomplished under simple radiological control by an insulated diathermy hook, which obviates the need to pass any endoscope large enough to take an electrode (Williams et al., 1974).

However, it is essential that the management of the infant with urethral valves is considered from all aspects—medical as well as surgical—and the process of investigation has to be integrated with the resuscitation often required for these sick infants.

If the child is admitted in good condition with a tense bladder and sterile urine, an indwelling 6F plastic urethral catheter will give good drainage for 24–48 hours, and during this time intravenous urography and urethrography can be undertaken so that there may be no delay in proceeding to valve ablation. If the child's condition shows evidence of dehydration and uraemia, this may well be correctable within the 48 hours by intravenous therapy and by a low-protein milk. Many of the children with renal failure are precipitated into the state of biochemical disequilibrium by cow's milk with its high protein and sodium content. If the child's urine is infected, he must be started on parenteral antibiotics immediately without waiting for the results of sensitivity tests, and currently gentamycin seems the best drug to use. More serious problems arise when the child's condition does not rapidly improve on rehydration, or when the infection is not brought under control in 48 hours by indwelling catheter and antibiotics. The biochemical problems encountered are sometimes of a temporary nature, due to over-hydration or to high potassium levels, and these may sometimes require a few days' peritoneal dialysis along with bladder drainage by urethral catheter. They may be less reversible due to the advanced state of renal deterioration, or due to a pyonephrosis in the obstructed kidneys. The latter cases are often best treated by immediate bilateral nephrostomy, which is the simplest method of obtaining free drainage direct from the kidneys. This may reveal a unilateral problem, with one kidney irreversibly damaged. Quite surprisingly often in the urethral valve cases one kidney is functionless and is better removed. Apart from this there are three forms of pathology to contend with: first of all there may be a secondary ureterovesical obstruction; secondly, there may be reflux; and thirdly, there may be a simple ureteric dysfunction resulting entirely from the degree of dilatation which precludes a propulsive contraction, and therefore allows stasis and complicating infection.

Secondary ureterovesicular obstruction may be due to the pressure from a massively hypertrophied detrusor muscle, but is more often the result of a para-ureteric saccule. It is recognized both from the local pathology and from the fact that, after removal of the urethral valves, dilatation persists or even increases in the upper urinary tract. Obstruction can be recognized by the pressure within the renal pelvis. In some cases we have a nephrostomy tube in situ, through which pressure measurements can be recorded during perfusion of the upper urinary tract, but even in the absence of nephrostomies, needle puncture of the kidney is possible and enables us to undertake these pressure studies. Re-implantation of the ureters with excision of the narrow segment and, if necessary, remodelling of the dilated segment, is effective and will produce a rapid improvement.

Reflux is common in urethral valve cases, and where it is unilateral it can be shown to be associated with very much more advanced renal destruction. The functionless kidneys are, in fact, usually refluxing ones. However, lesser degrees of reflux may well cease spontaneously after valve ablation; this occurred in approximately one-third of my cases. Persistent reflux can certainly be responsible for recurrent infection, though surprisingly a few cases continue with very few signs of trouble provided the original valvular obstruction has been adequately removed. Re-implantation of the ureters for reflux should not, therefore, be undertaken early in the course of the disease, particularly as the operation itself is not entirely without hazard, and it is more difficult to secure effective reflux prevention where the bladder is massively trabeculated and sacculated.

The remainder of the persistently dilated ureters are not evidently obstructed, nor do they allow reflux, and their management is problematical. Some urologists would prefer to re-model them all on the assumption that by narrowing the calibre the ureteric peristalsis will be rendered more efficient (Hendren, 1971). Others prefer conservative attitudes.

Even in addition to all the problems so far mentioned, there will be some urethral valve cases whose general condition is extremely poor, whose renal function does not improve on simple drainage, whose ureters are completely without propulsive function. In them, reconstructive surgery is unlikely to be effective, and their only hope of survival lies in long-term ureteric drainage on to the abdominal wall, in the hope that with the passage of months renal function will improve and ureteric peristalsis will reappear. Cutaneous drainage takes the form of some type of cutaneous ureterostomy: the simplest form is the loop, which, if placed high and well made, will give effective drainage without danger of stomal stenosis. It does, however, lead to complete defunctioning of the bladder, and some defunctioned bladders contract irreversibly. Moreover, since in many of these cases re-implantation of the lower ends of the ureters will be required, a difficulty arises at the time of reconstruction in loop ureterostomies, a simultaneous operation to close the loop and re-implant the lower end of the ureter endangering the blood supply of the segment in between. For this reason I now employ a ring ureterostomy, by anastomosing the afferent and efferent limbs of the loop; in this way, free drainage is still secured but a proportion of the urine enters the bladder to keep it functioning, and closure of the ureterostomy is very easily accomplished by excising the externalized part of the ring without interrupting the continuity of the internal part.

It will thus be clear that the treatment of urethral valves, as of many congenital obstructions, is a process which lasts many years and requires over this period both nephrological and urological supervision.

References

BERNSTEIN J. (1968) Developmental abnormalities of the renal parenchyma. *Pathol. Annu.* **3,** 213.

HENDREN W. H. (1971) Posterior urethral valves in boys. *J. Urol.* **106,** 298–307.

HODSON C. J., MALING T. M. J., MCMARAMON P. and LEWIS M. G. (1975) *Brit. J. Radiol.* Supplement. Intrarenal reflux.

LINCOLN K. and WINBERG J. (1964) Studies in urinary tract infection in infancy and childhood. *Acta Pediat. Scand.* **53,** 307–316, 447–453.

RICKHAM P. P. and JOHNSTON J. H. (1969) *Neonatal Surgery.* London, Butterworths.

ROLLESTON G. L., MALING T. M. J. and HODSON C. J. (1974) Intra-renal reflux and the scarred kidney. *Arch. Dis. Child.* **49,** 531–539.

SCOTT J. E. S. (1969) Results of anti-reflux surgery. *Lancet* **2,** 68–71.

WILLIAMS D. I. (1975) Surgery of the uretero-vesical junction. In: WILKINSON A. W. (ed.) *Recent Advances in Paediatric Surgery.* Edinburgh and London, Churchill Livingstone.

WILLIAMS D. I., BARRATT M., WHITAKER R. and KEETON J. (1974) Urethral valves. *Br. J. Urol.* **45,** 200–210.

YOUNG H. H., FRONTZ W. H. and BALDWIN J. C. (1919) Congenital obstruction of the posterior urethra. *J. Urol.* **3,** 289–354.

17

Diagnosis and Management of Skin Tumours

P. S. Boulter, FRCS, FRCSEd

More tumours occur in the skin than in any other organ of the body. Most of these are benign lesions which, while they may be unattractive, cause no other harm to the host. Some of them, however, can undergo malignant change. This is one of the aetiological factors that obtain in skin cancer, though not the most important. Most of the causative agents are related to the exposure of the skin to environmental hazards, both physical and chemical.

Aetiological agents in skin tumours

Some 90 per cent of skin cancers occur on the exposed surfaces of the body and here sunlight is clearly important. In addition, racial and genetic factors governing skin pigmentation play a complicating role in determining the geographical variance in skin cancer. In the USA a regular increase in skin cancer registrations in fair-skinned people is noted from north to south of the nation. The incidence rate for white people increases as their place of living becomes closer to the equator, with doubling of incidence for every 265 miles (Auerbach, 1961). There is relatively little correlation between latitude and skin cancer incidence in coloured people.

In Australia, particular attention has been focused on the causation of melanoma and here the latitude/incidence relationship is confirmed (Lancaster, 1956). The pale-skinned red-haired people of so-called Celtic stock who migrated to Australia from Ireland and Scotland have provided a high proportion of the cases of all types of skin cancer. There appears to be a true racial increase related, of course, to pigmentation and the historical and geographical accidents of emigration (Scott, 1972). While sunlight is the most important agent, others must be mentioned. Prolonged medication with arsenic can cause keratoses, and multiple squamous carcinomata may develop after many years. Tars and oils were incriminated two centuries ago in the chimneysweeps' cancers, and shale oil has been known for many years to be the agent responsible for other tumours.

Radiations other than the ultraviolet are of importance and the price paid by the early pioneers of radiology is well known. Similar post-irradiation dermatitis and subsequent malignancy is seen after therapeutic use of ionizing radiation. A time lapse of many years will often be noticed, as in the cases of squamous carcinoma of the forehead and scalp following radiation treatment of ringworm.

Similarly, old style cervical irradiation for tuberculous nodes, hyperthyroidism and other conditions has been followed by tumour development, perhaps here demonstrating a coincidental summation of the effects of therapeutic and ultra-violet radiation. Long-wavelength radiation is of little importance, though the Kangri cancer of Kashmir is a famous rarity, and cancer complicating erythema ab igne has been recognized. Skins which are scarred by chronic infection such as lupus, leprosy and the sinuses of osteomyelitis may undergo malignant change, and Marjolin's ulcer is a sequel of long-standing gravitational ulceration. Genetic predisposition to skin cancer is obvious where skin pigmentation is a factor and a special and dominant relationship is shown in xeroderma pigmentosum. Finally, viral infection causes warts and may cause keratoacanthoma.

Benign tumours

A multitude of unimportant benign tumours affect the skin and all its elements. The sweat and sebaceous glands, hair follicles, dermal blood vessels, nerves and connective tissues all have their own lesions. Only a few of these will be mentioned here and for a full account the reader is referred to Sanderson (1968).

Seborrhoeic keratoses

These verrucose areas of hyperkeratosis occur in the middle-aged and elderly.

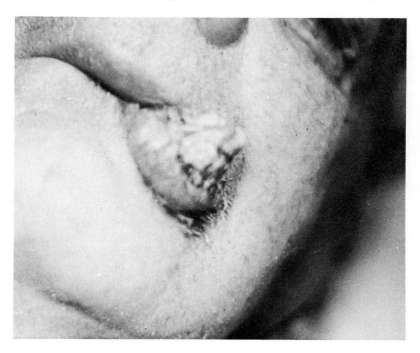

Fig. 17.1 Keratoacanthoma of lip. Note the keratin plug.

The majority of the lesions are on the face and back. They are rough to the touch and when scraped will shed a part of their surface. The apparent pigmentation is not melanin but a mixture of dirt and the discoloration of haemorrhage. When necessary, these lesions can be dealt with by softening with creams; excision or curettage is reserved for the more resistant and unsightly.

Keratoacanthoma

This is a benign, rapidly growing and disfiguring lesion which in appearance may simulate a keratinizing squamous carcinoma (Fig. 17.1). It is common in middle life, often occurs in exposed sites and is usually self-curing in weeks or months, leaving some scarring. The indications for treatment are therefore (1) cosmetic, and (2) to exclude the diagnosis of squamous carcinoma. The lesion is usually spherical with a surrounding smooth, pink, shiny and telangiectatic surface. There is a central horny plug which may become eroded to produce a crater. Treatment is by excision or curettage, though superficial radiotherapy has been used. If the lesion is not in an exposed situation and if it is rapidly evolving, then patience may triumph.

Cylindroma (turban tumour)

This is an uncommon, unsightly tumour of sweat gland origin, usually seen on the scalp and tending to appear in early adult life. The nodular masses may reach considerable size and dictate surgical treatment.

Dermatofibroma (histiocytoma)

This is a common lesion seen most often on the lower leg and upper arm. Some of these may be sclerosed haemangiomata, but others seem to occur in the sites of insect bites. The lesion is usually a hard circumscribed nodule in the skin which is slowly evolving and may undergo spontaneous diminution in size. The colour, at first pink, tends to fade. The indication for excision is usually cosmetic, though irritation may be considerable enough to justify operation.

Vascular tumours

These are common. Most are haemangiomata of various sorts and few require treatment. Congenital lesions tend to diminish in the first few years of life and surgery should be resisted until time has been given a fair trial. Radiotherapy, previously popular, is very rarely indicated as the tissues of a haemangioma are no more sensitive than those of the adjacent skin and damage is almost inevitable.

Pyogenic granuloma (granuloma telangiectaticum)

This pinkish vascular nodule often follows trivial injury and grows rapidly and sometimes painfully. It usually reaches its mature size in a week or two and remains until removed. Cosmesis, bleeding and odour will dictate treatment, which is by excision and curettage, usually with cautery of the base. It is occasionally confused with a rapidly evolving nodular melanoma and, while the resemblance is usually only superficial, the lesion should always be examined histologically.

Pre-malignant dermatoses

This diffuse assortment of conditions is united only by one characteristic—a tendency for invasive malignancy to supervene.

Solar keratoses

Solar keratoses are brown roughened areas seen in exposed sites. They are most often encountered on the face, scalp and hands and are exceptionally common in ageing fair-skinned individuals with a history of prolonged exposure. Both basal and squamous carcinoma may appear in the sites of keratoses. Post-irradiation keratoses are really a special variant of the solar form.

Arsenical and tar keratoses

These have much in common with solar keratoses and the appearance is very similar, though in arsenical keratoses the body surface may be very widely affected and, characteristically, multiple squamous carcinomata may supervene.

Cutaneous horn

This is usually seen in the elderly and comprises a narrow-based keratin horn which is often associated with surrounding desquamation and inflammation. Long neglect is occasionally followed by malignant change.

Leucokeratosis of lip

Leucokeratosis of the lip is a flat patch of thickened skin with a common preceding history of cigarette smoking. It is a precursor of squamous carcinoma and should be treated, preferably by cryosurgery.

Bowen's disease (Fig. 17.2)

This condition is of special interest. The lesion, slowly evolving and widely occurring on the body surface, is characterized by reddening, scaling and crusting of the surface with a surrounding micro-oedema of the skin. There are two interesting features of the condition. First, invasive skin cancer supervenes in some 50 per cent of observed cases and the lesion is most usually a squamous carcinoma. Secondly, visceral malignancy is found to occur in as many as 25 per cent of patients with Bowen's disease and these have included respiratory, gastrointestinal and genitourinary tumours (Graham and Helwig, 1959, 1964).

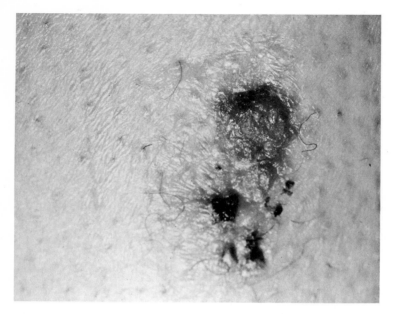

Fig. 17.2 Bowen's disease.

Erythroplasia of Queyrat

Queyrat's erythroplasia is a slightly raised reddened lesion on the surface of the glans penis or the foreskin. It is really Bowen's disease affecting the penis and is a precursor of carcinoma.

Extramammary Paget's disease and intraepidermal epithelioma of Jadassohn

These are histologically separate variants with similar local significance to Bowen's disease.

In general all these lesions should be dealt with by local irradiation or cryosurgery after appropriate biopsies. In extensive lesions more than one biopsy should always be done. Small lesions can of course sometimes be excised without trouble and where this is practical it is ideal for the patient. Queyrat's erythroplasia is an indication for circumcision. Because of the significance of Bowen's disease as a harbinger of both local and general malignancy, adequate investigation and effective follow-up are advisable.

Malignant tumours of the skin

Basal cell carcinoma (BBC)

This term should always be used and the synonym rodent ulcer should be forgotten. Too many practitioners fail to recognize the significance of the lesions of BCC in what may be a long period prior to ulceration. This tumour can occur at any age but is commoner with increasing years. Its incidence is high in areas with much sunlight, but even in temperate climates it is the commonest malignant tumour of the skin and indeed of the whole body. Basal cell carcinomata may be multiple, may show pigmentation and can occur anywhere on the skin, though the vast majority occur on the face, scalp and neck with the inner canthus, the eyelids and the temporal region especially common sites. The hands and fore-arms, back and upper chest are not infrequent places where BCCs may occur and here there is often an occupational factor—agricultural workers, fishermen and dedicated sunbathers being especially at risk.

Clinical features

The early lesions are usually only slightly raised, pinkish and give a naked-eye impression of thinned epidermis with telangiectasia. As the lesion develops it may

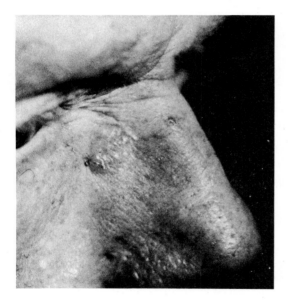

Fig. 17.3 Basal cell carcinoma. Note surface and lack of ulceration.

spread, with an appearance of skin atrophy and scarring in the less active areas; the characteristic pearly, raised and rounded edge becomes apparent later. In some cases considerable size (Fig. 17.3) may be reached without ulceration, while in others ulceration appears early (Fig. 17.4). Pigmentation is sometimes seen in parts or the whole of the tumour and the appearance of a superficial spreading melanoma may be simulated.

As the lesion increases and the growth rate appears to accelerate then ulceration and invasion of adjacent tissues occur. Because of the sites of the lesion, cartilaginous and bony involvement are common in neglected cases. It should be emphasized strongly, however, that for every classical ulcerated BCC there will

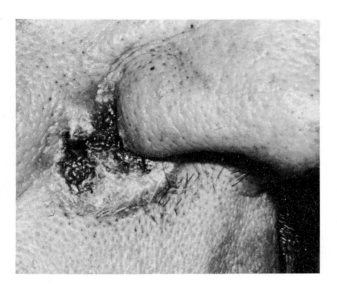

Fig. 17.4 Ulcerated basal cell carcinoma.

be many nodular and plaque-like lesions and some may be areas of little substance that simulate eczema or psoriasis.

While invasion is usual, metastasis is very rare though well documented cases do exist.

Treatment

The treatment of basal cell carcinoma is thus by effective and pathologically adequate local measures. The majority of cases are readily radiosensitive and carefully fractionated therapy produces good cure rates and a minimum of local deformity, though even the best result will be associated with some skin atrophy. The disturbance to the patient is minimal, and extensive and multiple lesions may readily be treated. Radiation, always after preliminary histological confirmation, is thus the treatment of choice in most patients. Contraindications to irradiation do exist. The tumour may be so small that biopsy and cure are identical. Adherence to bone or cartilage prohibits radiotherapy because of the high chance of subsequent necrosis. Exposure to extreme cold (as in Arctic regions) also is an indication for surgery as exposed irradiation scars are specially prone to frostbite. Lesions on the back of the hand are also best avoided by the radiotherapist. Finally, in BCC as in other tumours where a choice of treatment exists, social or geographical difficulty in follow-up may be indications for surgery. Previously it was felt that close proximity to the eye rendered irradiation undesirable, but increasing skill in shielding has made most periorbital tumours suitable for radiation.

Surgery

When surgical treatment is selected then excision must be adequate and the periphery of the tumour should be delineated carefully with a mapping pen. The lesion should be excised with a clear margin of at least 3–5 mm, and more where possible. Adequate excision should also take account of depth. Reconstruction may be by simple direct suture or may need the use of partial or full-thickness skin grafts. In larger, neglected and deeply invasive lesions, plastic reconstruction using rotation or pedicle grafts may be needed.

Sometimes combined therapy is of value when preliminary cleansing of extensive ulcers may be aided by fractions of radiotherapy prior to surgery and accompanying mechanical and antibacterial manœuvres. Finally, an absolute indication for surgery is recurrence of a previously irradiated tumour or the appearance of a new lesion closely adjacent to previously treated areas.

Lesser procedures have been advocated and are practised in places where multiple tumours are common. These consist of the following.

(1) Curettage followed by diathermy.

(2) Cryosurgical treatment is gaining favour and modern apparatus has rendered obsolete the old CO_2 snow methods.

(3) Local chemotherapy has been practised for some years and 5-fluorouracil cream is simple and effective, particularly in the flatter lesions.

With all these manœuvres the chance of local recurrence is higher than with more radical treatments, but this disadvantage can be tolerated when treatment of multiple lesions would transform the patient into a mosaic of scars. Effective follow-up is necessary in all cases and the less radical the treatment the more frequent should be the review.

Basisquamous carcinoma

This lesion is much less common than BCC but is a recognized variant when histological features of squamous carcinomatous change are seen often at the edge of a BCC. They seem to occur rather more often in recurrent lesions and in skin damaged by previous radiotherapy. The diagnosis is often suggested by a more necrotic, friable and moist edge to the lesion. Treatment is midway in aggressiveness between that of BCC and squamous cell carcinoma, and the possibility of lymphatic metastases should be remembered.

Squamous cell carcinoma (SCC)

This common skin tumour (formerly called epithelioma) can occur at any site in the skin, and aetiological factors have been described above. While sunlight is a factor, previous accidental or therapeutic x-radiation, chemicals and sepsis are much more important in this than in other skin tumours. There are only very few squamous tumours of skin where some previous exogenous cause of skin damage cannot be found. It is commoner with increasing age and the incidence rises sharply over the age of 60. Males are much more commonly affected than females and this is probably a reflection of their increased occupational exposure to environmental carcinogens. This tumour, unlike the BCC, can metastasize by lymphatics to the regional nodes, though in most sites node involvement is late and usually found only in neglected lesions. However, SCCs of the lip, pinna, penis and vulva tend to be more aggressive in their behaviour.

Clinical features

Most SCCs develop in damaged skin, and the first evidences of frank malignant change are usually induration and cracking. Surrounding hyperaemia is often seen, and bleeding and discharge may often be an early feature. As the lesion enlarges a tumour forms and will usually break down to form an ulcer (Fig. 17.5).

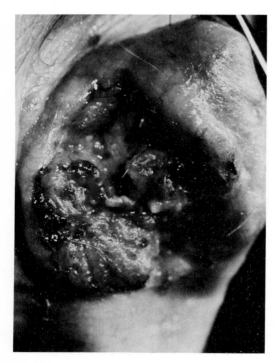

Fig. 17.5 Destructive squamous celled carcinoma of pinna.

Generally the course is more rapid than in BCC but much slower than in keratoa-canthomata. The anatomical site of development is less stereotyped than in BCC. In certain situations SCCs commonly develop where BCCs are rare. These places include the lip, pinna (where all lesions should be assumed to be SCCs until proved otherwise), genitalia and perineum.

Treatment

As in BCC, there is a choice of treatments available for the primary lesion. Most lesions are radiosensitive and, after adequate biopsy and histological proof, the majority can be managed by the radiotherapist. X-ray therapy, electron beams and local methods such as radium implants and moulds all have their place. There are certain sites, however, in which it is not advisable to use irradiation to the primary. These include the pinna, where radiation necrosis is a frequent and painful sequel. When the scalp is the primary site, wide depilation will follow adequate treatment and this will provide a cosmetic indication for surgery. Where surgery is chosen then excision should be wider in clearance than in the treatment of BCC. A margin of 1 cm or more is essential for all except the most trivial lesions, and wider margins may be required in large or rapidly growing tumours. Treatment of involved regional lymph nodes is by surgical block dissection except where gross neglect has allowed the patient to present with fixed and irremovable nodes. Here the radiotherapist may help considerably by preliminary therapy and block dissection may be carried out as a delayed measure. There is no indication for prophylactic block dissection in patients with SCCs other than those of the vulva. Elective dissection is required when nodes are involved on presentation or if they appear during follow-up, which should be conducted frequently at first and continued for the patient's lifetime.

Local cryosurgery and chemotherapy have their place in small lesions, particularly in those subjects with multiple tumours such as those arising in keratoses due to radiation or arsenic. Systemic chemotherapy has been used for some years and methotrexate has found a special place in the management of advanced or recurring squamous cell carcinoma. Given orally or parenterally, it retains its value in some advanced and recurrent lesions. Intra-arterial therapy which was tried with enthusiasm in the 1950s and early 1960s is but little used nowadays. In general the results of treatment of squamous cell carcinoma are very reasonable and 5-year cure rates are universally over 90 per cent.

Pigmented tumours other than melanomas

This large group includes lesions of more or less cosmetic importance but whose main import is their confusion with melanomata. As is mentioned later, an important cause of neglect in the management of melanoma is error in primary diagnosis and consequent delayed or incorrect treatment. Conversely, the mistaken diagnosis of melanoma may lead to unnecessary alarm in the patient and sometimes to excessively aggressive surgical treatment. Winkelmann (1972) has summarized the problem of differential diagnosis. Misdiagnosis is common but is diminished where combined clinical opinion from dermatologists and surgeons with an interest in such tumours is available. Epstein et al. (1969) in a survey of 559 pigmented lesions, found only 2·1 per cent to be melanomas; 12·9 per cent were pigmented basal cell carcinomas and most of the rest were pigmented naevi and seborrhoeic keratoses.

Seborrhoeic keratoses

Have already been described above.

Angiomata

Angiomata may be very darkly coloured and have surrounding melanin pigmentation in addition to their surface colour of haemosiderin and haemoglobin. Blanching on pressure and the soft consistency of these lesions are often a help in making the diagnosis.

Naevi (melanocytic naevi)

Melanocytic naevi are seen in three forms—junctional, compound and intradermal—and these are benign tumours of melanocytes with variable vascular elements and with hypertrophy of dermal tissues in the compound hairy naevi. They are all very common lesions and in the vast majority of patients are of no sinister significance. Up to one-third of melanomata, however, arise in pre-existing naevi, both junctional and compound, though one cannot rely on this figure too much. Some 'naevi' have in fact been slowly evolving melanomata or lentigos from the start. Cosmetic considerations or doubts in diagnosis may indicate the need for excision and biopsy and this is mandatory when any naevus enlarges, changes in colour, crusts, bleeds or itches.

Blue naevus

This harmless lesion is due to the presence of clumps of aberrant melanocytes in the dermis. The epidermis is normal, but through it a blue-grey colour will be seen and the lesion is quite often palpable. There is little need to treat blue naevi unless they are unsightly.

Pigmented BCC

Pigmented BCC has been mentioned previously. It may simulate melanoma very closely and is perhaps the lesion in which excision biopsy will most often be required.

Juvenile melanoma

This is a benign tumour of melanocytes occurring before puberty which is, for practical purposes, a vascular compound naevus. It may enlarge quite rapidly at first but ulceration is rare. Trauma will sometimes produce haemorrhage and crusting. As in angiomata, pressure will often produce blanching in these lesions. The main importance of the juvenile melanoma is the naked-eye and histological resemblance to true melanoma which can cause alarm to clinicians unacquainted with the lesion.

Other lesions

In addition, many other skin tumours may contain melanin or its presence may be simulated by vascular elements. They include pyogenic granulomas, glomus tumours, Kaposi's sarcoma, histiocytomas and keratoacanthomas. When doubt exists in the diagnosis, excision biopsy is indicated.

Melanoma

This lesion is almost a special subject. The earlier age of onset than is noted in other skin cancers, combined with its unpredictable course, has given it the title of the 'black sheep of malignancy' (Fitzpatrick and Clark, 1964). It is a less common tumour than either the BCC or the SCC, constituting only 1·5 per cent of skin cancers in Texas (Clark and MacDonald, 1953). In areas of lower solar irradiation the relative incidence is higher though the population incidence is lower, and in Sweden melanoma is reported as being 7 per cent of all skin cancers (Sylven, 1949). In malignant melanoma sunlight is the major carcinogen. In Australia the death rate in Hobart (43°S) is one-third of that in Brisbane (27°S) (Lancaster, 1956). In Queensland the annual incidence is 14 per 100,000 population and the factors which play a part have been analysed by members of the Queensland Melanoma Project (Beardmore, 1972). In most reported series of melanomas more females than males developed the disease, but the mortality rate is much higher in the males, particularly in younger patients, with the death rate becoming equal in old age (WHO, 1970). Malignant melanoma is very rare before puberty. The majority of melanomata arise in previously macroscopically normal skin, though up to one-third are said to arise in previous freckles and naevi and mechanical and chemical irritation has sometimes been blamed for malignant transformation.

Lentigo maligna (Hutchinson's freckle)

This condition is of very special interest. It is clinically a pre-melanomatous dermatosis but histologically is a melanoma in situ with junctional changes but not dermal invasion until it is transformed in part or in whole into a more active tumour. It was first described by Sir Jonathan Hutchinson (1892, 1894) and Dubreuilh (1912) gave a fuller description and indicated its malignant potentialities. The lesion of lentigo maligna starts as a small area of pigmentation, usually on the face of a middle-aged or elderly person and often in those who have been exposed to excessive sunlight. It spreads in the skin at a most variable rate and may come to enclose unpigmented areas. The oral mucosa and conjunctiva can be involved. When such lesions are watched there may be variation in intensity and distribution of pigmentation (Fig. 17.6), but the tendency is for steady centrifugal enlargement. Frank transformation into invasive malignant melanoma may occur at any time (Fig. 17.7). It is of interest that the melanomata arising in areas of lentigo maligna may show less aggressive behaviour than other melanomata (Clark and Mihm, 1969; Boulter, 1973). When the areas of lentigo maligna are recognized they should be treated by excision and grafting. Very small lesions have been dealt with by cautery and chemotherapy, but these methods deny

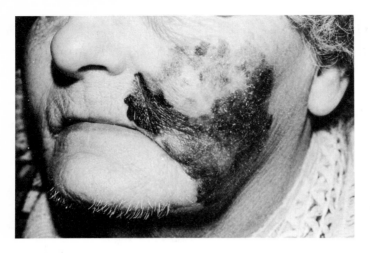

Fig. 17.6 Extensive lentigo maligna.

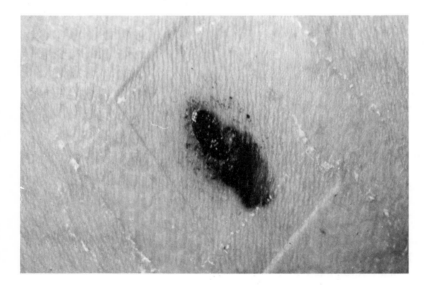

Fig. 17.7 Superficial spreading melanoma with adjacent strapping marks. N.B. Any pigmented lesion which the patient needs to cover with a dressing must be assumed to be a malignant melanoma.

the clinican the opportunity of proper histological assessment. Since lentigo spreads, the earlier the lesion is dealt with the better. The appearance of ulceration, bleeding and nodularity in an area of lentigo should be taken as positive evidence of malignant behaviour and energetic surgical treatment should be instituted without further delay.

Classification of melanoma

Three varieties of melanoma may be recognized clinically and the terminology used is that of Clark (1967).

Lentigo maligna melanoma (LMM)

Lentigo maligna melanoma is the least aggressive lesion, tends to occur in older patients and arises in areas of lentigo consequent often on prolonged solar irradiation. Most of these lesions are on the face.

Superficial spreading melanoma (SSM)

Superficial spreading melanoma is the next in order of increasing malignancy. The course is shorter before overt invasion occurs and it less often arises in obviously damaged skin. Exposure to sunlight is still, however, a potent factor. The age group is younger than in LMM, and a high proportion of these lesions are seen on the exposed parts of the limbs and on the back (Davis et al., 1966). Whether these lesions start in pre-existing moles or in apparently normal skin, the first symptom is usually an increasing area of discoloration with itching, bleeding or crusting. As time passes, nodularity and ulceration may be noted. Three varieties of SSM are seen: (1) ring melanoma often with adjacent depigmentation; (2) verrucose lesions; (3) plaque-like lesions.

Nodular melanoma (NM)

Nodular melanoma is the most aggressive form and is invasive from the start. Unlike the others it has initially little relationship to sunlight and can occur on

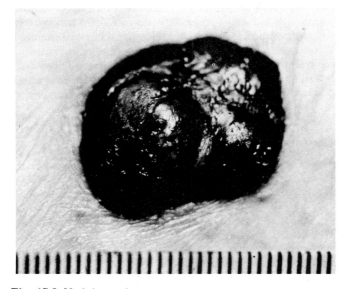

Fig. 17.8 Nodular melanoma.

any skin site. Nearly all mucosal, genital and anal melanomata are nodular *ab initio*. These lesions may be pigmented or non-pigmented and amelanotic forms are probably commoner in the more rapidly growing nodular melanomata (Fig. 17.8).

Behaviour of melanoma

Whichever variety of melanoma is being considered there are certain common factors. Enlargement occurs by surface spread, protuberance and invasion of the dermis and deeper structures. Pigmentation is variable and areas of surrounding depigmentation may occur. Within one tumour both deeply pigmented and non-pigmented areas may be seen. Metastasis by dermal lymphatics may lead to satellite nodules as well as to lymph vessel and node involvement. Blood-stream metastases may lead to pulmonary and other deposits. The prognosis of a patient with melanoma depends partly on what type of tumour he has and what stage of invasion it has reached before treatment is instituted. With increasing dermal invasion comes poorer prognosis, though immune responses may vary this. The histological appearance of a brisk leucocyte response at the base of a melanoma may be an observation of hopeful prognostic value.

Treatment of melanoma

Surgical excision of the primary lesion after appropriate histological confirmation is the treatment of choice. Traditionally incisional biopsy is frowned upon but may be unavoidable in certain larger lesions. Wherever possible frozen-section facilities should be available. The margin of excision recommended varies greatly. The size and behaviour of the lesion will in part dictate the extent of operation. A small lesion of dubious activity can well be excised with only a few millimetres of margin while a larger, more rapidly evolving or neglected lesion will demand wider margins of up to 5 cm. Here of course anatomical, cosmetic and surgical factors inevitably modify the operation. Adequate excision of most lesions will necessitate skin replacement either by split skin grafts or by flaps. In most cases the doctrine is accepted that the wounds of adequate removal can *not* be closed by simple suture.

Block dissection and its indications

Recent years have brought a more flexible attitude to block dissection in melanoma (Davis and MacLeod, 1971). Elective block dissection is advised:
    (1) when the regional nodes are involved clinically or suspect on lymphangiography;
    (2) when the primary lesion is so close to its regional lymph nodes that monoblock excision is both convenient and logical;
    (3) when the tumour is rapidly growing, nodular and when there is histological demonstration of invasion of dermal lymphatics; and
    (4) when follow-up is geographically difficult.
    Prophylactic block dissection, once very strongly urged, is now becoming much

less popular and the results of the recent European multi-centre trial give good support for a 'wait and see' policy (Szczygiel, 1974).

Lymphangiography

This has helped in the assessment of regional lymph nodes and is now frequently performed.

Endolymphatic therapy

This form of treatment is still under assessment but cannot yet be said to have a secure place in the therapy of melanoma. The technique is carried out in patients after surgery to their primary lesions. Distal lymphatic cannulation is performed and radioactive material such as ^{131}I and ^{32}P are injected with Ultra-Fluid Lipiodol as a vehicle. This visualizes the lymphatics and nodes and in some cases may improve the outlook by effective radiation of melanoma cells in sites reached by the agent (Edwards and Kinmonth, 1968).

Radiotherapy

Radiotherapy is usually reserved for lesions in sites unsuitable for surgery. Good results have, however, been reported by European radiotherapists and further work in this field is needed. Relative radioresistance and the more ready tendency to metastasize has combined to remove radiation therapy from the leading place it occupies in most other skin tumours.

Chemotherapy

Systemic chemotherapy is used in the management of advanced cases and the agents most commonly used include DTIC, BCNU and vincristine. Regional perfusion using melphalan and other drugs has been carried out extensively by American workers. Elective treatment of recurrent disease in limbs has given very encouraging results (Ryan et al., 1972). Less certain is the place of prophylactic regional perfusion as advocated by Rochlin et al. (1972). Isolated regional perfusion is not without risk, both anatomical and haematological, and should be reserved to metastatic disease not amenable to other methods of therapy.

Immunotherapy

There is evidence that melanoma is accompanied by immune responses in the host and various trials have been developed to exploit this phenomenon. Autoimmunization with irradiated cells, adaptive immunotherapy and non-specific stimulation have all been used. As yet such therapy is still at an experimental stage. Perhaps the only quasi-immunological method which is in regular use is the technique of direct inoculation of vaccinia virus into metastatic nodules (Hunter-Craig et al. 1970).

Spontaneous regression

Spontaneous regression is noted in malignant melanoma perhaps more often than in other skin tumours. Not infrequently the primary lesion may disappear while metastatic disease continues to flourish. Rarely, total remission can occur, attributed to immunological means, but this mechanism has never been proven.

Results of treatment

Since melanoma is not a homogeneous disease the results of treatment can only be talked of in rather general terms. An early lentigo maligna melanoma carries a 5-year cure rate of well over 90 per cent while a nodular melanoma of the same size may only have a 40 per cent 5-year survival. Lymphatic metastases on presentation suggest a poor prognosis, and indeed survival of more than 10 per cent of patients who present at such a stage of the disease is about the average.

The reticuloses and the skin

All the reticuloses can produce skin manifestations, with leukaemias and Hodgkin's disease doing so least commonly. Lymposarcoma and reticulum cell sarcoma do so more often and mycosis fungoides is primarily a disease of the skin. Treatment of these lesions is by permutations of irradiation and chemotherapy.

Kaposi's sarcoma

Kaposi's sarcoma is a cutaneous malignancy affecting skin capillaries and perivascular tissues. The lesions, usually multiple, are purple, circumscribed and may ulcerate. Some disappear spontaneously, but most develop and eventually are associated with systemic involvement. Treatment is by local radiotherapy and systemic chemotherapy.

Metastatic disease

Metastases from visceral tumours may present in the skin and probably the commonest primary is a bronchial carcinoma. Breast, gastrointestinal, thyroid and renal and indeed almost any neoplasms may be associated with skin metastases. Treatment of these lesions is thus an incident in the management of the disease and surgery, radiotherapy and chemotherapy may be indicated.

References

AUERBACH H. (1961) Geographic variation in incidence of skin cancer in the United States. *Public Health Rep.* **76,** 345–348.

BEARDMORE G. L. (1972) The epidemiology of malignant melanoma in Australia. In: MCCARTHY W. H. (ed.), *Melanoma and Skin Cancer*, Proc. Int. Cancer Conf. Sydney, Australian Cancer Society, pp. 39–64.

BOULTER P. S. (1973) Lentigo maligna and its relationship to invasive malignant melanoma. In: MCGOVERN V. J. and RUSSELL P. (ed.), *Proc. VIIIth Pigment Cell Conf., Sydney, 1972.* Basel, Karger; Chichester, John Wiley, p. 99.

CLARK R. L. and MACDONALD E. J. (1953) In: GORDON M. (ed.), *Pigment Cell Growth*. New York, Academic Press.

CLARK W. H. (1967) A classificiation of malignant melanoma in man connected with histogenesis and biological behaviour. In: MONTAGNA W. and HU F. (ed.), *Advances in Biology of the Skin*; Vol. 8, *The Pigmentary System*. Oxford and New York, Pergamon, pp. 621–647.

CLARK W. H. and MIHM M. C. (1969) Lentigo maligna and lentigo-maligna melanoma. *Am. J. Pathol.* **55,** 39–67.

DAVIS N. C., HERRON J. J. and MACLEOD G. R. (1966) Malignant melanoma in Queensland: analysis of 400 skin lesions. *Lancet* **2,** 407–410.

DAVIS N. C. and MACLEOD G. R. (1971) Elective lymph-node dissection for melanoma. *Br. J. Surg.* **58,** 820–823.

DUBREUILH M. W. (1912) De la mélanose circonscrite précancéreuse. *Ann. Dermatol. Syph.* **3,** 205–230.

EDWARDS J. M. and KINMONTH J. B. (1968) Endolymphatic therapy for malignant melanoma. *Br. Med. J.* **1,** 18–22.

EPSTEIN E., BRAGG K. and LINDEN G. (1969) Biopsy and prognosis of malignant melanoma. *JAMA* **208,** 1369–1371.

FITZPATRICK T. B. and CLARK W. H. (1964) Problems in the diagnosis of malignant melanoma. In: *Tumors of the Skin*. Chicago, Year Book Med. Publ., p. 169.

GRAHAM J. H. and HELWIG E. G. (1959) Bowen's disease and its relation to systemic cancer. *Arch. Dermatol.* **80,** 133–159.

GRAHAM J. H. and HELWIG E. G. (1964) Pre-cancerous skin lesions and systemic cancer. In: *Tumors of the Skin*. Chicago, Year Book Med. Publ., p. 209.

HUNTER-CRAIG I., NEWTON K. A. and WESTBURY G. (1970) Use of vaccinia virus in the treatment of metastatic malignant melanoma. *Br. Med. J.* **2,** 512–515.

HUTCHINSON J. (1892) Senile freckles. *Arch. Surg. (Lond.)* **3,** 319–322.

HUTCHINSON J. (1894) Lentigo-melanosis. A further report. *Arch. Surg. (Lond.)* **5,** 253–256.

LANCASTER H. O. (1956) Some geographical aspects of the mortality from melanoma in Europeans. *Med. J. Aust.* **1,** 1082–1087.

ROCHLIN D. B., WAGNER D. E. and ROCHLIN S. (1972) The therapy of malignant melanoma as treated by regional perfusion. In: MCCARTHY W. H. (ed.), *Melanoma and Skin Cancer*, Proc. Int. Cancer Conf. Sydney, Australian Cancer Society, pp. 443–451.

RYAN R. F., KREMENTZ E. T. and CARTER R. D. (1972) Treatment of malignant melanoma: a review of the Tulane experience. In: MCCARTHY W. H. (ed.), *Melanoma and Skin Cancer*, Proc. Int. Cancer Conf. Sydney, Australian Cancer Society, pp. 461–472.

SANDERSON K. V. (1968) Tumours of the skin. In: ROOK A., WILKINSON D. S. and EBLING F. J. G. (ed.), *Textbook of Dermatology*. Oxford, Blackwell Scientific Publ., pp. 1658–1748.

SCOTT G. (1972) Some sociological observations on skin cancer in Australia. In: MCCARTHY W. H. (ed.), *Melanoma and Skin Cancer*, Proc. Int. Cancer Conf. Sydney, Australian Cancer Society pp. 15–22.

SLVEN B. (1949) Malignant melanoma of the skin. Report of 341 cases treated during the years 1929–43. *Acta Radiol.* **32,** 33–59.

SZCZYGIEL K. (1974) Preliminary results of an international trial on prophylactic lymph node dissection. In: BUCALOSSI P., VERONESI U. and CASCINELLI N. (ed.), *Proc. 11th Int. Cancer Conf., Florence*. Amsterdam, Excerpta Medica.

WINKELMANN R. K. (1972) The differential diagnosis of melanoma. In: MCCARTHY W. H. (ed.), *Melanoma and Skin Cancer*, Proc. Int. Cancer Conf. Sydney, Australian Cancer Society, pp. 175–184.

WORLD HEALTH ORGANIZATION (1970) *Mortality from Malignant Neoplasms 1955–1965*, part 2. Geneva.

18

Benign Diseases of the Breast

G. J. Hadfield, TD, MS, FRCS

In this chapter I have selected for consideration some common conditions of the breast with a few of the less usual ones rather than a catalogue of all the possibilities. These less common conditions are included because, when they do occur, if they are not diagnosed correctly, they can be mismanaged. The subject is considered in a clinical manner in the way that the patients may present to us for advice in the outpatient department (Hadfield, 1974).

Patients who seek advice on account of a discharge through or near the nipple

First in this group we think of discharges that arise from disease of the nipple skin. The simplest of these is eczema often associated with poor personal hygiene. A loss of the nipple surface with scaling and a serosanguineous discharge may be caused either by Paget's disease or by an adenoma of the nipple (Handley and Thackray, 1962). The former is a well known neoplastic condition. The second is a little less well known condition where the substance of the nipple becomes cellular and normal architecture is lost. As a benign disease it is treatable by local excision.

Three main diseases give rise to a discharge from or near the nipple; namely, duct ectasia, mammillary fistula and papilloma.

Duct ectasia

Duct ectasia is the commonest of these conditions and presents as a nipple discharge of one or more varieties from one or more of the duct orifices (Fig. 18.1). It is caused by a generalized dilatation of the major duct system of the breast, with retrograde dilatation to the lobular ducts. These dilated ducts filled with secretion are easily identified at operation. The fluid within the ducts which causes the nipple discharge varies and may be coloured green or brown or it may be viscous and white in colour. This secretion is made up of amorphous debris and lipoid-containing macrophages and its viscosity is governed by the quantity of the solid element present.

The first recorded description of this condition was by John Birkett (1850).

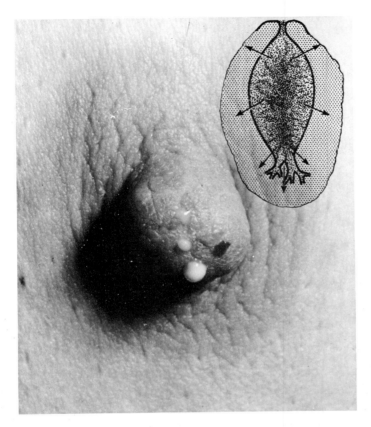

Fig. 18.1 Multiple points of discharge from the nipple taken from a patient with duct ectasia of the breast. Note that the discharges are of different characteristics and from several ducts. The diagram shows the mechanism of periductal mastitis by lipoid passing through the duct wall to cause a cellular reaction. (Reproduced from Hadfield, 1974, *Nursing Mirror* **138,** 68–70, by courtesy of the Editor.)

Since that time, other papers have confirmed and amplified his original observations and description (Sandison, 1962; Sandison and Walker, 1962; Hadfield, 1969 a, b).

This disease is often asymptomatic and so its incidence is difficult to determine as only those patients who have a copious or persistent nipple discharge or a swelling in the breast or para-areolar region seek medical advice. Figures of incidence from the study of post-mortem material should be the most reliable. There is, however, some discrepancy varying from 25 per cent in an autopsy study of 225 subjects (Frantz et al., 1951) to 72 per cent in a series of 800 autopsy examinations (Sandison, 1957).

In the author's series of 560 patients who had an excisional biopsy of an undiagnosed breast lump without a clinical nipple discharge, the breast tissue

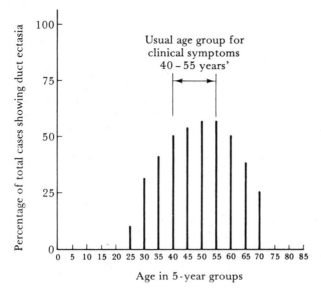

Fig. 18.2 The incidence of duct ectasia in 560 patients who had an excisional biopsy for an undiagnosed breast lump without a clinical nipple discharge.

surrounding the lump was studied for duct ectasia. Figure 18.2 shows the results of this enquiry, demonstrating that the main incidence of the disease was in the age group of 40–55 years. This agrees with our observations on another un-published but complementary series of patients operated on for a nipple discharge occurring from duct ectasia.

The diagrammatic part of Fig. 18.1 shows the pathological lesion in one of a series of dilated major ducts whose lining epithelium is atrophic and the lumen is filled with the secretion previously described. The disease is general to the whole dyct system, affecting it to a greater or lesser degree.

Around the dilated ducts there is a periductal mastitis, the cellular element of which is plasma cells (see Fig. 18.1). This is said to be caused by the leakage of lipoid through the thin duct walls and into the periductal tissue. The detailed pathology has already been discussed elsewhere (Hadfield, 1969a).

Occasionally, these periductal cellular areas become continuous and a mass of confluent periductal mastitis develops in the breast substance (see Fig. 18.4). This may be mistaken for an acute breast cancer, but the diagnosis can be estab-lished on needle biopsy. The treatment is conservative by rest and support, and in some cases a course of anti-inflammatory agents or steroids in the acute phase of the disease is required (Adair, 1933; Haagensen, 1971).

For the treatment of duct ectasia, surgery is advised when there is a copious and persistent discharge and when there is doubt in the diagnosis. Our preference in treatment is for excision of the major duct system (Hadfield, 1960, 1968). This operation removes the diseased major ducts but leaves the breast normal in size and shape.

Mammillary fistula

This uncommon condition is characterized by a chronic discharging fistulous track (Fig. 18.3) occurring unilaterally or bilaterally in the breasts of women in the middle 30s age group (Atkins, 1955). The diagram on Fig. 18.3 shows how this sinus communicates with one of the ducts of the major duct system to form a fistula. The surgical pathology of the condition has been described in detail elsewhere (Hadfield, 1969a). Briefly, the condition arises from two pathological lesions. First, the fistula originates from a single abnormal duct of the major duct system, the others being normal (Patey and Thackray, 1958). It may also arise from a major duct or ducts damaged by periductal mastitis, which, to a varying degree, affects all the other major ducts (Hadfield 1969a).

The choice of treatment lies between laying open the fistula and allowing it

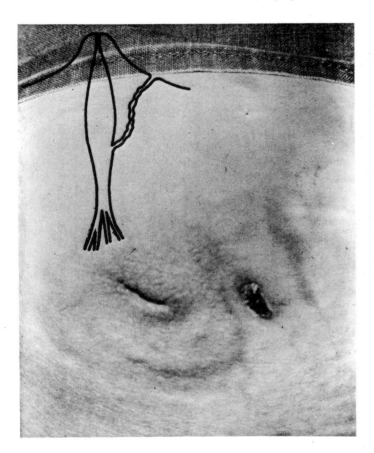

Fig. 18.3 A mammillary fistula. Note the opening of the fistula in the para-areolar region and the indrawn nipple which often occurs in this condition. The diagram shows the fistulous track and its communication with a major duct.

Table 18.1 Analysis of the main features of diseases of the major duct system of the breast

Disease	Age range in years	Presenting signs and symptoms	Histological features
Duct ectasia	40–55	A discharge from the nipple.	Duct dilatation with periductal cuffing by plasma cells. The duct lumina are filled with secretion.
		A discharge from the nipple with a lumpy breast.	
		A discharge from the nipple and a para-areolar swelling.	Duct dilatation—the periductal cuffing has become confluent.
Papilloma	40–69	A bloodstained or serosanguineous discharge from the nipple.	A single sessile papilloma confined to one duct. Variants depend on size and compression by the duct wall.
		The above discharges with a subareolar swelling.	(a) Showing marked fronds. (b) Compact type—fronds have fused to form a solid mass.
		A point of bleeding from one nipple duct with a green or white discharge from others.	Sessile papillomatous projections from the walls of several major ducts.
Mammillary fistula	25–38	A chronic para-areolar sinus.	A fistulous track opening at the areolar margin or through a Montgomery's tubercle and communicating with one duct of the major duct system which may be:
		A recurrent para-areolar abscess.	i. A congenitally abnormal duct in an otherwise normal major duct system. ii. A major duct previously damaged by periductal mastitis which has affected all the ducts.

Reproduced from Hadfield (1969) *Medical World* **107**, 12–14, by courtesy of the Editor.

to heal by granulation (Atkins, 1959) and excision of the major duct system with the sinus *en bloc* (Hadfield, 1960, 1968). Treatment by antibiotics has no effect on this condition. At one time the sinuses were thought to be tuberculous, but this is not so.

Duct papilloma

Medical advice is sought more urgently for this condition than the other two as it is characterized by a blood-stained discharge from the nipple. Formerly, it was commonly believed that a blood-stained discharge from the nipple was a sure sign of cancer (Holleb and Farrow, 1966). While it is not disputed that it can occasionally occur in breast cancer, it is more often associated with benign papilloma or duct ectasia. Often the discharge is not present on examination but can be obtained by radial pressure along the lines of the major ducts in the direction of the nipple.

Treatment is either by excision of the single damaged duct (Atkins, 1955) or, when the disease is more widespread or recurrent, by excision of the major duct system (Hadfield, 1960, 1968).

Occasionally a blood-stained discharge complicates breast-feeding and the fear of cancer may arise. In the majority of these cases, the cause is multicentric, papillomatous lesions of the major ducts (Hadfield, 1969b). These regress spontaneously with the cessation of lactation (Sandison and Walker, 1968). They are therefore likely to be a hormone-stimulated lesion.

The main clinical and pathological factors of these three conditions are summarized in Table 18.1.

Patients presenting with a solitary lump in the breast

An adequate history and examination may be sufficient to make a diagnosis in this group between the possibilities of fat necrosis, chronic abscess, confluent periductal mastitis, sclerosing adenosis, fibroadenoma and breast cysts. Often, however, the final diagnosis is only made when the lump is excised and submitted to histological examination, often by frozen section at the time of operation.

Fat necrosis (Hadfield, 1926) can arise from injury to the breast by an external blow or by injections into the breast substance (Adair and Munzer, 1947). A history of trauma is not always obtainable, but excisional biopsy will confirm the diagnosis.

The solitary breast lump of a chronic breast abscess will usually be supported by the history of acute inflammation treated late by antibiotics alone or with incomplete drainage.

Confluent periductal mastitis has already been referred to in the section on duct ectasia and its management discussed. Figure 18.4 is a photograph from a patient suffering from this condition.

When sclerosing adenosis presents as a solitary hard lump in the breast, this can be confirmed on biopsy and, as it is a benign lesion, adequately treated by local excision.

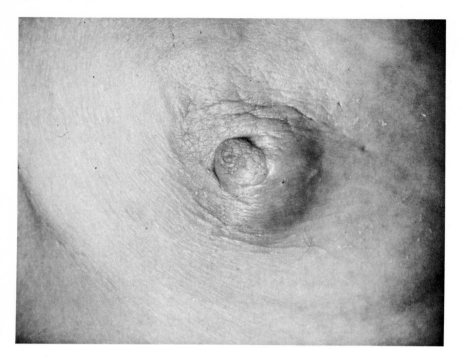

Fig. 18.4 Confluent peri-ductal mastitis presenting as a painful mass in the medial part of the right breast of a woman aged 38 years. The overlying skin was red. The diagnosis was made on needle biopsy.

The physical signs and pathology of fibroadenoma are well known. The characteristic small mobile tumour presents little problem in treatment by simple excision. Occasionally, the tumour may be massive and the patient alarmed by the size and the fear that it may be a cancer.

Breast cysts present as single or multiple lumps of varying size (Handley, 1969). We have recently reviewed (previously unpublished data) a group of 300 patients treated in our clinic over a 15-year period. The majority of our patients were about the age of 40 years and presented with a painless discrete lump in the breast substance or the peri-areolar region. In about one-quarter of the patients, pain was the first symptom. The duration of the history was from weeks or months, depending on the patient's disposition. Many of the patients stated that there appeared to be a change in size of the lump with their monthly periods while others described previous lumps which had disappeared spontaneously.

Cysts in our series were located equally in either breast, the majority occurring in the upper and outer quadrant.

At first examination, about 10 per cent of the patients had more than one cyst in the same breast. In the patients previously treated for a cyst, over one-third had developed another cyst at a different site in the breast on follow-up. The diameter of the cysts has varied from a few millimetres up to 3–4 cm. Previously, the majority of breast cysts were treated by local excision, but this involves an operation which is likely to be recurrent and will damage the breast shape and leave a scar. We consider that most cysts can be adequately treated by aspiration, a simple outpatient procedure which leaves neither scar nor deformity (Rosemond et al., 1955; Rosemond, 1963; Hadfield, 1974).

Our clinic routine is to examine the breast after aspiration, and as long as the lump has disappeared completely we review them after a 6-week interval. Cytological examination of the aspirated fluid is rarely informative and we do not use it as a routine.

In a small number of patients, surgical excision of the breast lump is indicated: first, when a dry tap is obtained and the lump remains and a solid tumour can be expected; secondly, when blood-stained fluid is obtained, and here cytological examination may be useful as this suggests a neoplasm in a cyst; thirdly, where a lump recurs following aspiration.

Breast cysts occurring in the menopausal patient (Handley, 1969) should be treated with caution as they may be associated with an undetected neoplasm.

From time to time, doubt is expressed on the safety of needle puncture of possible malignant conditions of the breast. There is no known evidence to prove that this procedure has any danger in this respect in breast lesions.

Patients with a discrete lump in a nodular or granular breast

In this group there are two main divisions of patients presenting for advice. First, there are those whose lesion can be described as adenosis and epitheliosis or chronic mastitis. Our policy here is to aspirate all discrete lumps. If they persist then we would excise them and examine by frozen section, carrying out definitive treatment at the same operation.

Secondly, and in some ways a more difficult group of patients to treat, are those with papillary lesions presenting with a single recurrent, or more than one, lump in the substance of the breast. Many patients present in their early 20s with these lesions, which may be multiple and are often recurrent at another site in the breast after excision.

At first excision of a solitary lump in the breast of these patients, the histologist has to decide between a papilloma and papillary carcinoma. The histological criteria on which this diagnosis is based were laid down by Kraus and Neubecker (1962) (see Table 18.2).

After the excision of a single tumour of this sort, the appearance of further similar tumours in the same or the opposite breast is likely and their management poses a difficult clinical problem. Multiple repeated excisions are unacceptable to the young woman and damaging to a potentially functioning breast. Many of the lesions give a positive result on thermography, suggesting actively growing tissue and are therefore suspect.

The management of these patients remains a matter of choice. Considering all the problems, our plan is to excise and examine histologically the first lump. Thereafter, further lumps are examined by needle or drill biopsy and, occasionally, mammography. Further excision is decided on the results of these tests.

Table 18.2 Papillary breast tumours: a comparison of the histological features

Papilloma	*Papillary Carcinoma*
Two types of epithelial cell.	Single type of epithelial cell.
Nuclei normochromatic.	Nuclei hyperchromatic.
Apocrine metaplasia present.	Apocrine metaplasia absent.
Complex glandular pattern.	Cribiform pattern.
Prominent connective tissue stroma.	Delicate or absent connective tissue stroma.
Periductal fibrosis with epithelial entrapment.	Epithelial invasion of stroma.
Intraductal hyperplasia in adjacent ducts.	Intraductal carcinoma in adjacent ducts.
Sclerosing adenosis sometimes present in adjacent breast tissue.	Sclerosing adenosis generally absent in adjacent breast tissue.

Reproduced from Kraus and Neubecker (1962) *Cancer* **15,** 444–455, by courtesy of the authors and the Editor.

In patients over the age of 45 years with recurrent peripheral papillary lesions of the breast, we recommend a subcutaneous mastectomy and the insertion of a prosthesis. The breast tissue after removal is subjected to strict scrutiny for breast cancer.

Haematoma of the breast

This condition can occur spontaneously or in patients on anticoagulant therapy. Treatment consists of supporting the breast, giving an agent which aids haematoma absorption and stopping anticoagulant therapy. Aspiration may be valuable if there is a large collection present. Incision may occasionally be required but is rarely of real value as the collection of blood is throughout the substance of the breast rather than in a localized site.

Patients complaining of a lump in the breast but the lesion is not in the breast

This group, which might be called 'the non-breast lumps', is more common in woman who practise self-examination of the breast. Patients with prominent and easily palpable lower ribs form the majority of people in this group. Other causes are tumours of the ribs such as chondroma or calcified haematoma, lesions of the lungs, mediastinum and pleural sac pointing through the chest wall, as well as parasternal nodes forming a parasternal dome-shaped tumour or cold abscess of the sternum.

Patients presenting with enlargement of the breast disc

This may vary in size and be unilateral or bilateral, symmetrical or asymmetrical. Mastitis may occur in breast-fed infants of both sexes. It is transient and disappears with weaning or spontaneously. Enlargement of the breast disc in young girls before puberty may sometimes be asymmetrical. In the large majority of instances this evens out and requires no treatment.

Gynaecomastia in boys and men may have an endocrinological basis and can be managed accordingly; if the breast becomes large and unsightly, it can be removed by operation. The idiopathic group, at one time thought to be due to irritation by clothing to form a fibrous tissue swelling, is now thought to be due to a genuine growth of the breast tissue as demonstrated by thick section techniques (Parks, 1959). These patients require investigation for a possible endocrine factor or, in some cases, for an occult cancer of the lung or contralateral breast. Removal of the breast may be necessary if it is large and painful or if the pathology is in doubt (Stokes, 1962).

Aids to diagnosis

On evidence obtained from the trio—a careful history, a full physical examination and histological examination of material obtained at biopsy—the majority of breast diseases are diagnosed. Aids to diagnosis can be useful, however, in cases of difficulty and doubt.

The technique and use of radiological methods has been described fully by Evans and Gravelle (1973). Anything less than good quality mammograms are not only useless but also potentially dangerous and misleading. In the benign group of these lesions, the greatest value lies in aiding diagnosis in multiple breast lumps and indefinite areas of breast thickening.

The duct system of the breast can be demonstrated by injection of contrast medium through the ducts as they open on the nipple and taking an x-ray of the breast. This examination is of value in duct ectasia where it will show up the nature and extent of the disease. Furthermore, it will demonstrate a space-occupying lesion in a duct from a papillary tumour and is useful when there is a history of a blood-stained discharge by the patient but no discharge can be demonstrated at examination.

Thermography is complementary to but gives a different type of information from mammography. The mammogram accurately demonstrates the lesion; the thermogram demonstrates its activity.

Pathology has a great deal to offer the clinician in diagnosis, either by frozen section of the lump, histological scrutiny of the whole breast specimens, and histological examination of drill or needle biopsy material. Cytological examination of discharges from the nipple and the contents of the aspiration of breast cysts, while occasionally helpful, is of doubtful value for routine use unless clinically indicated.

References

ADAIR F. E. (1933) Plasma cell mastitis. A lesion simulating mammary carcinoma. *Arch. Surg.* **26,** 735–749.

ADAIR F. E. and MUNZER J. T. (1947) Fat necrosis of the female breast. A report of 110 cases. *Am. J. Surg.* **74,** 117–128.

ATKINS H. J. B. (1955) Mammillary fistula. *Br. Med. J.* **2,** 1473–1474.

BIRKETT J. (1850) *The Diseases of the Breast and their Treatment.* London, Longmans.

EVANS K. T. and GRAVELLE I. H. (1973) *Mammography, Thermography and Ultrasonography in Breast Disease.* London, Butterworths.

FRANTZ V. K., PICKREN J. W., MELCHER G. W. and AUCHINCLOSS H. (1951) Incidence of chronic cystic disease in so-called 'normal breasts'; a study based on 225 postmortem examinations. *Cancer* **4,** 762–783.

HAAGENSEN C. D. (1971) *Diseases of the Breast,* 2nd edn. Philadelphia and London, Saunders.

HADFIELD G. (1926) Fat necrosis of the breast. *Br. J. Surg.* **13,** 742–745.

HADFIELD G. J. (1960) Excision of the major duct system for benign disease of the breast. *Br. J. Surg.* **47,** 472–477.

HADFIELD G. J. (1968) Further experience of the operation for excision of the major duct system of the breast. *Br. J. Surg.* **55,** 530–535.

HADFIELD G. J. (1969a) The pathological lesions underlying discharges from the nipple in women. *Ann. R. Coll. Surg. Engl.* **44,** 323–333.

HADFIELD G. J. (1969b) Discharges from the nipple in women. Significance and management. *Medical World* **107,** 12–14.

HADFIELD G. J. (1974) Benign disease of the beast. *Nurs. Mirror* **138,** 68–70.

HANDLEY R. S. (1969) Benign breast disease: surgical aspects. *Proc. R. Soc. Med.* **62,** 722–724.

HANDLEY R. S. and THACKRAY A. C. (1962) Adenoma of nipple. *Br. J. Cancer* **16,** 187–194.

HOLLEB A. I. and FARROW J. H. (1966) The significance of nipple discharge. *CA* **16,** 182–186.

KRAUS F. T. and NEUBECKER R. D. (1962) The differential diagnosis of papillary tumors of the breast. *Cancer* **15,** 444–455.

PARLS A. G. (1959) The micro-anatomy of the breast. *Ann. R. Coll. Surg. Engl.* **25,** 235–251.

PATEY D. H. and THACKRAY A. C. (1958) Pathology and treatment of mammary duct fistula. *Lancet* **2,** 871–873.

ROSEMOND G. P. (1963) Differentiation between cystic and solid breast mass by needle aspiration. *Surg. Clin. North Am.* **43,** 1433–1437.

ROSEMOND G. P., BURNETT W. E., CASWELL H. T. and MCALEER D. J. (1955) Aspiration of breast cysts as a diagnostic and therapeutic measure. *Arch. Surg.* **71,** 223–229.

SANDISON A. T. (1957) A postmortem study of the adult breast. M.D. thesis, University of St Andrews.

SANDISON A. T. (1962) An autopsy study of the adult human breast with special reference to proliferative epithelial changes of importance in the pathology of the breast. *Natl. Cancer Inst. Monogr.* **8,** 1–145.

SANDISON A. T. and WALKER J. C. (1962) Inflammatory mastitis, mammary duct ectasia and mammillary fistula. *Br. J. Surg.* **50,** 57–64.

SANDISON A. T. and WALKER J. C. (1968) Diseases of the adolescent female breast. A clinico-pathological study. *Br. J. Surg.* **55,** 443–448.

STOKES J. F. (1962) Unexpected gynaecomastia. *Lancet* **2,** 911–913.

Index

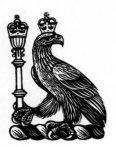

Current Surgical Practice Volume 1

From lectures given at the Royal College of
Surgeons of England.

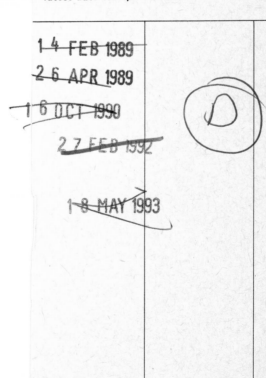
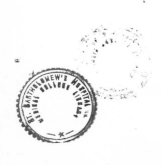